2nd EDITION

GROWTH and DEVELOPMENT Across the Lifespan

A Health Promotion Focus

Gloria Leifer, RN, MA, CNE

Professor, Obstetric and Pediatric Nursing

Riverside City College

Riverside, California

Eve Fleck, MS, ACE GFI, ACE PT, NASM CPT

IDEA: Author and Presenter

ELSEVIER

ELSEVIER
SAUNDERS

3251 Riverport Lane
St. Louis, Missouri 63043

ISBN: 978-1-4557-4545-6

GROWTH AND DEVELOPMENT ACROSS THE LIFESPAN: A HEALTH PROMOTION FOCUS, ed 2

Library of Congress Cataloging-in-Publication Data
Leifer, Gloria.
Growth and development across the lifespan : a health promotion focus/Gloria Leifer, Eve Fleck. – 2nd ed.
p. ; cm.
Includes bibliographical references and index.
ISBN 978-1-4557-4545-6 (pbk. : alk. paper)
I. Fleck, Eve. II. Title.
[DNLM: 1. Human Development–Nurses' Instruction. 2. Health Education–methods–Nurses' Instruction. 3. Health Promotion–methods–Nurses' Instruction. 4. Personality Development–Nurses' Instruction. WS 103]
613–dc23

2012025727

Vice President and Publisher: Loren Wilson
Executive Content Strategist: Teri Hines Burnham
Senior Content Development Specialist: Tiffany L. Trautwein
Publishing Services Manager: Jeff Patterson
Senior Project Manager: Anne Konopka
Design Direction: Jessica Williams

Printed in China
Last digit is the print number: 9 8 7 6

Dedicated to the memory of

Sarah Masseyaw Leifer,
a nurse, humanitarian, and mother,

and

Daniel Peretz Hartston, MD,
a pediatrician, husband, and world traveler,

and to the honor of
Heidi, Paul, Ruby,
Barnet,
Amos, Thuy, Spencer,
Eve, David, Zoe, Elliot, and Ian,
who acquaint me with the beauty, joys, and challenges of my lifespan voyage.
~ Gloria Leifer Hartston

To Mom, for her endless guidance, encouragement, support, and love.
~ Eve Fleck

Ancillary Writers

Anna Allen Hamilton, RN, BSN, MS
Former Instructor
McLennan Community College
Waco, Texas
Test Bank

Charla K. Hollin, RN
Allied Health Division Chair & ARNEC Program Chair
Director of Nursing Programs
Rich Mountain Community College
Mena, Arkansas
TEACH Lesson Plans

Laura Travis, MSN, BSN, RN
Health Careers Coordinator
Tennessee Technology Center at Dickson
Dickson, Tennessee
Answers and Rationales for Review Questions
Answer Guidelines for Critical Thinking Questions
TEACH Lesson Plan Pretests

Reviewers

Holly Burch, RN, BSN

PN Instructor, Practical Nursing
Hillyard Technical Center
St. Joseph, Missouri

Carolyn McCune, RN, MSN, NP (Women's Health)

Director, PN Program
Columbiana County Career & Technical Center
Lisbon, Ohio

Odia Obadan, MBBS, MS/IHPM

Harmony Healthcare Institute
Merrimack, New Hampshire

Terry Pope, MSN, RN

Faculty, PN Training Program
Ohio Hi Point Career Center
Bellefontaine, Ohio

Marjorie Sanfilippo, PhD

Associate Dean of Faculty and
Associate Professor of Psychology
Eckerd College
St. Petersburg, Florida

Maggie Thomas, PT, MA

Physical Therapist Assistant Program Director
Allied Health Department
Kirkwood Community College
Cedar Rapids, Iowa

Debbie Yarnell, RN, BSN

Program Coordinator, Practical Nursing Program
Eldon Career Center
Eldon, Missouri

Preface

Understanding growth and development at each age and stage of the life cycle is a valuable tool for the health-care worker when assessing, planning, and implementing health care and education for patients. This text enables the study of growth and development in a continuum across the entire lifespan and integrates concepts related to changes that normally occur in each stage of the life cycle.

Promoting healthy behaviors and healthy lifestyles is an integral part of improving the quality of life. Today, people want more control over their health care and want to be part of the decision-making process concerning their health-care needs. The emergence of complementary and alternative medicine (CAM) reflects trends toward self management and preventive care. The numbers of health-related publications, internet resources, health spas, and self-help groups have increased rapidly over the past 10 years. This also reflects people's growing interest in and concern with health and healthy behaviors.

The future brings possibilities of increased population growth, intensified international conflict, and advanced scientific achievements, all of which can influence the world's social, economic, and health environments. Our abilities to improve health, enrich the quality of life, and lengthen the lifespan may become even more important as the future unfolds.

Disease prevention and health promotion are complementary but distinct activities. *Disease prevention* is disease specific and involves early detection, early preventive measures (such as immunization programs), and environmental regulatory measures (such as maintaining a clean environment to prevent exposure to toxic agents that may cause cancer). *Health promotion* is not disease specific and involves developing healthy behaviors that increase the quality of life, such as eating a healthy diet and engaging in regular appropriate physical exercise. Today, health is defined not only as the absence of illness, but as a multidimensional state of being that includes physical, mental, social, and emotional health with associated environmental, economic, and cultural factors that enable and promote healthy behaviors that improve the quality of life.

Many researchers and theorists have charted the course of growth and development and have formed frameworks for understanding lifespan development. This text reviews these theories and concepts and discusses typical physical and behavioral changes that occur at each stage of the life cycle. When a health-care worker is familiar with normal developmental stages, aberrations can be identified, and typical patterns can be noted when designing individual approaches to care.

The fundamental patterns of growth and development are universal, including physical, mental, social, emotional, and moral growth, as well as changes that are influenced by biology, individual experience, environment, and health. Demographic changes toward a more ethnically diverse population evidences the need for health-care workers to provide culturally sensitive and culturally competent care across the lifespan. This text integrates information concerning *growth and development* and *healthy behaviors* with a discussion of the influence of *culture* and *family* on perceptions and practice.

In addition to addressing cultural differences, the text takes into account health-care strategies for handling patients of different age groups. The text explains concepts and theories about physical, cognitive, social, and personality development at each stage of the life cycle from conception to death. It also provides an explanation of normal development, behavior, skills, and limitations at each life stage and presents a discussion of external influences, such as culture, family, and environment, on normal development.

Each chapter provides information that helps students identify teaching strategies that incorporate personal priorities, skills, and limitations that characterize each stage of life. For example, teaching strategies or techniques that a health-care worker would use for a young child would be different from the strategies used to teach an adolescent. Because children are unencumbered by experiences, their processing and interpretation will be different from those of adults. The approach to working with young adults would also differ from working with a family mourning the death of a relative, even though the shared goal of teaching may be to enhance the healing process and to promote healthy behaviors.

As mentioned earlier, health promotion has the power not only to *increase* the quality of life at all stages but also *decrease* health-care costs. This, therefore, is an essential strategy basic to the national health plan. All health-care workers need to employ health promotion knowledge, skills, and attitudes in a variety of settings, including acute care, home care, and chronic care.

Healthy People 2020 provides a list of goals for health-care workers related to providing care to a diverse population across the lifespan in a variety of settings. The goals of *Healthy People 2020* are integrated throughout the text.

Health-care workers must develop culturally competent and age-appropriate education and care plans designed to meet the unique needs of the individuals they serve. Teaching skills can help health-care workers to educate at-risk populations about healthy diets, exercise, mental health, and lifestyle choices. Using every teaching opportunity in a culturally sensitive and developmentally appropriate manner will maximize learning and is the heartbeat of *Healthy People 2020.*

In summary, this text provides a comprehensive review of concepts of growth and development from conception to death, integrated with the goals of *Healthy People 2020* concerning promotion of healthy behaviors, and it is supplemented by an introduction to the influence of culture and family on perceptions and practices at each age level, which can be used by health-care workers in achieving their professional objectives.

ACKNOWLEDGMENTS

The birth of a book is a team effort. The authors express sincere appreciation to those who contributed materially, as well as to those whose support and encouragement were vital to the outcome of the project.

Terri Wood, former Senior Nursing Editor at Elsevier, seeded the vision and expressed confidence and support in the efforts of the authors to complete this text. Our sincere appreciation is extended to the many reviewers who shared their expertise and provided constructive comments. We especially thank Dr. Marjorie Sanfilippo, Associate Dean of Faculty and Associate Professor of Psychology at Eckerd College in St. Petersburg, Florida, for her detailed review of Chapter 5 and for her helpful suggestions. The able assistance of the Elsevier nursing editorial staff, including Teri Hines Burnham, Executive Content Strategist; Tiffany Trautwein, Senior Content Development Specialist; and Anne Konopka, Senior Project Manager, provided the necessary tools and helpful guidance and support throughout the publication process.

Professor Barnet Hartston deserves special thanks for his encouragement, support, and motivational ideas. Several of our photographic models, Zoe, Elliot, and Ian Fleck; Ruby Epstein and Spencer Hartston; and Sofia Augusta, added sparkle to many of the illustrations that appear in this text; their patience is appreciated. The authors express appreciation to each other for the support and mutual respect generated by this collaboration.

Last, but not least, gratitude is extended to our students from Hunter College of New York, California State University at Los Angeles, California State University at Northridge, and Riverside City College for helping us understand their learning needs and for inspiring us to continue the professionally challenging and personally rewarding careers of teaching and writing.

The use of information contained in this book is not dependent on scope of practice, so the text can be helpful to those studying within multidisciplinary health-related fields, such as nursing, psychology, counseling, early childhood education, or any field where understanding the needs, risks, and challenges of a specific age group influences a positive outcome to the interaction. We hope that the information contained in this text will provide the reader with tools to enhance communication and to develop effective plans of care for individual patients and their families.

Gloria Leifer Hartston, RN, MA, CNE
Eve Fleck, MS, ACE GFI, ACE PT, NASM CPT

Contents

CHAPTER 1

Healthy People 2020

http://evolve.elsevier.com/Leifer/growth

OBJECTIVES

1. Describe what *Healthy People 2020* is and what it is meant to do.
2. List public health issues defined by *Healthy People 2020.*
3. Discuss how the health status of a population is measured.
4. State one health issue or goal for each stage of the life cycle.
5. Discuss the role of the health-care worker in achieving *Healthy People 2020* objectives.
6. Discuss the role of the health-care worker in worldwide health improvement.

KEY TERMS

behaviors
biology
determinants of health
health status
Healthy People 2020
infant mortality rate
Leading Health Indicators
life expectancy
physical environment
social environment

DEFINITION

What *Healthy People 2020* Is

Healthy People 2020 is an evidence-based 10-year report card describing health-care accomplishments within the United States from the years 2000 to 2010. It is also a prescription for what needs to be done between now and the year 2020. The overarching goals of the *Healthy People 2020* plan are to enable the nation to achieve health equity, to eliminate disparities, and to create a social and physical environment that promotes good health, quality of life, healthy development, and positive health behaviors across all life stages. *Healthy People 2020* is "firmly dedicated to the principle that regardless of age, gender, race or ethnicity, income, education, geographic location, disability, or sexual orientation, every person in the nation deserves equal access to comprehensive, culturally competent, community-based health care systems that are committed to serving the needs of the individual and promoting community health" (*Healthy People 2020*).

Published by the U.S. Department of Health and Human Services (USDHHS) in 2011, *Healthy People 2020* is currently considered by many to be the most important document regarding health in the United States. First written in 1979, *Healthy People* is the work of more than 350 governmental agencies, organizations, and experts in the health-care field.

By analyzing current statistics every 10 years, *Healthy People* provides a snapshot of progress, trends, and issues, and it highlights future needs in health care by identifying specific goals. Goals and objectives are revised periodically based on accomplishments and needs.

Healthy People 2020 lists 42 topic areas (general categories) with more than 600 objectives (statements of movement toward targets), including more than 1200 measures to be achieved by the year 2020. Health problems and suggested improvements in health practices are designed according to evidence-based knowledge. The document groups four major age groups: (1) infants, (2) children, (3) teens and young adults, and (4) older adults and the geriatric population.

What *Healthy People 2020* Does

The *Healthy People 2020* guidelines established in 2011 focus on the larger social picture surrounding health-care outcomes than those presented in *Healthy People 2010.* Social issues, preparedness, and global health have been included for the first time. Eight *new topic areas* include:

1. Adolescent health including blood disorders and safety.
2. Early and middle childhood, genomics.
3. Global health; health-care associated infections.
4. Health related quality of life, including gay, lesbian, and transgender health.
5. Older adults, including those with dementia.
6. Preparedness.
7. Sleep health.
8. Social determinants of health.

Aspects of the goals and objectives of *Healthy People 2020* will be integrated throughout the chapters in this text. Specific tasks or risk factors will be identified, and health care interventions such as suggested age-appropriate exercise activities will be presented to promote a healthy lifestyle that leads to normal growth and development through the life cycle.

Leading Health Indicators

Health indicators are measurements of health-related concepts. Leading Health Indicators are selected high-priority issues for the current 10-year period. The leading health indicators for 2020 are:

1. Access to health services, including the availability of a primary-care provider for people with or without medical insurance.
2. Clinical preventive services, including recommended vaccines and immunizations (Figure 1-1).
3. Environmental quality, including air quality inside and outside the home.
4. Injury and violence, including unintentional fatal injuries and homicide.
5. Maternal, infant, and child health, including preventing prematurity and infant deaths.
6. Mental health, including preventing depression and suicide.
7. Oral health, including increasing the number of people older than 2 years who use the oral-care health system each year.
8. Reproductive and sexual health, including sexually active females who use reproductive health services and access to care for persons with HIV.

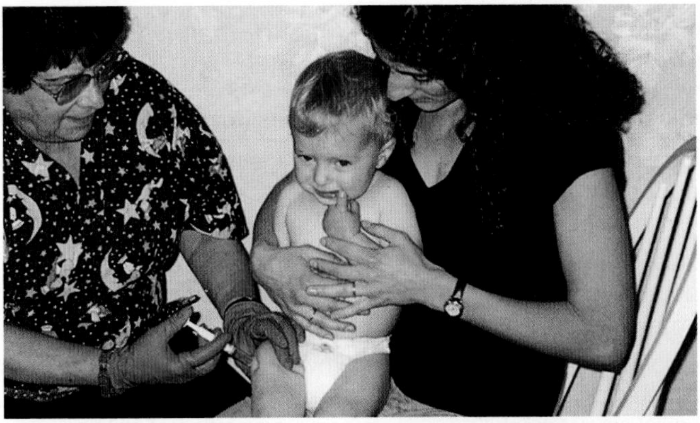

Figure 1–1 A mother holds her child in the "hug position" during immunization. Scheduled immunization programs for infants and children are listed in Appendix A.

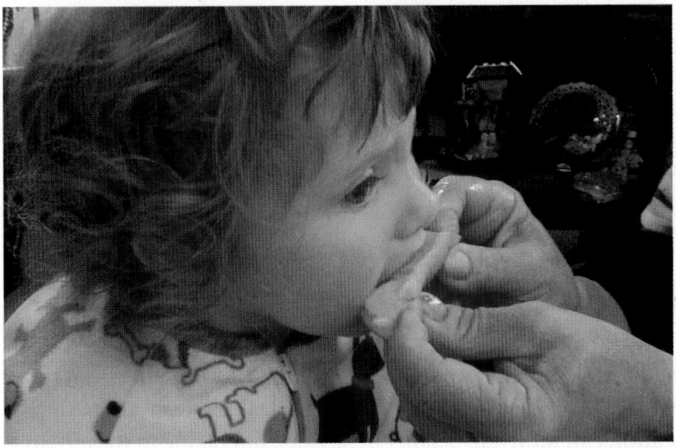

Figure 1–2 A child begins to learn about healthy food and nutrition early in life by developing a taste for fresh vegetables and fruits provided as daytime snacks.

9. Nutrition, physical activity, and obesity, including increasing the number of persons who meet federal guidelines for aerobic physical activity and increasing the consumption of vegetables (Figure 1-2).
10. Social determinants, including increasing the number of students who graduate with a regular diploma 4 years after ninth grade.
11. Substance abuse, including decreasing the number of adolescents and adults who abuse alcohol or illicit drugs.
12. Tobacco, including reducing adolescent and adult use of tobacco.

A sample chart showing how the topics, indicators, and objectives of *Healthy People 2020* are integrated and tracked is shown in Table 1-1. Preparedness is not yet listed as a leading health indicator because of a lack of literature in which to identify evidence-based practices, but the topic may be included as a leading indicator later in the decade.

Determinants of Health

Determinants of health are the range of social, economic, and environmental factors that influence health status. These can include individual behavior and biological and genetic factors.

TABLE 1-1 Sample Tracking of Relationships Among *Healthy People 2020* Topics, Indicators, and Objectives

Topic	Indicator	Objectives (for Action Planning)
Access to health care	Actual proportion of population with access to health care	Increase the number of people with access to medical and preventive care
Injury and violence	Actual proportion of population experiencing injury/violence	Reduce the occurrence of fatal and nonfatal injuries
Social determinants	Proportion of population experiencing a healthy social environment	Improve environmental health literacy Improve proportion of children ready to participate in elementary school Increase educational achievement of adolescents and young adults
Health-related quality of life	Proportion of population engaging in healthy behaviors, such as good nutrition and physical exercise	Increase participation in quality physical activity at all ages Reduce occurrence of obesity Promote healthy diets

Data from U.S. Department of Health and Human Services. Healthy People 2020 Objectives (2011). Retrieved from www.healthypeople.gov/2020/topicsobjectives2020/pdfs/HP2020objectives.pdf

Behavior and biology are interrelated. A disease affects biology, but behaviors can make a person susceptible or resistant to a disease. Social and physical environments impact behavior. For example, education can motivate healthy behaviors, but ozone in the environment can have a negative impact on biology (genetics). Policies and access to health care also figure prominently into this cycle. Therefore, personal health behavior is closely related to the general environment in achieving the *Healthy People 2020* goals (Figure 1-3).

Biology refers to the individual's genetic makeup (those factors with which he or she is born), family history (which may suggest risk for disease), and the physical and mental health problems acquired during life. Aging, diet, physical activity, smoking, stress, alcohol or illicit drug abuse, injury or violence, or an infectious or toxic agent may result in illness or disability and can produce a "new" biology for the individual.

Behaviors are individual responses or reactions to internal stimuli and external conditions. Behaviors can have a reciprocal relationship to biology (i.e., each can react to the other). For example, smoking (behavior) can alter the cells in the lung and can result in shortness of breath, emphysema, or cancer (biology) that then may lead an individual to stop smoking (behavior). Similarly, a family history that includes heart disease (biology) may motivate an individual to develop good eating habits, avoid tobacco, and maintain an active lifestyle (behaviors), which may prevent his or her own development of heart disease (biology).

Personal choices and the social and physical environments surrounding individuals can shape behaviors. The social and physical environments include all factors that affect the life of individuals, positively or negatively, many of which may not be under their immediate or direct control.

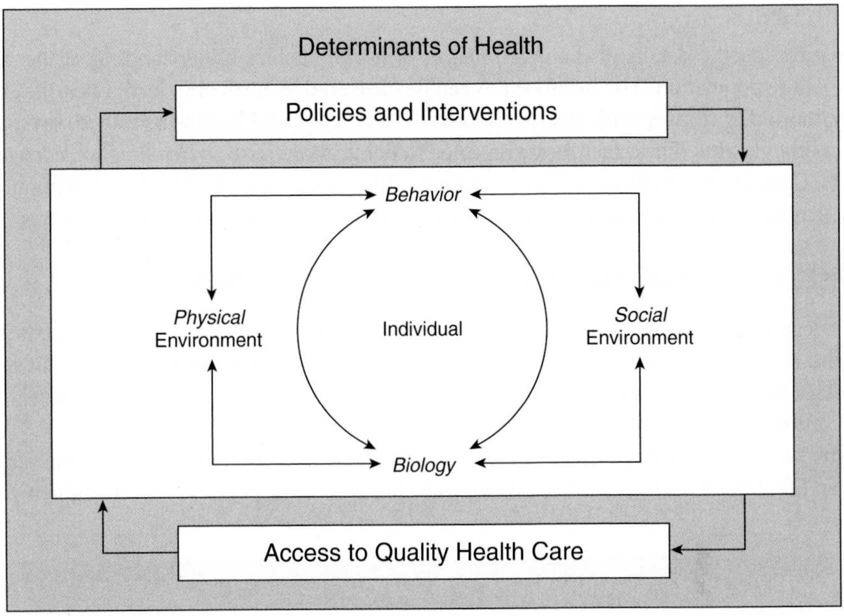

Figure 1–3 Determinants of health. *(From U.S. Department of Health and Human Services (2000). Healthy People 2010. McLean, VA: International Publishing, Inc.)*

Social environment includes interactions with family, friends, coworkers, and others in the community. It also encompasses social institutions, such as law enforcement, the workplace, places of worship, and schools. Housing, public transportation, and the presence or absence of violence in the community are among other components of the social environment. The social environment has a profound effect on the health of the individual and the larger community and is unique because of cultural customs, language, and personal, religious, or spiritual beliefs. At the same time, individuals and their behaviors contribute to the quality of the social environment.

Physical environment can be thought of as that which can be seen, touched, heard, smelled, and tasted. However, the physical environment also contains less tangible elements, such as radiation and ozone. The physical environment can harm individual and community health, especially when individuals and communities are exposed to toxic substances, irritants, infectious agents, and physical hazards in homes, schools, and worksites. The physical environment also can promote good health by providing clean and safe places for people to work, exercise, and play.

Policies and interventions can have a powerful and positive effect on the health of individuals and the community. Examples include health promotion campaigns to prevent smoking, policies mandating child restraints and safety-belt use in automobiles, disease prevention services (e.g., immunization of children, adolescents, and adults), and clinical services (e.g., enhanced mental health care). Policies and interventions that promote individual and community health may be implemented by a variety of agencies (e.g., transportation, education, energy, housing, labor, justice, and other venues), places of worship, community-based organizations, civic groups, and businesses.

Health Status

Evaluating specific details of the *determinants of health* enables understanding of the health status of the population. The health status can be measured by birth and death rates, life expectancy, morbidity from specific disease, access to health care, and health-insurance coverage, as well as other factors. These factors are reported in publications such as *Healthy People Review* or *Health, United States*. In these publications, the health status is described for the total population of the United States. The leading causes of death across the life span are presented in Box 1-1.

PROGRESS AND GOALS YET TO BE ACHIEVED

Each decade, when the goals and objectives of *Healthy People* are identified, communities and health-care professionals are expected to develop action plans to help achieve and maintain healthy behaviors and lifestyles, thus enabling access to and use of federal, state, and community programs and resources.

One example of the goals of *Healthy People 2020* is to increase quality and years of human life. Life expectancy is the average number of years a person born in a given year is

BOX 1-1 Leading Causes of Death by Age Group*

YOUNGER THAN 1 YEAR
- Congenital anomalies
- Disorders related to premature birth
- Sudden infant death syndrome
- Maternal pregnancy complications
- Sepsis, respiratory distress

1–4 YEARS
- Unintentional injuries
- Birth defects
- Homicide
- Cancer

5–14 YEARS
- Unintentional injuries
- Cancer
- Homicide, suicide
- Heart/respiratory disease

15–24 YEARS
- Unintentional injuries
- Homicide
- Suicide
- Cancer
- Heart disease

25–34 YEARS
- Unintentional injuries
- Suicide
- Homicide
- Cancer
- Heart disease

35–44 YEARS
- Unintentional injury
- Cancer
- Heart disease
- Suicide

45–54 YEARS
- Cancer
- Heart disease
- Unintentional injury
- Suicide

55–64 YEARS AND OLDER
- Cancer
- Heart disease
- Respiratory disease
- Unintentional injury
- Diabetes mellitus

OVER 65 YEARS
- Heart disease
- Cancer
- Respiratory disease
- Stroke
- Dementia

Data from Minino, A., Xu, J., Kuchanek, K. (2008). Deaths: Final Data for 2008 NVSR Vol 59 #2 December 9, 2008S.
*Listed in order of prevalence within each age group.

expected to live. In 1900, the life expectancy was 47.3 years. In 2009, the life expectancy was 75.6 years. These statistics show definite improvement; however in 2009, many countries had better life expectancy rates than the United States (Table 1-2).

Life-expectancy statistics can further be analyzed in terms of gender (women live an average of 6 years longer than men), race (white women have a greater life expectancy

TABLE 1-2 Life Expectancy at Birth by Country

Rank	Country	Life Expectancy in Years	Rank	Country	Life Expectancy in Years
1	Monaco	89.68	29	Jordan	80.18
2	Macau	84.43	30	United Kingdom	80.17
3	Japan	83.91	31	Greece	80.05
4	Singapore	83.75	32	Saint Pierre Miquelon	80.00
5	San Marino	83.07	33	Austria	79.91
6	Andorra	82.50	34	Faroe Island	79.85
7	Guernsey	82.24	35	Malta	79.82
8	Hong Kong	82.12	36	European Union	79.76
9	Australia	81.90	37	Luxembourg	79.76
10	Italy	81.86	38	Belgium	79.65
11	Liechtenstein	81.50	39	Virgin Islands	79.47
12	Canada	81.48	40	Finland	79.41
13	Jersey	81.47	41	South Korea	79.30
14	France	81.46	42	Turks and Caicos Islands	79.26
15	Spain	81.27	43	Wallis and Futuna	79.12
16	Sweden	81.18	44	Puerto Rico	79.07
17	Switzerland	81.17	45	Bosnia and Herzegovina	78.96
18	Israel	81.07	46	Saint Helena, Ascension, and Tristan da Cunha	78.91
19	Iceland	81.00	47	Gibraltar	78.83
20	Anguilla	80.98	48	Denmark	78.78
21	Netherlands	80.91	49	Portugal	78.70
22	Bermuda	80.82	50	United States	78.49
23	Cayman Islands	80.80			
24	Isle of Man	80.76			
25	New Zealand	80.71			
26	Ireland	80.32			
27	Norway	80.32			
28	Germany	80.19			

From Central Intelligence Agency. Country Comparison: Life Expectancy at Birth. *The World Factbook.* Retrieved March 8, 2012, from www.cia.gov/library/publications/the-world-factbook/rankorder/2102rank.html.

than other racial groups in the United States), and education status and income (a higher-income person may live 3 to 7 years longer than a lower-income person). Life-expectancy statistics from other countries may reflect the quality of health care in that country or the endemic prevalence of high infection, mortality, or HIV/AIDS infections (CIA, 2011; Ezzati, Friedman, & Murray, 2009).

Progress toward stated goals has been seen in several areas since the inception of *Healthy People* in 1979, but much remains to be done. Another important indicator that measures the status of the nation's health is the infant mortality (death) rate. The infant mortality rate is the number of deaths that occur before 1 year of age per 1000 live births. In 1975, the infant mortality was 15 per 1000 live births. In 1997, the number decreased to 7.2 deaths per 1000 live births (USDHHS, 2000). However, according to the National Center for Health Statistics (NCHS), in 2009 the U.S. infant mortality rate was 6.8 per 1000 live births.

The 1998–1999 review of the *Healthy People 2000* goals showed that about 15% of the objectives were met in the areas of nutrition, maternal–child health, heart disease, and mental health. More than 40% of the objectives were achieved in areas such as immunizations, breastfeeding, and breast-cancer screening between the years 2000 and 2010.

ISSUES AND GOALS RELATED TO PHASES OF THE LIFE CYCLE

Prenatal and Infant Health

Maternal and infant health is the core of the health status of the next generation. The U.S. infant mortality rate has declined steadily since 1979, but as of 2008, 28 countries have a lower infant mortality rate than the United States (CDC, 2008). The leading areas of progress between the years 2000 and 2010 include reducing sudden infant death syndrome (SIDS) with the back-to-sleep educational program that urges parents to place infants on their backs rather than on their abdomen when putting their infants down for a nap or for the night, and promoting the use of folic-acid supplements early in pregnancy to reduce congenital malformations such as spina bifida. Guidelines for "Baby Friendly" hospitals have been established to increase breastfeeding during the first year of life.

Childhood Health

The overall goals for this population are to increase health literacy and to improve the quality, availability, and effectiveness of community-based programs designed to prevent disease and to improve health. Health issues should be added to school curricula, teachers should be well informed, and school nurses should be available in all schools. Completion of high school should be encouraged to provide the education necessary for understanding the importance of healthy lifestyle choices. The target is that 90% of persons will receive a regular diploma 4 years after entering the ninth grade and that the United States will have the highest proportion of graduates in the workforce by the year 2020 (Obama, 2011). Encouraging school attendance, home schooling during prolonged illness, and school counseling services aid in achieving these goals. Increasing access to quality education, preparing students for college, providing early education (in the form of Head Start) programs, helping children with special needs, and using innovative strategies to help achieve positive student outcomes are also current objectives for *Healthy People 2020*.

School health services were established more than 100 years ago to reduce absenteeism caused by communicable diseases. Current school health programs reflect the concept that physical health and mental health are related to academic and social success. School nurses assess development, screen for specific health problems, refer to community agencies, and provide immunization clinics.

Adolescent and Young-Adult Health

In 2006, the adolescent death rate was 64 per 100,000 (MMWR, 2008). The *Healthy People 2020* goal is to reduce the death rate by increasing the proportion of schools that provide comprehensive health education in order to prevent health problems related to injuries, violence, suicides, tobacco and drug use, unintentional pregnancy, STDs, and unhealthy diets and activity lifestyles.

Older Adult Health

Although the life expectancy has increased, the problems related to maintaining an independent lifestyle remain a challenge. Goals for older adults include improving health, function, and quality of life. The goals of increasing physical activity, self-management of chronic diseases, use of health services, and training of caregivers will aid in achieving these objectives.

Geriatric Adult Health

Goals for the geriatric phase of life include: (1) reducing the number of illnesses and deaths related to vaccine-preventable illnesses by increasing the number of adults over age 65 who receive annual vaccines against influenza and pneumococcal pneumonia, (2) reducing the number of hip fractures (more than 75% of which occur in elderly females), and (3) increasing the availability of diagnostic tools that can decrease the number of undiagnosed dementia cases.

ROLE OF THE HEALTH-CARE WORKER IN ACHIEVING *HEALTHY PEOPLE 2020* GOALS

Health care workers play an important role in helping to achieve the goals of *Healthy People 2020* at all phases of the life cycle by:

- Increasing the use of prenatal services, which reduces the occurrence of low-birth-weight newborns and prematurity.
- Promoting breastfeeding, which increases the health of the newborn and bonding between mother and infant.
- Educating the school-age child about nutrition, diet and exercise, smoking and drug use, and healthy lifestyles.
- Promoting health through employer-sponsored programs.
- Providing health-education services to patients in managed-care organizations.
- Identifying health risks through screening programs, which can lead to early diagnosis and treatment of disease.
- Encouraging older adults to participate in at least one organized health-promotion activity.

Future health care reform may enable all people to be covered by some type of health-care insurance, which will increase accessibility and aid in achieving the stated goals of *Healthy People 2020.*

WORLD HEALTH

At the same time as *Healthy People* was being initiated and developed, efforts toward worldwide health improvement were also initiated by the World Health Organization (WHO). In 1978, the International Conference on Primary Health Care was held in Alma-Ata, Kazakhstan. The world community was urged to protect and promote the health of all people of the world, and a list of world-health goals was developed. A charter for health promotion was adopted at an international conference in 1986 in Ottawa, Canada. This charter defined world-health promotion as "those processes that enable people to increase control over and improve their health" (WHO, 1986). As a result of meetings held in various locations around the world in the 1990s, objectives were developed for improving the environment; eliminating poverty; and providing reproductive health services, adolescent health, women's empowerment, human rights, and tobacco control.

Progress has been made in improving world health by decreasing infant mortality rates, increasing access to immunizations, and providing areas of safer environmental sanitation. However, much work has yet to be completed. In September 2000, the United Nations adopted a "UN Millennium Declaration" that stated a series of goals and targets and indicators related to health and the alleviation of poverty. In 2005, these goals were restated at a meeting with WHO and the World Bank, where specific steps were recommended to speed achievement of the worldwide goals (Kubiszewski, 2008). A core principle of the Millennium Declaration was that human development is a shared responsibility. WHO will monitor the progress, which will be reported by the National Health Information System.

The current targets to be achieved by the year 2020 include halving the proportion of people who suffer from hunger and poverty, ensuring primary education for all children, and reversing the spread of HIV/AIDS, malaria, and other major diseases. In developing countries, progress has been slow and education is an important first step. WHO uses these goals and targets to focus on collaborative programs to improve global health care.

An outline of some effective interventions is available on *Evolve.* The current Millennium Declaration goals for global health include:

- Eradicating extreme poverty and hunger.
- Promoting gender equality and empowering women.
- Reducing child mortality.
- Improving maternal health.
- Combating HIV/AIDs, malaria, and other endemic diseases.
- Ensuring environmental sustainability.
- Establishing a global partnership to achieve the goals.

Global health efforts are necessary, because health problems are no longer confined to local areas. Outbreaks of illness in one area of the world can quickly spread to other areas of the world because of increased use of airline travel. Improvement in technology is not the key to improvement in health—*prevention* is. Prevention of illness through education and access to early health care is essential. The cultural competence of health-care workers and their willingness to be change agents for the traditional health-care delivery system is also essential.

Health-care workers must work with the local community and form partnerships for health. Improving prenatal care, nutrition, exercise, and access to children's health care all over the world are important beginning efforts toward improving world health. The health-care team can build a bridge of health that extends around the world. Providing culturally competent care in the local community is the starting point for that bridge. Working with organizations, political groups, and government agencies to help form legislation for policies and practices relating to health care is the responsibility of the individual as a health care worker, as well as the individual as a citizen.

KEY POINTS

- *Healthy People* is a 10-year report card issued by the USDHHS concerning what has been accomplished in the area of health care in the United States and what is yet to be accomplished.
- *Healthy People 2020* identifies leading health indicators that are of priority concern in health maintenance.
- The *overreaching goals* of *Healthy People 2020* are to enable the nation to achieve health equity, to eliminate disparities, and to create social and physical environments that promote good health, quality of life, healthy development, and positive health behaviors across all life stages.
- *Topics* are general categories addressed by *Healthy People 2020.* There are 42 topic areas with 600 related objectives in the current document.
- *Objectives* are statements of movement toward a target, such as "the number of days the air quality index is above 100."
- *Indicators* are high-priority issues that measure progress toward objectives.
- *Determinants of health* are the range of social, economic, and environmental factors that influence the health status, such as genetics, biology, policy, and law.
- *Health status* is measured by statistics, such as birth rates, death rates, and life expectancy.
- Global efforts are necessary to improve health care, because problems are no longer confined to local areas.
- The UN Millennium Declaration (updated in 2005) identifies worldwide goals.
- Providing culturally competent health care increases compliance with healthy lifestyles and can help in meeting the goals of *Healthy People 2020.*

Critical Thinking

School nurses and health care workers, working as a team, can contribute to the goals of *Healthy People 2020* by teaching relevant health topics to students. A school nurse or health care worker is assigned to teach one class to a group of elementary-school children and one class to a group of high-school students. List two topics for each class that would be age appropriate and relevant to the goals of *Healthy People 2020.*

REVIEW QUESTIONS

1. **The health status of a population is measured by:**
   a. the number of health facilities available.
   b. the number of people in a country.
   c. statistics, such as birth and death rates.
   d. membership in HMO organizations.

2. **Health care is best improved by:**
   a. increased number of doctors available.
   b. coordinated worldwide efforts.
   c. local health-department programs.
   d. statewide programs.

3. ***Healthy People 2020* is:**
   a. a report card on the progress of health care and identification of priority future needs.
   b. a list of laws that concern health-care requirements.
   c. a list of mandates related to medical practice.
   d. a list of health-care facilities that will be available by the year 2020.

4. **Health care workers play an important role in helping to achieve the goals of *Healthy People 2020* by:**
   a. treating the poor population who are ill.
   b. promoting breastfeeding and early prenatal care.
   c. working overtime to meet patient needs.
   d. working in community-based clinics.

5. **Leading health indicators include:**
   a. physical activity, mental health, access to health care, and environmental quality.
   b. reduction in birth rates, death rates, and morbidity.
   c. health-care conferences held locally and worldwide.
   d. the number of new policies and laws related to health care.

CHAPTER 2

Government Influences on Health Care

http://evolve.elsevier.com/Leifer/growth

OBJECTIVES

1. Trace the history of government involvement in health care.
2. Analyze health-care legislation and its influence on health-care delivery.
3. Discuss current health-care policy issues, including health-care reform.
4. List some factors that influence the cost of health care.
5. Describe two types of health-care delivery systems.
6. Identify future trends in health care.
7. Discuss the nurse's role in political activity related to health care.

KEY TERMS

accreditation
Federal Register
health maintenance organizations (HMOs)
homeopathy
informed consent
managed care organizations (MCOs)
Medicaid
Medicare
nurse practice acts
Nursing Licensure Compact (NLC)
Occupational Safety and Health Act (OSHA)
plan of care
political action committees (PACs)
preferred provider organizations (PPOs)
scope of practice
standards of practice

THE IMPORTANCE OF UNDERSTANDING THE ROLE OF GOVERNMENT IN HEALTH CARE

The government plays a key role in promoting the health and well-being of Americans, and understanding its contributions and influences on health care is important. This brief chapter presents a history of government involvement in heath care in the United States as well as current and potential future trends. This knowledge allows consumers and health-care workers to have an understanding of and an informed say (vote) in developing new legislation.

HEALTH-CARE LEGISLATION

In the past, monarchs, the church, or people with specific knowledge or expertise made health-care decisions for the entire population of a locality or a country. These decisions evolved into judgments based on individual case decisions. From repeated judgments, laws were developed that became part of a system of rules. In the United

States, as time passed, legislative groups or bodies were added to the lawmaking process, and eventually the congressional system was formed. A system of courts and legislative bodies are organized around three levels of government: the federal, state, and local sectors. Most lawmakers are elected by the people to represent the needs of their communities.

Laws originally revolved around individual rights and property rights, but in the nineteenth century, laws concerning health care were developed based on the fundamental principles of health-care leaders such as Hippocrates, Dorothy Dix, Clara Barton, and Florence Nightingale. The efforts of these and other leaders in the field of health care led to the development of standards of practice, which were the foundations of laws related to consumer protection.

The first legal health-care issues concerned the definition of health related to the ability of slaves to work. Early court decisions influenced the methods of health-care delivery systems and the providers within these delivery systems. Patient-care problems included infected wounds, trauma care, and care for specific age-related diseases. Most of the caretakers were self taught, and the health-care needs of most patients were often attended to by family members. As health-care needs increased, and care became more complex, experts were called in for consultation. In 1750, the first hospital for the poor was established in Philadelphia.

HOSPITALS AND NURSING SCHOOLS

In 1873, the Bellevue Hospital School of Nursing was established in New York as a proponent of the Nightingale principles of nursing care. Clara Barton founded the American Red Cross in 1881, which focused on community health needs. In 1887, the Mayo brothers in Minnesota established the concepts of private-office health-care practice and then group clinics. The formation of the American Medical Association and philanthropic organizations, such as the Rockefeller Foundation and the Carnegie Foundation, advocated professional care, and self care was devalued. By the end of the nineteenth century, three schools of nursing existed in the United States. A group of nurse leaders formed the American Society of Superintendents of Nurse Training Schools, which adopted a code of ethics based on the Nightingale pledge. The structure was similar to the American Medical Association in elevating professional care.

By 1903, licensure by a state government agency was required to practice nursing, and the original Society for Training Schools evolved into the National League for Nursing (NLN). In 1911, school alumnae formed the American Nurses Association (ANA). Gradually the belief that nurses needed higher education and increased theoretical knowledge led to the opening of a program at Columbia University in New York to train teachers of nursing. The founders of this program for nurse educators, Isabelle Hampton Robb and Mary Adelaide Nutting, advocated the professionalism of nursing.

Hospitals gradually became the centers for health care, because they had more resources for care than a private doctor's office. Health centers developed and specialization increased. Specialty service units appeared in hospitals, including medical, surgical, and obstetrical units. One of the earliest pieces of governmental legislation concerning hospitals was the Hill-Burton Hospital Construction Act of 1946, which provided grants to states for the purpose of building new hospitals.

Although nursing as a career flourished with the establishment of the Army Cadet Nursing Corps to care for military personnel, nursing in civilian life did not receive the respect it deserved until later. Most schools of nursing were managed in hospital settings, but in 1965, the ANA advocated that nursing education take place in a college setting, and a respected profession of nursing was reborn. A standardized national competence examination was determined to be a requirement for nursing licensure, and today almost all registered nurses earn their nursing degrees in college institutions.

The federal government provided funds to train vocational nurses who cared for patients in the community setting. Vocational nursing programs were about 13–18 months in length and focused on skills and theory correlated with clinical practice. Today many licensed practical/vocational nurse programs are based in community-college settings.

THE MULTIDISCIPLINARY HEALTH-CARE TEAM

Health care soon grew into an industry that depended on multidisciplinary providers, such as doctors, nurses, laboratory technicians, X-ray technicians, social workers, and others. The goals of the team are to ensure the optimum physical, social, and mental well being of the patient, and members work together to provide comprehensive care. Communication among team members and the patient is vital. The plan of care was developed as a tool for this communication and can be an individual patient plan of care, a family plan of care, or a hospital care path that outlines the needs of the patient and the planned approach to meet these needs.

Standards of care provided by nurses and other members of the multidisciplinary team were developed by professional organizations to ensure quality care for patients.

NURSE PRACTICE ACTS

States have government-established nurse practice acts, which define the scope of practice for nurses within that state. The scope of practice is the identification of and legal limitations to the usual and customary skills practiced by a professional. Usual and customary practices are determined by the educational preparation for that profession. Currently each state has its own nurse practice act with some variations in scope of practice, and nurses are responsible for knowing the nurse practice act(s) of the state(s) in which they practice.

The National Council of State Boards of Nursing has designed a broad model Nurse Practice Act that serves as a multistate licensing arrangement (i.e., the Nursing Licensure Compact [NLC]), which enables traveling nurses to function in multiple states (NCSBN, 2008). As of 2011, there were 24 states in which nurses could hold multistate licenses without additional application procedures or fees. The mobility of nurses, the growth of traveling-nurse programs, and the use of Internet services have led to the need for interstate licensing of nurses.

PATIENT'S BILL OF RIGHTS

The President's Advisory Commission on Consumer Protection and Quality in the Health Care Industry adopted a Consumer Bill of Rights and Responsibilities in 2009. This report stressed the importance of the relationship between the health-care provider and the patient and stipulated that the health-care system:

- Is fair and meets patients' needs.
- Gives patients a way to address problems.
- Encourages patients to take active roles in health care.

The key areas in the Consumer Bill of Rights includes the rights of the consumer to:

- Have choice of providers.
- Have access to emergency services.
- Take part in treatment decisions.
- Receive respect and nondiscrimination.
- Maintain confidentiality of health-care information.
- Have resources for complaint and appeal.

Minnesota was the first state to establish a Bill of Rights for Patients as a state law in 1973, and the American Hospital Association (AHA) updated *The Patient Care Partnership: Understanding Expectations, Rights, and Responsibilities* in 2003 (Box 2-1). One of the most important rights of patients is the right of informed consent, and the nurse is responsible to sign as a witness that a patient has received information regarding risks, advantages, and alternatives available for a planned procedure in a language that can be understood by the patient.

The U.S. government mandates provision of health-care services to physically handicapped persons, mentally handicapped persons, and pregnant women. These rights must be upheld if the hospital is to remain accredited or approved. Accreditation is the process by which an institution is recognized as meeting specific predetermined standards of care. Although the government does not accredit hospitals, a hospital that is not accredited by any group may not be eligible to receive state or federal funding assistance. The AHA adopted criteria for hospitals for the pursuit of excellence (Box 2-2). Many of these criteria are assessed when the hospital seeks accreditation by various accrediting groups.

BOX 2-1 The Patient Care Partnership: Understanding Expectations, Rights, and Responsibilities

When you need hospital care, your doctor and the nurses and other professionals at our hospital are committed to working with you and your family to meet your health-care needs. Our dedicated doctors and staff serve the community in all its ethnic, religious, and economic diversity. Our goal is for you and your family to have the same care and attention we would want for our families and ourselves.

The sections explain some of the basics about how you can expect to be treated during your hospital stay. They also cover what we will need from you to care for you better. If you have questions at any time, please ask them. Unasked or unanswered questions can add to the stress of being in the hospital. Your comfort and confidence in your care are very important to us.

WHAT TO EXPECT DURING YOUR HOSPITAL STAY

High-Quality Hospital Care

Our first priority is to provide you the care you need, when you need it, with skill, compassion, and respect. Tell your caregivers if you have concerns about your care or if you have pain. You have the right to know the identity of doctors, nurses, and others involved in your care, and you have the right to know when they are students, residents, or other trainees.

A Clean and Safe Environment

Our hospital works hard to keep you safe. We use special policies and procedures to avoid mistakes in your care and keep you free from abuse or neglect. If anything unexpected and significant happens during your hospital stay, you will be told what happened, and any resulting changes in your care will be discussed with you.

Involvement in Your Care

You and your doctor often make decisions about your care before you go to the hospital. Other times, especially in emergencies, those decisions are made during your hospital stay. When decision-making takes place, it should include:

Discussing Your Medical Condition and Information about Medically Appropriate Treatment Choices. To make informed decisions with your doctor, you need to understand:

- The benefits and risks of each treatment
- Whether your treatment is experimental or part of a research study
- What you can reasonably expect from your treatment and any long-term effects it might have on your quality of life
- What you and your family will need to do after you leave the hospital
- The financial consequences of using uncovered services or out-of-network providers

Please tell your caregivers if you need more information about treatment choices.

Discussing Your Treatment Plan. When you enter the hospital, you sign a general consent to treatment. In some cases, such as surgery or experimental treatment, you may be asked to confirm in writing that you understand what is planned and agree to it. This process protects your right to consent to or refuse a treatment. Your doctor will explain the medical consequences of refusing recommended treatment. It also protects your right to decide if you want to participate in a research study.

Getting Information from You. Your caregivers need complete and correct information about your health and coverage so that they can make good decisions about your care. That includes:

- Past illnesses, surgeries, or hospital stays
- Past allergic reactions
- Any medicines or dietary supplements (such as vitamins and herbs) that you are taking
- Any network or admission requirements under your health plan

Understanding Your Health-Care Goals and Values. You may have health-care goals and values or spiritual beliefs that are important to your well-being. They will be taken into account as much as possible throughout your hospital stay. Make sure your doctor, your family, and your care team knows your wishes.

Understanding Who Should Make Decisions When You Cannot. If you have signed a health-care power of attorney stating who should speak for you if you become unable to make health-care decisions for yourself, or a "living will" or "advance directive" that states your wishes about end-of-life care, give copies to your doctor, your family, and your care team. If you or your family need help making difficult decisions, counselors, chaplains, and others are available to help.

Protection of Your Privacy

We respect the confidentiality of your relationship with your doctor and other caregivers, and the sensitive information about your health and health care that are part of that relationship. State and federal laws and hospital operating policies protect the privacy of your medical information. You will receive a Notice of Privacy Practices that describes the ways that we use, disclose, and safeguard patient information and that explains how you can obtain a copy of information from our records about your care.

Help When Leaving the Hospital

Your doctor works with hospital staff and professionals in your community. You and your family also play an important role in your care. The success of your treatment often depends

(Continued)

BOX 2-1 The Patient Care Partnership: Understanding Expectations, Rights, and Responsibilities—cont'd

on your efforts to follow medication, diet, and therapy plans. Your family may need to help care for you at home.

You can expect us to help you identify sources of follow-up care and to let you know if our hospital has a financial interest in any referrals. As long as you agree that we can share information about your care with them, we will coordinate our activities with your caregivers outside the hospital. You can also expect to receive information and, when possible, training about the self care you will need when you go home.

Help with Your Bill and Filing Insurance Claims

Our staff will file claims for you with health-care insurers or other programs such as Medicare and Medicaid. They also will help your doctor with needed documentation. Hospital bills and insurance coverage are often confusing. If you have questions about your bill, contact our business office. If you need help understanding your insurance coverage or health-care plan, start with your insurance company or health benefits manager. If you do not have health-care coverage, we will try to help you and your family find financial help or make other arrangements. We need your help with collecting needed information and other requirements to obtain coverage or assistance.

From the American Hospital Association. (2003). *The Patient Care Partnership: Understanding Expectations, Rights, and Responsibilities.*

BOX 2-2 AHA Criteria for Hospitals in Pursuit of Excellence

Care Coordination – Involves coordinating the multidisciplinary team and multiple facilities in providing seamless care.

Efficiency – Defined by the Institute of Medicine (IOM) as activities that involve reducing quality waste by utilizing best practices and reducing administrative and production costs.

Health-Care–Acquired Infections – Includes provisions for reducing health-care associated infections.

Health-Care Equity – Includes expansion of programs to support the development of interdisciplinary community-based links that target underserved communities.

Health Information Technology – Promotes use of electronic health records to centralize health-care delivery and to link providers and patients with information in a timely manner.

Medication Management – Includes reducing medication errors by educating patients to participate in care, and to improve labeling, dispensing, and information sheets.

Payment Models – Hospitals should devise alternative payment systems and should reward providers for improving care.

Patient Input – Includes improving patient flow throughout all areas of the hospital and avoiding delays that may jeopardize patient safety.

Workforce and Culture – Includes improving participation of staff to implement performance excellence, use evidence-based practices, and provide culturally competent care.

Adapted from Health Research & Educational Trust. *Hospitals in Pursuit of Excellence*. 2010. Retrieved July 12, 2012, from http://www.hpoe.org/topic-areas.

THE GOVERNMENT'S ROLE IN HEALTH CARE

The Constitution of the United States, Article 1, section 8, states that a role of the federal government is to provide for the general welfare of the people and provides the spending power to do so. Therefore, the government can act to protect the health, welfare, and safety of the people. For example, to protect the health of the community, the government requires specific immunizations for schoolchildren before they are allowed to enter school.

The involvement of government in health care began gradually. The Children's Bureau, established in 1912, studied the needs of children, established agencies to provide services (e.g., Woman, Infants, and Children program [WIC]), and defined essential community health and nursing responsibilities. The Sheppard-Towner Act of 1921 influenced social welfare policies. President Roosevelt's New Deal, designed to revive the country from the Great Depression, provided government spending for health care. The National Insurance Plan proposed by Mayor Wagner of New York, combined with the passage of the Social Security Act of 1935, were the sparks that ignited expanded government involvement in public health care. In 1937, the Unemployment Compensation and Old Age Benefit laws were passed.

United States Department of Health and Human Services

Originally established in 1939 as the Federal Security Agency, the United States Department of Health and Human Services (USDHHS) was renamed in 1980. *Healthy People 2020,* published by the USDHHS, is considered by many to be the most important document concerning health in the United States today (see chapter 1). Under the guidance of this department, the three levels of government (local, state, and federal) provide direct services, financing, information, and setting of policy.

Direct Services

Direct services include providing health care to Native Americans, military personnel and their families, and prisoners. It is also concerned with managing screening clinics for diseases, such as tuberculosis, and managing immunization clinics for children.

Financing

The government funds health education programs and finances health care through Medicare, Medicaid, and Social Security programs (Box 2-3). The government also provides grants for medical and nursing research and education.

BOX 2-3 Medicare and Medicaid

Medicare is a type of insurance program in which benefits are received after contributions are made through payroll deductions.

Medicaid is similar to a welfare program in which benefits are provided on a basis of need or poverty.

These programs determine physicians' fees using a complicated formula.

Many services may not be covered or may require a copayment at the time services are rendered.

Information

Government agencies, such as the National Institutes of Health (NIH) and the Centers for Disease Control and Prevention (CDC), write periodic reports concerning vital statistics, census data, and results of health surveys. Information is published in *Health, United States,* an anuual report that provides a snapshot of the health status of U.S. residents.

Policy Setting

Most health-care legislation in the United States is delegated to the USDHHS, although specialties such as environmental health or occupational health may have separate agencies to focus on those specific areas. The Public Health Service sector of the USDHHS, which oversees the health care of U.S. citizens, has a Bureau of Professions responsible for the Division of Nursing, Division of Dentistry, Division of Medicine, and so on.

Federal legislation concerning health care (Table 2-1) is recorded and published in the Federal Register. Revisions of various regulations are based on research findings and public input, and periodic hearings are held. When a law is passed, monitoring of the private sector for compliance occurs.

TABLE 2-1 Examples of Federal Legislation Related to Health Care

1798	The Marine Hospital Service Act provided medical care to merchant marines (eventually became U.S. Public Health Service).
1878	The Port Quarantine Act prevented people with infectious diseases from entering the United States.
1879	A National Health Department was established.
1901	The Pure Food and Drug Act monitored the manufacture, labeling, and sale of food and drugs (later became the Food and Drug Administration [FDA]).
1912	The Children's Health Bureau established and implemented child labor laws. The bureau meets every 10 years to focus on children's needs.
1921	The Sheppard-Towner Maternity-Infant Care Act provided funds for health and welfare of mothers and children.
1935	The Social Security Act passed Title VI to assist states in providing public health services. Enabled development of Medicare and Medicaid programs.
1939	The Federal Security Agency combined health, education, and welfare services.
1940	The Communicable Disease Center (now known as the Centers for Disease Control and Prevention [CDC]) was established in Atlanta, Georgia.
	The Nurse Training Act provided funds to encourage nursing education.
1944	The Public Health Act consolidated public health legislation into one law.
1945	The McCarran-Ferguson Act gave state governments the right to regulate health insurance plans.
1946	The Hill-Burton Act provided for new hospital construction with provisions for care of the uninsured.
1947	The Army Nurse Corps was established.
1948	The National Institutes of Health (NIH) was established.

1954	The Taft Sanitary Engineering Center was established to improve environmental health.
1955	The U.S. Medical Library was formed to provide access to medical literature.
1964	A health amendment provided increased funds for nursing education.
1965	The Title VIII Social Security Amendment created Medicare to care for older adults and the disabled. Title XIX provided access to health care for the poor via Medicaid.
1970	The Occupational Safety and Health Act (OSHA) focused on workplace and environmental health.
1971	The Environmental Protection Agency was formed to monitor all environmental programs.
1972	The National Security Act was amended to encourage health maintenance organizations (HMOs) and preferred provider organizations (PPOs) to manage health care. Provided grants for HMO development.
1973	The Health Maintenance Organization Act required employers to offer federally qualified HMO coverage for employees and mandated state supervision.
1980	Infant Formula Act required standards for the manufacture of infant formulas.
1981	The Omnibus Budget Reconciliation Act provided money for grants for various health promotion projects, such as nursing homes, skilled nursing facilities, and home health agencies.
1982	The Tax Equity Fiscal Responsibility Act (TEFRA) amended the Social Security Act establishing the diagnosis-related group (DRG) system, which changed health care radically by establishing strict rules for reimbursement.
1985	The Consolidated Omnibus Reconciliation Act (COBRA) ensured continuation of health insurance for a time after loss of coverage due to job termination.
1989	Reimbursement of nurse practitioners for care provided was approved.
1990	The Health Objectives Planning Act resulted from the 1979 *Healthy People* report, which identified and monitored the nation's health-care goals. Established *Healthy People 2000* and *Healthy People 2010.*
1996	The Health Insurance Portability and Accountability Act (HIPAA) enabled portability of health insurance, privacy of medical information, and coverage for preexisting conditions.
1997	The Welfare Reform Act regulated restrictions for Aid to Families with Dependent Children (AFDC).
2002	Laws prohibit smoking in some public buildings.
	The use of mercury alloys in dental amalgam for certain patients, and the use of mercury in medical devices such as blood pressure machines, were prohibited.
	Asbestos abatement programs for school buildings were created.
	Lead and chemical poisoning prevention and screening programs were established.
	The Homeland Security Act addressed the public health and safety of the nation in the event of a terrorist attack.
2003	HIPAA regulations were enforced nationwide.

(Continued)

TABLE 2-1 Examples of Federal Legislation Related to Health Care—cont'd

2005	Public Readiness and Emergency Preparedness Act (PREPA) encouraged rapid production of vaccines to protect Americans in case of a public health emergency threat.
	Patient Safety and Quality Improvement Act (PQIA) encourages reporting to a database to monitor adverse events, near misses, and dangerous conditions.
2009	Health-Care Recovery and Reinvestment Act. A stimulus package provides for adoption of health information technology, confidentiality of health-care records, and provides new funding for Medicaid and health care for the poor. Promotes prevention and wellness initiatives and provides for medical research.
	Family Smoking Prevention and Tobacco Control Act. Passed in 1990, authorized the FDA to regulate the manufacture, marketing, and distribution of tobacco products, including Bidid, Ktetek, and will include electronic cigarettes, smokeless tobacco, and Hookah. It also prohibits distribution of samples and sponsorship by tobacco companies of school, athletic, or social events. It also prohibits sale of tobacco products in community vending machines (Chen, 2011).
2010	Patient Protection and Affordable Care Act. Extended health-care coverage to 32 million Americans who would otherwise have been uninsured. Medicare payroll taxes were slated to pay for services. Set limits on insurance companies' power to deny coverage to individuals and families. Passed into law by a narrow margin, became a political issue, and may be revised by future political administrations before it is fully implemented.

Although an individual U.S. citizen has the right to privacy and freedom, a federal law can mandate quarantine if it is deemed necessary to protect the health or welfare of individuals in a community (e.g., from tuberculosis or smallpox infections). State laws can also mandate specific health-related actions. For example, some states require all college students to be covered by health insurance, which may be paid for by student fees.

Occupational health is regulated by the federal Occupational Safety and Health Act (OSHA), which requires standards of safety be maintained by employers to protect the health and safety of employees and mandates the reporting of injuries sustained by workers. Workers have the right to know if they are working in a toxic environment. Workers injured on the job also have the right to receive health-care and financial compensation for any life-altering injury that occurs while on the job. State laws license and certify home care and hospice facilities and can also regulate, to some extent, insurance companies and labor unions.

Some federal laws can affect the social development of young adults. For example, 18- to 25-year-old men must register with Selective Service. In the event of a crisis requiring a military draft, these men may be called into active service in a sequence based on a random lottery number and the date of birth, which may interrupt career or marital plans. Both federal and local laws regulate the age at which one can drink alcohol, drive a car, and work.

The government also defines the age at which senior citizens are eligible for full Social Security benefits. This age has been designated as 65 years but may be changed to 67 or 68 years of age in the future to help reduce costs.

There are also governmental influences on the family, including tough divorce laws in some states and lenient divorce laws in other states. Most states currently have lenient abortion laws and favor the concept of giving custody of children to the biological parent whenever possible in an effort to provide caregivers who will consistently meet the developmental needs of children.

THE RISING COSTS OF HEALTH CARE

Health Care Delivery Systems

The cost of health care in the United States has steadily increased in recent history and continues to rise. Public health benefits (Medicare and Medicaid) were introduced, but increasing costs threaten their survival. Maintaining quality care while ensuring cost containment is a major challenge in health care today. Cost controls involve addressing issues such as national health goals, entitlements, the right to health care, use of available resources, and identification of the changing health-care needs of the people.

The National Committee for Quality Assurance was established to review and accredit managed care organizations (MCOs), which attempt to standardize and control costs of health care. Health maintenance organizations (HMOs) provide care for prepaid members, and preferred provider organizations (PPOs) contract with professionals to provide care to a specific group of patients at an agreed-on fee-for-service rate. Savings realized from government-sponsored health-care programs could be used for other government-sponsored programs or to help reduce the federal budget deficit; therefore, the costs of health care are of interest to all people in the United States.

Private Health Insurance

Increasing health-care costs have also led to higher premiums for membership in private health-care insurance plans. Part of the health insurance costs may be the responsibility of employers who then recoup their costs by increasing the cost of their consumer product, which in turn may raise the cost of living.

Health Promotion

Prevention and early intervention seem to be the keys to reducing health-care costs and are the core of *Healthy People 2020* (see Chapter 1). The Human Genome Project (see Chapter 6) gives health-care providers the potential to predict, detect, and treat illnesses before they become expensive, chronic problems. The information gained from this project may be used effectivey in the future to decrease the occurrence of chronic health-care problems.

Health-Care Reform

Historically, people in the United States oppose the government becoming involved in health-care programs and generally resist "socialized" medicine. Any effort to reform health care must involve managing costs, promoting access, and identifying payors. However, the potential for rationing care and limiting coverage for specific problems are two of consumers' major worries regarding the future of health care. Health care reform has become a major political issue, and laws and policies passed by one political party may be overturned when another is elected into power.

Resurgence of Self Care

The focus on illness prevention and early detection and intervention increasingly leads health-care delivery from inpatient to outpatient care settings where education can help to increase healthy behaviors and prevent illness. Self care is a valuable adjunct to health-care reform, as the focus of health care continues to shift from treatment to prevention of illness and from hospital-centered to community-based care. Self care is not a new concept. Midwives and lay practitioners were popular in the eighteenth and nineteenth centuries. In the 1830 s and 1840 s, the interest in self care peaked, and hydrotherapy (therapy using water) and homeopathy (the use of minute portions of naturally occurring chemicals for their healing powers) flourished.

In 1959, Dorothy Orem developed the self-care model related to nursing practice. In the 1960s, Martha Rogers, a nursing theorist, proposed a holistic view of health care, and in 1989 another theorist, Jean Watson, focused on the value of the nurse-patient relationship in the promotion of health. Today the desire of the individual to have control over their body has resulted in a resurgence of self care. Many health-care organizations, such as Kaiser Permanente Foundation Health Plan, distribute self-care guides to all members. Self care, nutrition, and exercise classes are all readily available and are in popular use.

Complementary and alternative medicine (CAM) is practiced by individuals in the community, and many applications have been adopted in traditional care settings (Hollenberg, 2007). Health-care agencies depend on self-care education to promote health and prevent disease because it is an effective cost-containment technique. Outreach programs target local populations for screening and education based on needs assessments of the community. Providing safe environments in educational institutions and including self-care health concepts in school curricula are essential elements of modern health-care reform. Nursing education programs are increasing students' experiences with healthy individuals in community-based settings. Culturally competent care of a diverse population is being integrated into medical and nursing school programs. Occupational health programs, in the form of supporting employee health, and websites for dissemination of health-care information are also important to the future of health care.

GLOBAL HEALTH

In 1945, the United Nations (UN) was formed by the joining of many nations for the promotion of common goals, including human rights, peace, and the economic and social advancement of all people. The UN headquarters is located in New York City and meets annually with the World Health Organization (WHO), which was created in 1946 to establish worldwide policies and services to promote health and health research (see Chapter 1).

THE FUTURE OF HEALTH CARE

Federal legislation and funding serve to increase the involvement of government in health care. The increasing health-care costs, the increasing need for health care, and the growth of various health-care delivery systems have also resulted in the need for continued federal intervention. Public health programs have the potential for improving health and reducing health-care costs through the early detection of and the intervention in diseases. Government agencies provide vital statistics that aid in identifying areas of need and in developing intervention strategies.

Political influence is promoted by political action committees (PACs). PACs influence legislation by offering monetary contributions to legislators who support their needs and by providing lobbying efforts to create an awareness of needed legislation. The ANA and other medical organizations have PACs to represent the needs of nurses and patients. Many nurses serve as elected public officials, and nurse legislators help in interpreting health-care issues.

Nurses play a key role in the future of health care by supporting and educating patients; providing cost-effective, quality care; and becoming involved in the legislative decisions of local, state, and federal governments. Nurses realize that the role of government related to health care influences the delivery of health care. For that reason, nurses need to be active in the political arena to ensure that the needs of nurses and patients are considered when discussing, creating, and passing laws related to health care.

KEY POINTS

- The role of the government in health care was established in article 1, section 8, of the U.S. Constitution, which provides spending power to promote the general health, welfare, and safety of the people.
- Standards of health care practice are the foundation of health-care legislation.
- The Hill-Burton Hospital Construction Act of 1946 provided funding to build new hospitals.
- The Army Cadet Nurse Corps was established to care for military personnel, and nursing as a career began to flourish.
- The multidisciplinary health-care team includes doctors, nurses, lab technicians, X-ray technicians, social workers, and others.
- Local governments established guidelines for nursing practice that defined the scope of practice for each level of professional nursing.
- Twenty-four states participate in the NLC multistate nurse licensing partnership.
- Minnesota was the first state to establish the Patient's Bill of Rights as law.
- A hospital that is not accredited may not be eligible to receive state or federal funding assistance.
- The Social Security Act of 1935 expanded government involvement in public health care.
- The Department of Health and Human Services of the federal government provides direct services, information, and health-care legislation.
- The United Nations meets annually with the World Health Organization to establish worldwide health policies, services, and research.
- Federal legislation that is passed is published in the Federal Register.
- Occupational health is regulated by the Occupational Safety and Health Association (OSHA), which sets standards of health and safety in the workplace.
- The federal government provides legislation and funding to support the goals of *Healthy People 2020.*
- Political influence is promoted by political action committees (PACs), in which nurses can advocate for patient needs and interpret health-care issues.
- The Patient Protection and Affordable Care Act of 2010 addressed the problem of accessability of health care for all Americans but passed by a narrow margin. It may be revised by future administrations that are elected by the people.

Critical Thinking

Nurses and other health-care workers may have the opportunity to join political action committees to assist in increasing awareness of the need for health-related legislation. Discuss two topics currently relevant to health-care reform that this committee might promote.

REVIEW QUESTIONS

1. **The purpose of the Nurse Practice Act is to:**
   a. define the scope of practice for each level of professional nursing.
   b. define the length of nursing education programs.
   c. determine criteria for licensing nursing schools.
   d. license nurses to practice.

2. **Most schools of nursing are currently located in a(n):**
   a. hospital.
   b. high school.
   c. independent occupational setting.
   d. college.

3. **The right of the government to play a role in health care originates in:**
   a. the U.S. Constitution.
   b. laws decided by local courts.
   c. the Democratic Party.
   d. an annual vote by the people.

4. **The functions of the U.S. Department of Health and Human Services (USDHHS) include:**
   a. writing licensing exams for health-care professionals.
   b. prioritizing medical practices.
   c. operating clinics for the indigent population.
   d. setting policy, providing information, and financing health-care programs.

5. **Political Action Committees (PACs) influence health care by:**
   a. writing health-care laws.
   b. supporting legislators who vote on health-care policies.
   c. studying the needs of local communities.
   d. promoting higher salaries for nurses.

Cultural Considerations Across the Lifespan and in Health and Illness

CHAPTER 3

http://evolve.elsevier.com/Leifer/growth

OBJECTIVES

1. Define culture and its expression.
2. Describe the difference between beliefs and values.
3. Identify various beliefs and values in today's adult population.
4. Discuss the impact of culture and personal values on everyday life and healthy behaviors.
5. Explain the relationship of culture and values to health-promotion teaching.
6. Define complementary and alternative therapies.
7. Discuss the role of the government in promoting culturally competent health care.

KEY TERMS

acculturation
alternative medicine
beliefs
complementary medicine
cultural awareness
cultural care
cultural competence
cultural interventions
cultural sensitivity
cultural stereotyping
culture
ethnicity
ethnocentric
stereotyping
values

Cultural aspects of growth and development for each phase of the life cycle are integrated in the specific chapters later in this text. This chapter is designed to provide some specific illustrations of how understanding the cultural needs of others can improve health-promotion services and outcomes, enhance cost effectiveness of health care, reduce errors, and increase compliance to healthy behaviors, which will aid in achieving the goals of *Healthy People 2020.*

DEFINITION

Culture is defined as a set of learned values, beliefs, customs, and behaviors that is shared by a common social group and is passed down through generations of family. Culture can influence food choices, parenting styles, and preferences for treatment measures. Health-care workers can demonstrate cultural sensitivity by observing and demonstrating knowledge of culturally appropriate verbal language, body language, use of personal space, and gestures of respect toward family members. Religion is closely related to culture, and religiously appropriate interventions should be integrated sensitively to meet the spiritual needs of patients and their families.

Cultural competence is the awareness of, acceptance of, and respect for beliefs, values, traditions, and practice that are different from one's own. The ability to adapt health care so that it does not violate the culture or religion of the patient is at the core of cultural competence. Achieving cultural competence is aided by knowledge, skills, and encounters with others of different cultures.

Health-care workers must remember that there are always individual differences among people in cultural groups. Individual members of a culture group may not each strictly adhere to all traditions of the culture (see Chapter 4. The assumption that all the people of one culture behave the same way and believe the same thing is called cultural stereotyping and can be offensive. It is particularly important to be sensitive to individual differences when working with a diverse population.

Beliefs are cultural teachings of practices and values that are handed down for generations and determine how one behaves and responds to daily life and health-care practices. Values are deep feelings about what is right or wrong, good or bad. Most personal values are learned in childhood and are well established by 10 years of age (Wold, 2008). Values are influenced by culture, and some behaviors that may be valued and encouraged by Western culture may be looked down on by another culture.

It is often a challenge for new immigrants to assimilate into the American culture without losing some cultural values and practices. Ethnicity is a cultural pattern shared by people with the same cultural heritage. Language, preferred diet, specific customs, family roles, and religious beliefs are often shared among those with the same ethnicity. Cultural awareness means recognizing the history of patients' ancestry or culture and how their customs influence the handling of problems, issues, or teachings. Health-care workers should be careful not to be ethnocentric, believing their culture, beliefs, and values to be superior to others. Health-care workers must apply the patients' cultural beliefs, values, and practices to each situation when planning care and health-promotion activities but should avoid stereotyping the patient, which is assuming that all people from a specific cultural or ethnic group behave or believe the same way. Often, acculturation, the adjustment to a new culture, results in differences in practice within the same cultural group. Cultural assessments should be completed on all patients as they enter the health-care system in order to affect a positive outcome.

Cultural care consists of health-promotion activities initiated by a culturally competent health-care worker who enables a patient to modify health behaviors toward beneficial outcomes while respecting the patient's cultural values, beliefs, and practices (Kavanaugh, 2004). Cultural interventions are achieved when health-care information is presented in a way that includes specific cultural styles, colors, pictures, symbols, and so forth, that add credibility to the content by reflecting cultural values. Health-care information should be presented in the language of the recipient, using interpreters whenever necessary.

Often, some of the patient's traditional practices can be incorporated into the care plan. For example, an Asian woman who refuses to eat or take oral medication after giving birth may not have been offered the culturally appropriate hot foods and may have been expected to drink ice water with her oral medication. In this example, the care provided conflicted with the woman's cultural practices. However, offering hot soup to eat and room-temperature water without ice with her medications easily solves the problem.

Two important factors for consideration when providing culturally competent care are:

1. *Communication* – Obtain interpreters to aid in data collection and in providing information in the patient's native language. Gestures and body language are important. Some cultures value eye-to-eye contact, whereas others tend to avoid direct eye contact.
2. *Personal space* – In American culture, an intimate zone is considered to be up to 1.5 feet, personal distance is 1.5 to 4 feet, social distance is 4 to 12 feet, and public distance is 12 feet (Hall, 1963). Comfortable personal space may differ among individuals and cultures.

See Table 3-1 for examples of variations among selected cultural groups.

TABLE 3-1 Variations of Selected Cultural Groups

	African American	Asian	Hispanic	Native American
Verbal communication	Asking personal questions of someone met for the first time is seen as improper and intrusive	High respect for those in position of authority	Expression of negative feelings is considered impolite	Speaks in a low tone of voice and expects listener to be attentive
Nonverbal communication	Direct eye contact is often considered rude	Direct eye contact with superiors is considered disrespectful	Avoidance of eye contact is a sign of attentiveness and respect	Direct eye contact is considered disrespectful
Touch	Touching another's hair is considered offensive	Touching the head of a newborn is considered bad luck. Prefers not to shake hands with opposite sex	Touching is common between two people during conversation	A light touch of a person's hand rather than a firm handshake is used when greeting a person
Family organization	Women play key roles in health-care decisions	Emphasis may be on family needs rather than individual needs. The opinion of the elder is sought	All members of the family may be involved in health-care decisions	Emphasis tends to be on the family rather than on individual needs
Alternative healers	"Root doctor," "voodoo priest," spiritualist	Accupuncturist, accupressurist, herbalist	Curandero, espiritualista, yerbo	Medicine man, Shaman

Modified from Cherry B, Jacob S: *Contemporary nursing: issues, trends and management*, ed 5, St Louis, 2011, Mosby.

CULTURE AND PREGNANCY

The cultural background of the family may strongly influence family members' view of the birth experience. An appropriate approach to determine what the pregnant woman considers normal practice is to ask the following questions:

1. Is pregnancy viewed as a healthy time, a vulnerable time, or an illness?
2. Is the birth process viewed as dangerous?
3. Is birth a public or private experience?
4. What type of help is needed/accepted?
5. What is the expected role of the family?

Some cultures restrict the behavior of the husband during the perinatal phase. In *Native American* culture, the husband avoids eating meat while the woman is in labor and delivery. In *Arabic*, *Chinese*, *Cuban*, and *Ethiopian* cultures, the husband remains in control of decisions but does not otherwise participate during birth. In the *Orthodox Jewish* religion, the husband may not participate in prenatal classes or during labor, and he may not view the infant during the birth process. Only verbal encouragement is usually allowed. In *South American*, *Vietnamese*, and *West Indian* cultures, the husband is expected to be nearby. Most other cultures allow the husband to be present and to participate during the birth process.

Many non-Western cultures expect the woman to have at least 20 to 40 days of bedrest after giving birth. *Southeast Asian*, *Hispanic*, *African-American*, and *Chinese* cultural practices usually avoid full washing of the hair or body until lochia has ceased. Because pregnancy, labor, and delivery are considered "cold" conditions, air-conditioned rooms and cold fluids are avoided.

Cambodian women often discard colostrum and do not eat vegetables during the first week after delivery. Traditional Japanese cultural practices dictate bathing the newborn twice a day for a week with loud noise and music playing to ward off evil spirits. In the United States, the baby is the focus of gift giving following birth, whereas in many non-Western cultures, the mother is the focus of attention. A patient's perspective in research on intercultural caring in maternity care can be accessed at www.ncbi.nih.gov/pmc/articles/pmc2879866.

CULTURE AND THE CHILD

Cultural practices can influence the timing of developmental stages. For example, the development of initiative may be later for children in families that practice an authoritarian style of parenting, because these families place great value on obedience and conformity in children.

CULTURE AND THE ADOLESCENT

Independence in adolescents is not valued equally by all cultures. Some *Chinese* cultures, for example, do not recognize adolescence as a period of development. There is no word for adolescence in their language.

Adolescents understand abstract thinking, and traditional religious practices and symbols help stabilize the adolescent's developing identity. Many cultures practice specific rituals that recognize passage of the individual from childhood to adulthood. These practices can be symbolic rituals or celebrations, such as a bar mitzvah in the *Jewish* religion, or can be an actual test that demonstrates mastery of specific survival skills to determine that the adolescent is ready to take on adult responsibilities, such as is practiced in some native African cultures.

Adolescents or young adults who try to seek recognition or wish to express rejection of society's culture will promote unique changes in styles, thoughts, and practices that can collide with family values and beliefs. Changes in taste for music, clothing styles, and use of social media influence living styles, and often the changes in practices for the younger age group may be quite different from their cultural background. The changes may take the form of an interim "fad," or they may persist and affect the following generation's practices and values.

CULTURE AND THE ADULT

In *Jewish* religious culture, women are considered to be in a state of impurity during menstruation and after giving birth. Very religious husbands may not touch their wives during these times. Health-care workers can inquire about and be sensitive to this cultural practice and can provide physical assistance when needed, such as after a cesarean section.

In many religions, birth control is not encouraged. The *Roman Catholic Church* and the *Mormon Church* (Latter-Day Saints) allow only natural family planning, using abstinence as the technique of choice. The *Christian Science* religion approaches health care with a spiritual framework, and adherents may decline preventive medicines, although some required vaccinations or personal birth-control drugs may be accepted. The *Unitarian Universalist Association* advocates birth-control practices and supports the woman's choice related to abortion. The *Islamic* culture permits contraception but forbids abortion.

Different cultures place different emphases on women's experiences of menopause. In cultures where age is revered, menopause may be a nonevent. In the United States, where a high value is placed on youth, sex appeal, and physical beauty, menopause and related body changes may challenge feelings of self-worth.

CULTURE AND THE OLDER ADULT

A positive attitude toward life and health is encouraged for older adults in most cultures. Most cultures look to elders as a source of wisdom, and often elders play a major role in raising or disciplining grandchildren. In many cultures, elders are also welcomed as the preferred babysitters and parenting consultants. Many older patients who are confined to wheelchairs or nursing homes may have limited contact with family but may place a high value on any available assistance in accessing family contact.

CULTURE AND HEALTH BELIEFS

Many non-Western cultures believe that balances between hot and cold affect health and illness. This belief is known as the humoral theory. *Latin American, African, Hispanic, Haitian,* and *Chinese* cultures have traditional cold remedies to treat hot diseases and hot remedies to treat cold diseases. Cold illnesses or conditions include pregnancy, earache, chest pain, paralysis, gastrointestinal diseases, rheumatism, and tuberculosis. Hot illnesses include dental problems, sore throat, rashes, and kidney disorders. In *Asian* cultures, the forces of yang (light heat or dryness) and yin (darkness, cold, or wetness) influence the balance and harmony of a person's state of health. Yin (cold foods) includes fruits, vegetables, cold liquid, and beer. Yang (hot foods) includes meat, eggs, hot soup, cantaloupe, and fried foods.

Foods are classified as hot or cold according to their effects on the body when metabolized rather than their thermal temperature.

The *Native American* culture defines wellness as harmony in body, mind, and spirit. A holistic approach to healing is valued.

CULTURE AND ILLNESS

Specific holidays may involve some restriction of activity. *Orthodox Jews* do not turn electricity, such as lights or television, on or off, nor do they use the telephone from sunset Friday night to sunset Saturday. During times of culturally restricted behavior, medical appointments or procedures should be postponed if delay is possible without endangering the patient. Shaving can be done with an electric razor if a beard must be removed, but a razor blade must not touch the skin.

In the *Roman Catholic* and many other Christian faiths, a sacrament is offered to the seriously ill person. To enable this practice, the health-care worker should notify the priest, if possible before the patient loses consciousness. Abstinence from solid food is required for at least 15 minutes before clergy offers the consecrated host to people receiving communion. Rosary beads or religious medallions may be pinned to the gown or to the bed of the ill person. *Mennonite* women may wear head coverings during hospitalization. Persons of the *Christian Science* faith often decline medications or psychotherapy. For *Jehovah's Witnesses*, receiving blood transfusions or medications containing blood products violates religious guidelines. However, today there are some alternatives to blood transfusions, such as plasma expanders and autologous transfusions.

Religious *Mormons* wear a sacred undergarment that should not be removed unless an emergency occurs. Patients of the *Islamic* faith may request that the Koran be kept at the bedside and that nothing be placed on top of it. Religious jewelry or prayer strings should not be removed from the body unless medically necessary.

Buddhist and *Hindu* cultural beliefs suggest that illness is the result of sins committed in a previous life or for the atonement of sins in the present life. Time for concentrated meditation (yoga) may be requested or viewed as required for healing.

Social behavior consistent with the "sick persons' role" may vary from being demanding to silent passivity depending on the cultural background and other personal variables of the patient.

CULTURE AND DEATH

The Self-Determination Act of 1991 granted patients in the United States the legal right to full disclosure of medical information to allow individuals to participate in their own care. In some non-Western cultures, information is released to the patient at the discretion of family members. In most Western cultures, a high value is placed on individual life. In many non-Western cultures, the welfare of the family is primary, and life-and-death decisions are made by group approval.

Judaism and some other cultures believe that dying persons must have someone with them as their soul leaves the body. Traditionally the body is not left alone until burial, which must occur within 24 hours (or as soon as possible) after death. The body is dressed in a shroud, and no metal objects, including nails, may be in the coffin. No flowers are permitted during the funeral or for the 7 days of mourning immediately following. Mirrors are covered, and immediate family may sit on low, hard benches during the mourning period.

Last rites are obligatory for many *Christian* cultures. The *Unitarian Universalist* faith prefers cremation to burial. The *Islamic* culture requires the body to be placed in a position facing Mecca. According to the Islamic culture, persons do not own their bodies, and so cremation, autopsy, and organ donation are prohibited.

A *Hindu* priest may place a thread around the neck or waist of the deceased as a blessing before cremation, which is preferred over burial. *Buddhist* culture teaches acceptance of the inevitability of death and believes the person's state of mind at the moment of death influences rebirth. Suicide, violent death, or the death of a child may require special rituals because the state of mind at death may not have been optimal. Buddhist culture also considers it bad luck for a pregnant woman to attend a funeral.

In *Native American* cultures, a dying person may be surrounded by a positive celebratory atmosphere of family and children. Some *African Americans* believe that dying in the home brings bad luck to the house. They prefer that death occur in a hospital and may prefer that professionals prepare the body for burial.

In *Central American* cultures, death with dignity in the home setting is preferred over a hospital setting, because death is considered a spiritual event.

The *Hmong* culture suggests a person must be well dressed at the time of death. A health-care worker may inform the family if the patient's death is imminent, so that the family can bring the desired clothing to the hospital. Internal metal objects, such as plates, bullets, or medical devices, must be removed from the body before burial, and metal objects such as zippers or buttons are prohibited from touching the body after death.

CULTURE AND TEACHING

In the United States, the myriad of cultures creates an opportunity for misunderstandings and misinterpretations of health-care teachings. People from cultures that place a high value on pleasing others may answer questions with information they think others want to hear to maintain a harmonious relationship. To collect accurate data, questions should be phrased in a neutral fashion. *Asian*, *Native American*, and *Muslim* patients consider direct eye contact impolite and may stare at the floor as a symbol of respect during contact with the health-care worker, which should not be misinterpreted as not paying attention. *Hispanic* patients may view extended eye contact as related to the evil eye, which will bring bad luck. Many *Asians* believe the head is sacred and therefore must not be touched or patted. Palpating the fontanel of an infant may be interpreted as a disrespectful action unless the medical procedure is properly explained and is accepted by the parents. *Native American*, *Chinese*, and *Japanese* cultures suggest that silence indicates respect for another person, whereas *Russian*, *French*, and *Spanish* cultures may interpret silence as agreement with the speaker. Yet other cultures make every effort to fill silent moments with conversation. These factors should be considered and interpreters used when appropriate. Whenever possible, family members should not be used as interpreters when embarrassing or confidential issues are discussed.

CULTURE AND FOOD

Many cultures and religions include specific foods as an integral part of holiday celebrations and may restrict consumption of specific foods. For example, *Mormons* do not consume alcohol or any beverage containing caffeine, and many Mormons fast on the first Sunday of each month. The *Hindu* culture prohibits consumption of all meats, whereas *Islamic* culture specifically prohibits pork. The heatlh-care worker should be aware that some gelatin preparations and medications with a gelatin base might contain pork products. Mixing dairy and meat products at the same meal is prohibited in the *Jewish* religion. Also in the Jewish religion, pork is avoided, all meats must be specially prepared or koshered, and only fish with scales are permitted. The *Seventh Day Adventist* religion encourages a vegetarian diet. *Hispanic* diets incorporate the concept of cold foods, such as vegetables, fruits, and dairy products, and hot foods, such as garlic, grains, and selected cuts of meat.

COMPLEMENTARY AND ALTERNATIVE THERAPIES AND CULTURE

For many years, Western medicine treated and provided medicines and therapy to the patient in the hospital setting, and the patient had little input regarding the plan of care (which was mostly curative rather than preventive). A growing desire for control of one's own body and health-care decisions, and a desire for consideration of family, cultural beliefs, and values, motivated a self-care movement that is bringing health care out of the hospital and into the community and home (Nash, 2009). The focus continues to shift to health promotion and maintenance of wellness, and the health-care provider is more often considered a facilitator for the consumer to choose options that best meet personal needs and cultural values. The emphasis on self care, health promotion, and disease prevention is clearly reflected in the *Healthy People 2020* goals.

Complementary and alternative medicine (CAM) has become increasingly popular. Alternative medicine are those therapies that are used *instead* of Western medical care. Complementary medicine are those therapies used *together with* Western therapies. Many CAM practices, such as acupressure during labor and the use of antinausea bracelets for chemotherapy, have been adopted as valid Western health-care practices (Figure 3-1). Self care, wellness, and illness prevention are the core aspects of CAM therapy, which considers the whole physiological person as well as social, cultural, and spiritual aspects.

Every patient should be assessed for CAM therapy use, because some therapies might interact negatively with medications prescribed during an illness. Some CAM therapies have their roots in "folk medicine" or ancient, time-tested remedies practiced in many countries and passed down through specific cultures. CAM therapies include massage, energy healing, acupuncture and acupressure, reflexology, homeopathy, biofeedback, aromatherapy, guided imagery, herbal remedies, and others.

THE GOVERNMENT'S ROLE IN PROMOTING CULTURALLY COMPETENT CARE

The National Center for Complementary and Alternative Medicine (NCCAM) is an agency of the National Institutes of Health (NIH) that conducts research on the effectiveness of specific CAM therapies and documents their findings in medical journals. The United States Department of Health and Human Services Office of Minority Health and Cross Cultural Health Care has a specific Agency for Healthcare Research and Quality (AHRQ) that promotes behaviors and policies related to cultural competence in health care. The U.S. Office of Minority Health provides information concerning culturally and linguistically (language) appropriate health services (CLAS). One recommended standard of CLAS includes promoting attitudes, behavior, knowledge, and skills necessary to work effectively in a culturally diverse work

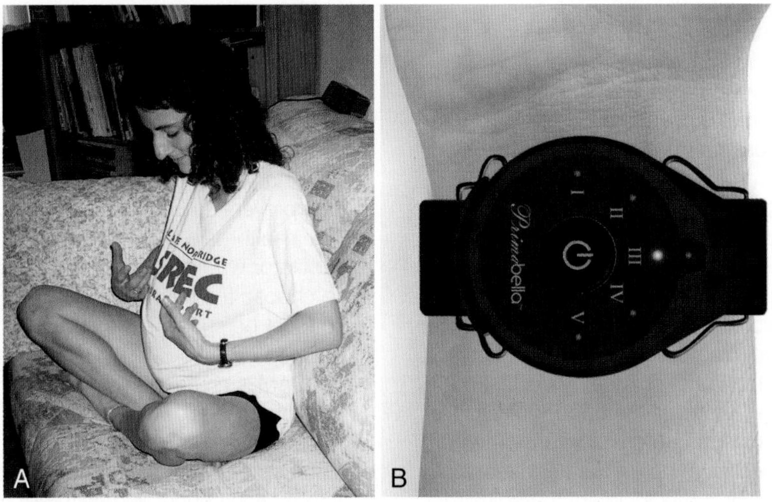

Figure 3–1 **A,** *Effleurage* involves the slow massage of the abdomen in a circular motion using the fingertips to stimulate large diameter nerve fibers, thus interfering with the transmission of pain sensations. Pressure should be firm enough to avoid a tickling sensation. This form of CAM therapy is used effectively during the active phase of labor. This therapy involves the gate-control theory of pain relief. **B,** The *PrimaBella* is a non-invasive transdermal device cleared by the FDA for treatment of pregnancy-induced nausea and vomiting (morning sickness). The device is applied to the ventral side of the wrist where the median nerve is closest to the surface of the skin. It emits a programmed pulse that stimulates the nerve to create electrical signals that travel to the central nervous system to restore normal gastric rhythm. It is a form of CAM therapy involving transcutaneous electrical nerve stimulation. (Photo courtesy Neurowave Medical Technologies.)

environment. Culturally competent care can improve communication, enhance education, and aid in achieving the established goals of *Healthy People 2020*. See Appendix B for a multilingual glossary of symptoms for health-care workers to use until an interpreter becomes available.

In the year 2000, racial and ethnic minorities comprised 25% of the U.S. population. It is predicted that by the year 2050 the proportion of ethnic minorities will increase to 50% (Office of Minority Health, 2011). Culturally diverse membership of managed Medicaid programs already has reached 15%. This trend cannot be ignored, and health-care workers must implement CLAS and provide culturally competent care. Understanding culture as related to health care will:

- Improve services and health-care outcomes.
- Enhance cost effectiveness of health care.
- Reduce errors caused by misunderstandings.
- Assist in reaching *Healthy People 2020* goals.

Further information concerning cultural practices can be found throughout the text and in the Bibliography.

KEY POINTS

- Culture is defined as patterns of values, beliefs, and practices that are handed down through generations.
- Ethnicity is defined as a cultural pattern shared by a group of families that have a shared cultural heritage.

(Continued)

- Cultural values are established in childhood and are evidenced by 10years of age.
- Cultural awareness means learning patients' cultural beliefs, practices, and values and understanding how they differ from one's own.
- Cultural competence is the ability to adapt health care so that it does not violate the cultural beliefs or practices of the patient.
- Effective communication and sensitivity to personal space are two important factors in providing culturally competent care.
- The myriad of cultures in the United States provides the opportunity for misunderstanding, misinterpretation, and errors in health care and teaching.
- Alternative medicine are therapies that are used instead of traditional Western medical therapies.
- Complementary medicine are therapies that are used together with traditional Western medical therapies.
- The focus of health care is shifting from the hospital to the home and community with a focus on wellness and prevention of illness.
- The health-care provider is considered a facilitator who empowers the consumer to choose the best available options to meet personal needs and cultural values.
- NCCAM is an agency of the National Institute of Health that researches the effectiveness of CAM therapies.
- The Office of Minority Health provides information concerning culturally and linguistically (language) appropriate services (CLAS).

Critical Thinking

You are assigned to assess a patient whose culture is different from your own. Describe factors you would consider in planning your approach.

REVIEW QUESTIONS

1. A person's culture includes:
   a. age.
   b. genetic predisposition.
   c. handicap.
   d. customs.

2. Culturally competent care is provided by:
   a. using scientific evidence.
   b. following all orders written by the health-care provider.
   c. involving the patient and family in developing the plan of care.
   d. researching folk laws and remedies from the cultural background of the patient.

3. If a patient refuses to take his vitamin pill because he believes the gelatin base is unhealthy, the nurse should:
   a. challenge his belief.
   b. educate him concerning the need and value of that vitamin pill.
   c. obtain the help of a clergyman to persuade him to take the pill.
   d. respect his belief and find another vitamin preparation.

4. When providing health-care information, the health-care worker should *(Select all that apply)*:
   a. speak only with the patient.
   b. include the family member who is the decision maker of the family.
   c. always provide instructions clearly written in English.
   d. include resources to call if there are further questions.

5. In the American culture, personal space is an intimate zone that is considered to be:
   a. up to 1.5 feet.
   b. 4 feet.
   c. 12 feet.
   d. more than 12 feet.

CHAPTER 4

The Influence of Family on Developing a Lifestyle

http://evolve.elsevier.com/Leifer/growth

OBJECTIVES

1. Define the various types of family structures.
2. List the developmental stages of a family.
3. Define family systems theory.
4. Give examples of family system stressors.
5. Discuss the effect of the family lifestyle on child development.
6. State three childrearing styles.
7. List three developmental theories.
8. List the effects culture has on personal values, beliefs, and behaviors of family members.
9. Define what makes a family dysfunctional.
10. Discuss one positive and one negative influence of technology and electronic media on the family and child development.
11. Understand the effects of a disaster on the family and development.
12. State the effect of the community on the family and child development.

KEY TERMS

blended family
cultural assimilation
cultural relativism
culture shock
developmental stage
developmental task
dysfunctional family
Facebook depression
family
family systems theory
posttraumatic stress disorder (PTSD)
sexting
sibling rivalry
theory

DEFINITION

The family has been defined as a basic human social system that involves commitment and interaction among its members. This commitment includes a responsibility for the physical and emotional well-being and successful development of the children in that family. For most people, the family is the strongest and most influential group to which a person belongs. A healthy family is not necessarily a family where all members are at the optimum level of health. A healthy family is one that can successfully adapt to crises, challenges, and changes during the life cycle. The role of the nurse or health-care worker is to help the family adapt to these challenges. Health-care workers must understand the many factors that influence family functioning and child development. Comprehensive care involves the patient and the family unit.

Family Structure

Family composition and cultural backgrounds have changed dramatically in the United States during the last 40 years. The traditional nuclear (two-parent) family, where the father works outside the home and the mother remains at home to care for the children, has given way to many other variations. The number of married couples with children under the age of 18 has declined from 26.4 million in the year 2000 to 23.9 million in the year 2011, only 20% of households (Census Bureau, 2011). The daily availability of the father to the children is often decreased because of the demands of the workplace. The father may leave the house to travel to work before the child awakens and may return after the child is asleep at night. Flexibility is needed to maintain paternal role modeling, mutual respect, and equality of involvement in childrearing.

Dual-career families, in which both parents work outside the home, have become the norm in modern America. Conflicting demands among work responsibilities, continuing education for career advancement, and the demands of childrearing often create pressures that require careful scheduling, close communication, flexibility, and mutual support. Children of dual-career families are often expected to be more independent at an earlier age, and parents tend to overestimate the ability of the child to manage without direct supervision. Acute illness, chronic illness, or discipline and behavior problems can create additional stresses in this type of family structure (Box 4-1).

All family variations have some form of influence on childrearing and development. Table 4-1 lists the types of family structures found in the United States. An essential core of parenting within any family structure is commitment to the child. The parenting arrangement may be challenged by divorce, environmental poverty, or illness or death of a parent. Communication between parent and child helps the child adjust to a specific lifestyle that may be different from his or her peers. Children need to have a sense of belonging, support, and consistency in their lives to achieve optimal development (Figure 4-1, A).

EFFECT OF FAMILY ON GROWTH AND DEVELOPMENT OF THE CHILD

There are many factors within the family structure, including interactions and lifestyles, that can affect the growth and development of a child. The more common aspects of family variations are discussed in this chapter.

BOX 4-1 Ten Potential Challenges in Dual-Career Families

1. Need for child-care arrangements.
2. Time to participate in children's activities.
3. Time to support and encourage academic achievements.
4. Time to support and encourage peer interaction.
5. Time for child-focused family activities.
6. Need for close scheduling and travel away from home on the part of family members.
7. Lack of energy for home and child-care activities.
8. Difficulty with unexpected illness or injury management.
9. Increased need for child to self manage.
10. Maintaining healthy nutrition options at mealtimes.

TABLE 4-1 Various Types of Family Structures

Type of Family*	Description
Nuclear	Traditional—husband, wife, and children (biological or adopted)
Extended	Grandparents, parents, children, and relatives
Single parent	Women or men establishing separate households through individual preferences, divorces, death, or desertion
Foster parent	Parents who care for children who are sent to them via the court system because of dysfunctional families, absent families, or individual family problems
Alternative	Communal family
Dual career	Both parents work because of desire or need
Blended	Mother or father, stepparent, and children
Polygamous	More than one spouse at the same time
Homosexual	A single homosexual person or two persons of the same sex who may have children from a previous relationship, who have adopted children, or have children via artificial insemination
Cohabitation	Heterosexual or homosexual couples who live together with their children but remain unmarried (a type of cohabitation may be experienced by college students who live in a dormatory or in off-campus school housing with men and women sharing facilities)

Modified from Leifer G: *Introduction to maternity & pediatric nursing*, ed 6, Philadelphia, 2011, Saunders.
*Not all may be legally sanctioned.

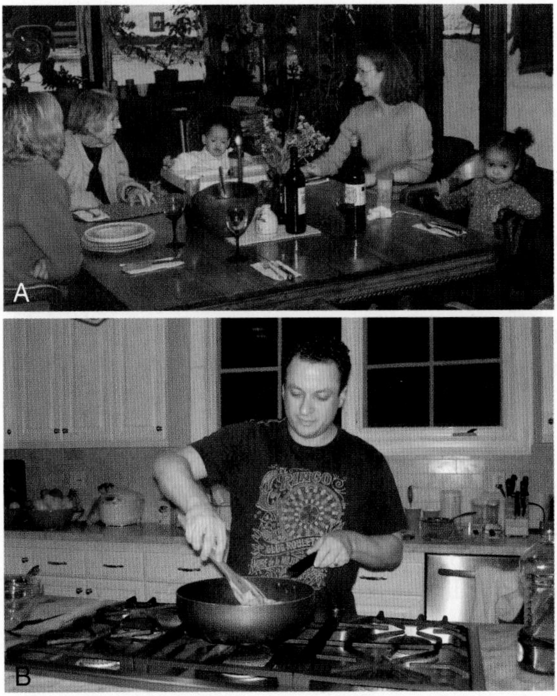

Figure 4–1 **A,** Several generations gather around the table for celebrations. Such activities strengthen the family structure. **B,** Healthy eating starts with freshly cooked nutritious food.

Size of Family

The interpersonal relationship between siblings is unique. The presence of a brother or sister in a family group helps provide support and gives early experience in developing the skills necessary for social interaction. Older children can help younger siblings grasp language skills, but the firstborn or only child may have a longer, more intense verbal interaction with the parent. This one-to-one relationship may result in the development of a wider vocabulary and better conversational skills at an earlier age. Although social experiences may be limited for the single child, the popular use of day care and preschool can provide an opportunity to develop social skills and can decrease the feeling of loneliness for an only child.

Spacing of Siblings

The age of the older child at the time of the birth of the sibling contributes to the response of the older child. When the new baby arrives, a 1-year-old child may whine and cling, whereas a 2-year-old child may regress in toileting or feeding behaviors, and a 4-year-old may develop temper tantrums. A child older than 5 years may feel protective of the new arrival. Shared experiences among siblings with fewer than 4 years difference in age increase the likelihood of sibling rivalry. Sibling rivalry is a competition or struggle between two or more children in a family. It can contribute positively to child development by offering the opportunity for children to develop interpersonal skills and to handle conflict, but it can also cause stress and chaos in a family.

Divorce

The psychological health and development of the child may be affected by the divorce of his or her parents. The child may be thrust into a single-family home or a newly blended family if remarriage occurs. Children of divorce often have a higher incidence of behavioral or learning difficulties later in life (Kim, 2011). The effect of joint custody on the child is partially determined by the motivation for such an arrangement. The best motivation would be to ensure continuing relationships with both parents, but other reasons often include convenience or lack of commitment by one or both parents. The presence or absence of hostility between the parents is an important factor that influences the psychological adjustment of the child regardless of the type of custody arrangements made.

The child should be prepared for the divorce and assured he or she had no role in the breakup of the marriage. However, self blame is common despite assurances. Children should be told how the divorce will affect them and their needs, as well as what they can expect in terms of living arrangements and continued relationships with both parents. Children need permission to continue to love both parents and to feel free to express these feelings. Table 4-2 shows typical responses to divorce according to age group and developmental level and related guidance or interventions that can be offered by the nurse and the health-care team.

TABLE 4-2 Responses to Divorce by Age Group

Age Group	Signs and Symptoms	Interventions Needed
Preschool	Regression Returns to thumb sucking Intensified fears Sleep disturbances Fear of abandonment	Maintain household routines Reassure love of child Spend added time with child Establish and maintain bedtime rituals
School age	Shows open grieving Feels rejected Fears being replaced by absent parent Difficulty in concentrating, resulting in poor grades Fears expressing emotions	Allow child to love both parents Help child move from parent to parent Diminish worry about present and future Attend school events Do not use child as confidant or as spouse substitute
Adolescent	Worry about fate of own future marriage Must rethink values and morality of the world May become depressed or suicidal May be expected to assume greater family responsibilities	Avoid delegating too much home responsibility Encourage discussion with neutral party Encourage pursuit of own interests Help in use of support systems
Adult	Increased dependence on eldest child Open expression of fears, anxieties, and anger Inability to focus on needs of children	Counsel to join a single-parent support group Encourage professional counseling Refer to social or financial-aid resources
Geriatric	Depression, loneliness, helplessness, bitterness Increased dependence on children and grandchildren	Encourage joining groups Increase activities that are of personal interest

Stepchildren and Foster Children

A blended family is one in which one or both spouses bring children from a previous relationship into a new family unit. The children may have to adjust to a new home and school environment with new rules and new roommates (stepsiblings) who are strangers. This often accompanies a dilution of attention from the biological parent, who must divide attention among a larger family group. Resentment between stepsiblings may occur. A stepparent may be given a name other than "mother" or "father" if the children feel guilty that the stepparent is replacing the biological parent.

Children who enter foster care must face a strange environment without the support of even one biological parent. There is added uncertainty regarding the length of placement, which can result in insecurity and lack of trust in others. In 2010, there were more than 408,000 children in foster care in the United States (Needell, 2011). Federal legislation in

1980 and 1995 promoted family reunification as the goal for all foster care, so that relatives are now sought first as caregivers for children displaced from biological families before the children are placed in foster care.

Chronic Illness

Having a child, parent, or dependent relative with a chronic illness can strain sibling relationships and exact tolls on the emotional, psychological, and economic resources of the family. The healthy child may be expected to be more independent, to carry more responsibilities, or to step into a caregiver role that may keep him or her away from normal activities with peers. Although some healthy children may react with anger at the ill family member, many children develop a greater capacity for empathy because of their experiences with the person who is chronically ill (Table 4-3). Communicating the needs, limitations, and feelings of the ill relative and acknowledging the needs and feelings of caregivers and the impact on the family can make the crucial difference between resentment and attachment for each member of the family. Caregiver group support may be available in local communities.

The death of a child in the family may cause a parent to become overprotective of the surviving children, thus depriving them of normal independence and interaction with their peers. The nurse can explain and discuss terminal illness and its developmental and behavioral consequences by identifying family strengths, coping styles, and strategies. A comprehensive plan for care, continuing education, and promotion of optimal growth and development can then be designed and implemented by the health-care team.

The family that has a newborn child with a chronic illness or deformity goes through a grieving process. This process includes shock, disbelief/denial, anger, depression, withdrawal, adaptation, and adjustment. Any new crises can cause setbacks to previous stages and delay the coping and adjustment of family members. The health-care worker must recognize these stages, determine the resiliency of the family to create a support network, and help them use resources within the family and the community.

Use of Child-Care Services

Individual child care or group day care is a replacement for direct care by a parent and is currently used more often than nannies, extended family members, sibling care, and private babysitters. More than 2 million families nationwide received federally funded

TABLE 4-3 Understanding Chronic Illness at Various Ages

Age	Concept of Illness
Preschool	Magical thoughts
Early school age	Concrete, rigid ideas
Late school age	Little comprehension, although can list symptoms
Adolescent	Child shows greater understanding of cause of illness
Adult	Understands abstract principles and concepts involved in the illness

day-care services in 2009 (CLASP, 2010). The terms *day care* and *child care* do not indicate details about services provided. Child-care services are regulated for health and safety by the American Public Health Association but vary widely in ability to nurture growth and development. High-quality day-care settings can contribute to cognitive development (see Chapter 8).

UNDERSTANDING FAMILIES THROUGH THEORIES

A **theory** is a group of concepts that forms the basis for understanding observations. An accepted theory is logical, consistent, and integrates past and current research. Theories provide a way to study family interaction or individual growth and development. The theories are useful because they help us understand why things happen the way they do and help us identify interventions needed for individuals or families that experience problems. Various theories of individual growth and development are discussed in detail in Chapter 5.

Family Systems Theory

Family systems theory is based on the understanding that family functions are interconnected. This means that what happens to one family member affects the entire family. No illness is seen as an isolated, individual event. Everything is viewed in the context of family interactions. For example, when a child has a problem such as anorexia, the entire family is affected. The problem of the child affects the family system, and the family system affects the general maintenance or recovery of the problem that the child is experiencing. Many problems of the individual, such as anorexia, can be manifestations of a dysfunctional family system. Therefore interventions, according to the family systems theory, must involve the whole family, not just the affected individual. Often, stabilizing the family group helps to stabilize the problem of the individual.

Murray Bowen, of Georgetown University, was one of the pioneers of the family systems theory, and Salvador Minuchin, of Argentina, first wrote about the values of family therapy in 1974. They stated that there are interactions among the biological, developmental, psychological, and social factors in the family that determine the individual behaviors of each family member. There is a natural tendency in families to seek a stable state. For example, if one child is very aggressive and constantly breaks rules, another child in the family will assume the role of the good child to maintain family stability. This process is called *family dynamics*. Child guidance worker John Bowlby (1951) was a pioneer in describing how a child's distress was a reflection of a family in distress, and treatment of both was essential to a return to optimal health. It is, therefore, important for health-care workers to understand the organization and communication within the family unit. Today, managed health care favors the treatment of the entire family rather than just the affected individual, because the results are quicker and longer lasting.

The Family Apgar

In 1978, Gabriel Smilkstein created the Family Apgar as a tool to assess family function (Box 4-2). It was initially used by physicians and psychologists to assess the family's ability

BOX 4-2 Family Apgar

Adaptation—Sharing of resources and helping of family members.
Partnership—Lines of communication and participation of family members.
Growth—How responsibilities are shared among family members.
Affection—Visible and invisible emotional interactions among family members.
Resolve—How time, money, and space are used for solving or preventing problems among family members.

Modified from Smilkstein G: The family apgar: a proposal for a family function test and its use by physicians. *J Fam Pract* 6:1231–1238, 1978.

to adapt, grow, develop, and resolve issues. The role of the health-care worker on the multidisciplinary health-care team is to observe a family's function and ensure that the needs of each family member are being met. Referral to available community resources, which may include social agencies, school professionals, psychologists, or pediatricians, can help identify problems and initiate appropriate early interventions. Accepting the nontraditional family and helping the adults care for their own physical and psychological needs are the first steps in helping the parents to care for their children and to promote optimal growth and development for the entire family unit (Figure 4-2).

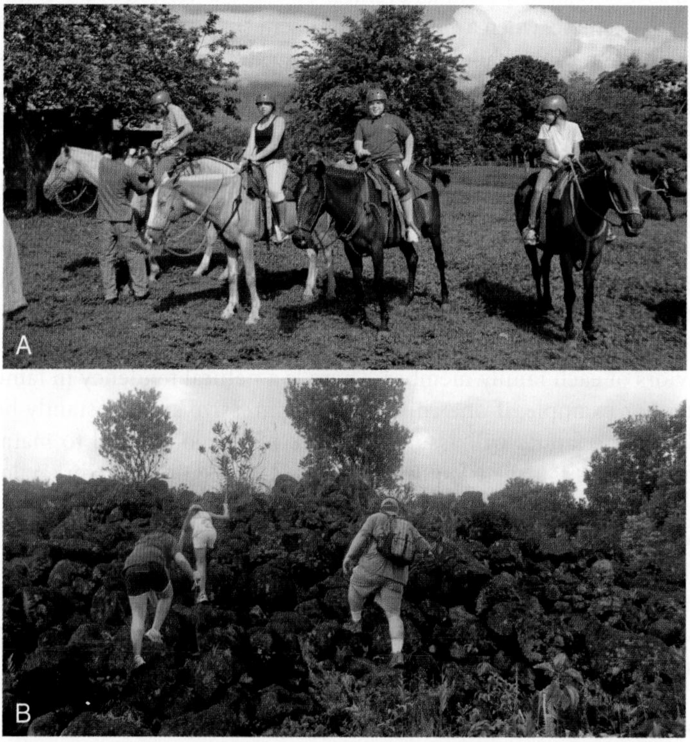

Figure 4–2 **A, B,** In accordance with the goals of *Healthy People 2020,* the family that exercises together, or engages in active recreational activities together, promotes positive attitudes about exercise throughout the life cycle. Healthy activity can take place inside or outside of the home setting.

Developmental Theories

There are various theories of growth and development (see Chapter 5), and each theory emphasizes specific areas of development, such as motor, cognitive, social, and so on. Piaget offers a developmental theory of cognition, whereas Freud's theories involve behaviors that are motivated by unconscious wishes. Because of the interactions between an individual and the environment, psychosocial theories of development are also important to understand.

Erik Erikson is one of the best known psychosocial theorists, and his concepts are presented in Chapter 5 and throughout this text. The growth and development of a parent in relation to Erikson's theory of development is described in Table 4-4. A developmental stage is defined as a period in life characterized by the mastery of specific skills or behaviors. Each stage incorporates achievements from the previous stage and contains skills, behaviors, or tasks necessary to enter and successfully master the skills, behaviors, and tasks of the next stage. Handling psychosocial conflicts using coping strategies and support systems or significant relationships has an important effect on the developing personality.

Robert Havighurst was a theorist who described a sequence for learning developmental tasks at each stage of development, including tasks of late adulthood and for the aged. His view emphasized that society determines the skills that need to be acquired at each stage of development, but he pointed out that readiness to learn and teachable moments for acquisition of these skills must be utilized, or difficulties in later life can occur.

Betty Neuman, a nursing theorist, believed that nurses and other health-care team members should care for the total patient and family needs, with special efforts directed toward maintaining the interaction of the family within their environment. Specific interventions to reduce stress and to achieve maximal wellness are the basis of the theory.

Evelyn Duvall, a family theorist, proposed specific stages of family development. Each stage of development is unique with new competencies to be mastered. Various stages of physical and psychosocial development occur concurrently, so all processes are integrated.

GROWTH AND DEVELOPMENT OF THE FAMILY

Developmental Tasks of the Family Life Cycle

The family has a life cycle of its own, which is described by events and is influenced by the environment (Table 4-5 on p. 48). Deviation from the smooth flow of the family developmental cycle can result in dysfunctions.

A **developmental task** is a competency or skill that helps a person cope with the environment or advance personal development. Tasks occur in sequence, and mastery of developmental tasks of one stage are usually required to master developmental tasks of the next stage of development. There are physical, cognitive, psychological, motor, and psychosocial developmental tasks. Both the individual and the family have developmental tasks to achieve at specific stages across the lifespan, such as the following:

- *Physical competencies,* which include functional abilities that result from motor and neurological development.
- *Emotional competencies,* which include self awareness, empathy for others, and using strategies to cope with stress or frustrations.
- *Social competencies,* which include the ability to form positive interpersonal relationships.

The concepts of several theorists are presented in Chapter 5 and in each chapter covering the life cycle. Refer to psychology or anthropology texts for other details concerning individual theorists.

TABLE 4-4 The Growth and Development of a Parent

Child's Tasks (Erikson's Stages)	Parent's Tasks	Nursing Interventions
FIRST PRENATAL TRIMESTER		
Growth	Develop attitude toward newborn: Happy about child? Parent of one disabled child? Unwed mother? These factors and others will affect the developing attitude of the mother.	Develop positive attitude in both parents concerning expected birth of child. Use referrals and agencies as needed.
SECOND PRENATAL TRIMESTER		
Growth	Mother focuses on infant because of fetal movements felt. Parents picture what infant will look like, what future he or she will have, and other ideas.	Parents' focus is on child care and needs and providing physical environment for expected infant. Therefore, information concerning care of the newborn should be given at this time.
THIRD PRENATAL TRIMESTER		
Growth	Mother feels large. Attention focuses on how fetus is going to get out.	Detailed information should be presented at this time concerning the birth processes, preparation for birth, breastfeeding, and care of siblings at home.
BIRTH		
Adjust to external environment	Elicit positive responses from child and respond by meeting child's need for food and closeness. If parents receive only negative responses (e.g., sleepy infant, crying infant, difficult feeder, congenital anomaly), development of the parent will be inhibited.	Encourage early touch, feeding, and other practices. Explain behavior and appearance of newborn to allay fears. Help parents to identify positive responses. (Use infant's reflexes, such as grasp reflex, to identify a positive response by placing mother's finger into infant's hand.)
INFANT		
Develop trust	Learn "cues" presented by infant to determine individual needs of infant.	Help parents assess and interpret needs of infant (avoid feelings of helplessness or incompetence). Do not let in-laws take over parental tasks. Help parents cope with problems such as colic.

TABLE 4-4 The Growth and Development of a Parent—cont'd

Child's Tasks (Erikson's Stages)	Parent's Tasks	Nursing Interventions
TODDLER		
Autonomy	Try to accept the pattern of growth and development. Accept some loss of control but maintain some limits for safety.	Help parents cope with transient independence of child (e.g., allow child to go on tricycle but don't yell "Don't fall," or anxiety will be radiated).
PRESCHOOL-AGE		
Initiative	Learn to separate from child.	Help parents show standards but "let go" so child can develop some independence. A preschool experience may be helpful.
SCHOOL-AGE		
Industry	Accept importance of child's peers. Parents must learn to accept some rejection from child at times. Patience is needed to allow children to do for themselves, even if it takes longer. Do not *do* the school project *for* the child. Provide chores for child appropriate to his age level.	Help parents to understand that child is developing his or her own limits and self-discipline. Be there to guide child, but do not constantly intrude. Help child get results from his or her own efforts at performance.
ADOLESCENT		
Establishing identity Accepting pubertal changes Developing abstract reasoning Deciding on career Investigating lifestyles Controlling feeling	Parents must learn to let child live his or her own life and not expect total control over the child. Expect, at times, to be discredited by teenager. Expect differences in opinion and respect them. Guide but do not push.	Help parents adjust to changing role and relationship with adolescent (e.g., as child develops his or her own identify, he may become a Democrat if parents are Republican). Expose child to varied career fields and life experiences. Help child to understand emerging emotions and feelings brought about by puberty.

Role of the Health-Care Worker

Understanding the developmental stages and tasks of families and individuals enables the health-care team to provide individualized care. Optimal growth and development results when the person or family masters each task in the various stages of the life cycle. When working with patients or families, health-care team members must consider the developmental stage of the family and the individual, as well as cultural influences, before designing or carrying out a plan of care that will meet comprehensive needs.

TABLE 4-5 Growth and Development of the Family

Stage of Development	Developmental Tasks
Marriage	Establish mutual goals and values Define roles and responsibilities Respect extended families
Childbearing	Adjust to intrusion of child Expand roles and responsibilities Meet the needs of the child without losing sight of each other
Childrearing	Meet own needs and continued achievements, as well as the needs of the children Establish a child-care philosophy
Child launching	Maintain a supportive home base while letting go of the children to encourage their own fulfillment Accept challenges to family values by children
Contracting family	Experience empty-nest syndrome as children leave home Reintegrate and rediscover marriage relationship Increase community involvement Adjust to the grandparent role
Aging family	Develop new roles and interests within limits of abilities Fulfill lifelong dreams Adjust to retirement Cope with loss and loneliness Adjust to declining income and energy Maintain positive self-esteem Maintain contact and relationship with children and grandchildren

From Duvall E, Miller B, *Marriage and family development*, ed 6, 1984, Adapted by permission of Pearson Education Inc., Upper Saddle River, NJ.
NOTE: Each stage of family development has its own set of phases within that stage of development.

Childrearing Styles

Various family styles of functioning can be adopted by a couple in the beginning phases of family development and may be influenced by their cultural backgrounds. Some parents implement an *autocratic style,* where decisions are made without the input of the children. Respect and obedience are expected without discussion. In the *democratic style,* children are encouraged to participate in decision making, and all members of the family exhibit mutual respect. This is the ideal childrearing style, because it nurtures positive self esteem in all family members. The *laissez-faire style* offers complete freedom for all members, with no rules, minimal discipline (if any), and no effort at impulse control. Whichever style of childrearing and family development is selected, consistency of that style by both parents is essential for the development of stable family dynamics.

A functional family is a stable unit (firmly established with constant members) with consistent rules whose members are able to deal with conflict, stress, and problems in a way that promotes the physical and psychological well-being of its members. A dysfunctional family is a family unit that does not offer consistency of members or rules, may exhibit poor interpersonal relationships among its members, deals poorly with conflicts and problems, and often cannot reach out to the community for help. Dysfunctional family styles often result in antisocial behaviors of family members, where behavior of individuals may violate the rights of others. Early referral by the health-care team can help family members recapture self esteem and break the cycle of family dysfunction in future generations.

When a family member has a problem, the health-care worker must determine how the problem is perceived by the family, if coping skills exist, and if support systems are available. This is the core of a family-care plan. The role of the nurse or health-care worker is to help the family manage the problem. Referring the family to available community resources as appropriate and providing follow-up care are important in the plan of care.

Cultural Considerations

Effect of Culture on the Family

Culture is defined as a set of learned values, beliefs, customs, and behaviors that is shared by interacting individuals, such as a family (see Chapter 3).

Cultural assimilation is a process by which members of a specific cultural group lose the characteristics of that group and adapt practices of another group. It is often referred to as "Westernization" of a culture when time spent in the United States results in the adoption of an Americanized view of family function and behavior.

Cultural relativism is the concept that normality comes from the standard social practices of a specific culture. What is normal practice in one culture may not be considered normal practice in another culture.

Culture shock is the effect of a sudden, drastic change in the cultural environment of an individual or family.

As people travel around the world with ease and frequency, and families relocate from continent to continent, different cultural groups interact. Cultural backgrounds affect methods of communication and perceptions and response to health and illness. For example, in one culture, the response to a disability may be to hide it, whereas in another culture reentry into society is the treatment goal.

Ethnocentrism is the belief that one's own culture is the standard of behavior and is better than other cultures. Health-care workers need to understand their own cultural beliefs and recognize how they may differ from their patients. It is unrealistic to expect the patient to change his or her cultural beliefs and practices. Health-teaching plans must be designed to avoid conflict with the cultural beliefs and practices of the patient and family. Methods of communication are related to cultural practices. Understanding the culture and knowing who to communicate with in the family is essential in providing effective health care.

Cultural competence involves cultural awareness, acceptance, and respect toward behaviors and practices that are different from one's own. Knowledge of various cultures and the ability to adapt the delivery of health care so that it does not violate the culture or religion of that group are the core of cultural competence. The health-care worker must overcome cultural barriers to communication and behavior to provide effective health care to a culturally diverse society. Some cultural beliefs and practices related to stages within the life cycle were discussed in Chapter 3. Cultural assessment includes values, socioeconomic status, communication patterns, nutrition, language, religious practices, health beliefs, and cultural aspects of the disease and illness.

INFLUENCE OF ELECTRONIC MEDIA AND TECHNOLOGY

Media include newspapers, magazines, music, videos, movies, websites, and television. Electronic media have enabled people to be in immediate contact with the thoughts and actions of others around the world, and the increased exposure of children to media can have positive and negative influences on children's development and behavior.

The optimal style of TV viewing is family viewing, with adults selecting the programs and sharing thoughts with the child about what they are watching; however, studies have shown that family viewing does not happen routinely (Kaiser, 2010). Many programs typically selected by children may be developmentally inappropriate for their ages. TV viewing is a passive experience, but the developmental stage of the child influences the ability to understand complex story plots that involve narration, cultural references, or interruptions in the continuity of the story.

Character movements, sound effects, animation, and high-pitched voices capture the attention of young children, and attention is maintained if the content of the program is understood by the child. Although some studies have shown that exposure to violent TV content can provoke aggressive acts in children who have a tendency for aggression, other authorities believe that desensitization may occur with repeated viewing of such content (Rupured, 2007). There are many divergent opinions concerning the long-term behavioral effects of viewing violence on TV.

The Children's Television Act of 1990 has defined prime time or family-viewing time for programs and has placed some controls on programs aired during the hours when young children are likely to be watching. The American Medical Association (AMA) has offered guidance for health-care workers in helping parents monitor their children's TV viewing habits as part of healthy living counseling (Box 4-3).

Violent video games are of more concern than violent TV programs. The interactive practice, imitation, repetition, reward, and reinforcement involved in the playing of a video game are the same basic elements involved in learning a behavior. Therefore learning and imitating aggressive behaviors is a definite risk of interactive violent video games. Some studies have shown that physiological changes occur during the interactive playing of video games. Release of a chemical called dopamine in the body increases, and dopamine is known to be related to learning, attention, and motor integration (Pagani, 2010). The lesson taught in some violent video games may be that violence is fun and rewarding. Associating violent acts with a pleasant experience may provide the basis for learning violent behavior.

BOX 4-3 Teaching Parents How to Manage Media

Monitor TV, video games, and websites (including social networking) that the child views.
Do not use TV or video games as babysitters (i.e., to keep the child quiet or entertained for long periods).
Develop family guidelines for movies that are allowed.
Help the child interpret commercials and other advertising.
Provide opportunities for active play and socializing in balance with media viewing.
Contact sponsors and TV stations and demand quality programming during hours when children are most likely to watch TV.

Because of the continued improvement in the realistic graphics of video games, further research concerning games' effects is needed. Most agree that video games should not replace other childhood activities such as athletics, chores, outside play, hobbies, reading, music, and homework (Graham, 2010). Some video games can be played real-time over the Internet with strangers around the world, which could lead to the development of unhealthy or dangerous relationships among participants. Often parents set limits on the time spent playing video games but do not restrict the type of game played and are often unaware of the violent nature of some video games. Parents need to be educated concerning the rating of video games and the amount of time the child should spend playing the games.

Video games can also have medical effects on players. The flicker frequency on the screen can trigger a seizure in a child who has photosensitive epilepsy. Also, an increase in blood pressure and oxygen consumption, breathing patterns, and adrenaline levels on a daily basis may contribute to heart disease later in life.

There are many positive outcomes of media use by children. *Sesame Street* is an example of a TV program that provides positive messages and education for young children. Video games can help increase hand-eye coordination, and many games are available without violent content. Computer games and websites can provide interactive stimulation that captures the attention and helps in developing processing skills and problem-solving abilities (Figure 4-3). Drills and repetition with periodic rewards can spark interest, maintain attention, and increase developmental abilities.

One danger in children's use of the Internet is the potential for sexual predators to obtain private information and arrange personal meetings. Also, the use of "cookies" to track interests and target the viewer for marketing ads requires parental supervision of the child's viewing choices to minimize negative outcomes.

Computer-assisted instruction is now offered in most schools and community libraries and is also accessible at home at minimal cost. Distance learning enables an adolescent or adult to obtain college credit for courses without leaving home. Attitude and behavior remediation in the form of online driving schools are also available and are popular.

The Internet is a source of seemingly endless information, but some critical thinking, in the form of evaluating the source of the information to determine validity, is important.

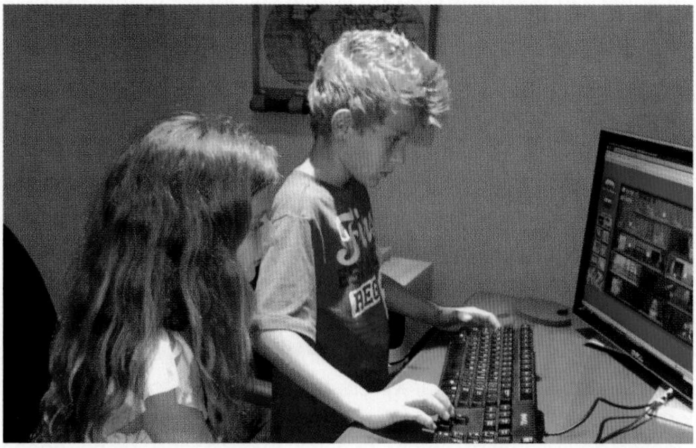

Figure 4–3 Computer games can provide interactive skills, and the Internet can offer a wealth of information to children and adults.

Computers and the Internet also allow accessibility to vitally important services and social interactions:

- Banking and other forms of financial activity can be accomplished online.
- Older adults can find information about a health concern, which can increase understanding of their own health problems and augment the teaching of the health-care team.
- Font size on the screen can be adjusted for the visually impaired.
- People for whom English is their second language (ESL) can have information translated into their native language to enhance their pleasure and understanding.
- Disabled persons confined to the home can enjoy personal contacts with the outside world.
- E-mail and programs such as Skype enable the elderly to maintain close communication with family and friends without the burden of taking pictures and writing and mailing letters.

The Growth of Social Networking Sites

Social media and networking sites (such as Facebook, Twitter, LinkedIn, YouTube, Pinterest, and many others) have become staples in everyday life because they allow people to communicate with each other, learn and gain information, share interests, and find support concerning personal illness or problems. Social networking has both positive effects and risks to the healthy growth and development of children. Facebook is designed for children over 11 years of age, but some younger children lie about their age to gain access.

The American Academy of Pediatrics (AAP) reported that more than half of adolescents log on to social networking sites once a day with many logging on more than 10 times a day (Gordon, 2011). Facebook depression is a common term used for the teen who overuses social networking to the point of altering sleep and eating habits and isolating himself from peers and family, eventually succumbing to general depression. Another negative effect of social networking is *cyber bullying*, which can have devastating effects on the immature mind.

Other types of technology also affect the interactions among children and adolescents. For example, sexting is the sending or receiving of sexually explicit text messages and pictures.

Parents need to learn the technology, monitor their child's activities, and share the journey by discussing networking experiences as they discuss the child's other daily activities. Health-care workers can guide parents toward resources that encourage proper use of technology and media so that they can reap the rewards and avoid the pitfalls (Box 4-4).

BOX 4-4 Resources for Internet Safety

www.i-safe.org – Founded in 1998 and endorsed by the U.S. Congress. The site is dedicated to protecting online experiences of children to make cyberspace a safe and educational place.

www.getnetwise.com – A public service sponsored by the technology industry to help guide intelligent use of the Internet.

www.ikeepsafe.org – The home of "Faux Paw, the Websurfing Techno Cat" is supported by a coalition of governors, their spouses, law enforcement, the AAP, and other associations to offer parents, educators, and caregivers guidelines and tools to ensure the safe use of technology.

www.onguardonline.gov – Offers safety tips for tweens and teens concerning social networking sites.

EFFECTS OF A DISASTER ON FAMILY AND DEVELOPMENT

Disasters are a part of life and can occur in the form of a natural disaster (e.g., hurricane, earthquake, or flood) or a human-made disaster (e.g., war or catastrophic oil spill). In the past, unless the family was personally involved at the location of the disaster, the event was soon forgotten and the impact thought to be minimal. However, with the current incorporation of media in daily life, disasters in every part of the world can be relayed in explicit detail.

In many homes, the tragic attack on the World Trade Center in New York City on September 11, 2001, was viewed as it was happening and was reviewed on TV for months and years afterward. This event brought terror into private homes and lives as it was occurring and demonstrated that the family does not need to be directly in the area of the disaster to experience such aftereffects. Witnessing the disaster on TV in the privacy of their homes and observing the responses of their parents makes children almost as vulnerable as the on-scene victims.

Studies have shown that children can suffer from posttraumatic stress disorder (PTSD) after witnessing parental violence or any event that causes upheaval or disruption of family life (Elhai, 2011). PTSD has been defined as the development of characteristic symptoms following an extreme traumatic stressor (APA, 2012). Some signs and symptoms of PTSD in children who have experienced a recent traumatic or abusive situation may be social withdrawal; appearing very serious (less playful) than other children their age; feelings of depression, anxiety, helplessness, or mistrust; giving up rather than displaying self-protective behavior; reacting quickly with fear; or having a dismal view of the future. Adults with PTSD, including adult survivors of childhood trauma, may display similar emotions and behaviors. They may also develop an expectation of abuse or negative experiences and sometimes may unintentionally make choices and have reactions that increase the risk of additional trauma. Symptoms of PTSD can be alleviated or prevented with psychotherapy.

Studies have shown that boys born during wartime had developmental delays that may have been caused by an overattachment to their mothers (Chartrand 2008). This overattachment resulted from an overprotective mother-child relationship that was directly influenced by the stresses of war. Emotional trauma from disasters can affect children and are influenced by parental reactions to the events.

Children respond to personal disaster by exhibiting anxiety, disorganization, confusion, inhibited activity, apathy, withdrawal, and sleeping and eating dysfunctions. These responses can affect school performance and appetite, which impacts growth and development. In response to a disaster event, school-age children may regress to earlier developmental abilities and behavior patterns. Phobias, flashbacks, and reenactments during play are also common. Adolescents may respond with an increase in sexual promiscuity, vandalism, or substance abuse.

These responses are the result of the child's perception of the disaster and the ability of the parents to cope as models of behavior. If a child is intimately involved in the disaster and strangers intrude in his or her life, these responses can intensify. Because children are dependent, they are more vulnerable to further trauma after a disaster occurs. If the community and the parents are personally affected, the child's functioning is disrupted. Symptoms of depression or stress that persist for more than a month after the disaster may warrant referral for a psychiatric evaluation.

Often parents are not aware of the child's responses, or parents tend to minimize the effect of the event on the child. The nurse and health-care worker should look for signs of PTSD when in contact with a child who is going through the aftermath of a disaster.

Children of rescue workers can develop anxiety concerning their parents' risky activities, and professional support may be indicated (as evidenced during the 9/11 disaster). Nurses, health-care providers, and teachers must advocate preparation and training for disasters and develop an awareness of risks in their own environment.

Role of the Health-Care Team

Professionals who care for children have a responsibility to understand and respect the opportunities that the fast-developing electronic media offer for learning and media's role in revolutionizing education. There is also a need to help the child self regulate choices of what to view and to help parents use media in a positive way to promote a well-balanced lifestyle. Educating the public about quality programming and working with professional groups, industry, and regulating agencies to decrease the violence, pornography, and other negative aspects, and to promote quality programs, are vital.

Nurses and health-care workers must recognize that the response to disasters is influenced not only by a personal threat of injury or being close to the area of the disaster, but can be influenced by parental response to the event. Parents should be guided to provide extra emotional support to children, to reassure them that their environment is safe, and to try to maintain a familiar and consistent daily routine. Parents should be urged to discuss the disaster in honest terms at a level appropriate to the child's age. Drawings and play can be used to help children express their feelings. Parents can review how family members can help each other. Coping abilities of the children and the family should be monitored and referral for professional help offered as needed.

EFFECT OF COMMUNITY ON FAMILY AND DEVELOPMENT

Initially the family is the center of relationships that influence the development of the child. As the child grows, relationships expand, and outside influences affect the family as well as the child's growth and development. Teachers, coaches, clubs, teams, and peers each place demands on the family unit and have an increased effect on growth and development of its members. Most outside influences aid in learning social rules of behavior, help develop a sense of belonging, and contribute to the development of a positive self-image. The effects of outside influences during the stages of the life cycle are discussed in the following chapters.

HEALTHY LIFESTYLE HABITS

Attitudes toward exercise and food are formed in the home, and the family plays a crucial role in the development of healthy lifestyle habits. Parents are role models for children and have a major part in determining what the child sees as normal. Active parents are more likely to involve their children in regular physical activities, whereas sedentary parents are more likely to create a more inactive environment for their children (see Figure 4-2). Replacing 60 minutes of television, computer, or video game time each day with fun family activities (such as taking a walk, playing catch, or bicycling) can foster healthy habits while also improving family relationships. Physically active children are much more likely to become physically active adults who are at decreased risk for disease and disability later in life.

Healthy food choices also begin at home. Parents and caregivers must set good examples by consuming mainly fresh foods and water and limiting intake of processed foods and sodas (see Figure 4-1, B). Children look to parents for the development of lifestyle habits, and adults need to teach by example.

FAMILY-CENTERED HEALTH CARE

In family-centered health care, the family is central to the plan of care for any individual family member. Identifying and valuing the strengths of the family network to cope, support, and assist in the care of a family member are essential. Today the family no longer hands over total responsibility of patients to health-care personnel. Expanded visiting hours in the hospital setting allow family members to participate in care. Home-care services have expanded to allow care of the patient in the home setting, with the family functioning as the experts and the nurse or health-care team functioning as consultants in a true partnership experience that empowers the family. To achieve family-centered care, the nurse and health-care worker must first listen to the family's perception of the problem and communicate the perception of the health-care team, identifying similarities and differences. Armed with cultural competence and an understanding of the family as a unit, nurses and health-care workers can provide meaningful, effective, family-centered health care.

KEY POINTS

- The family is a social system that involves interaction with and commitment to its members.
- Family structures include the nuclear two-parent family, the dual-career family, the extended family, the single-parent family, the blended family, and others.
- Traditional family development includes marriage, childbearing, childrearing, child launching, the contracting family, and the aging family.
- A family systems theory is based on understanding that what happens to one member of the family affects the entire family.
- The family lifestyle; size, number, and spacing of siblings; and family health all have an effect on the growth and development of the child.
- Childrearing styles can be classified as autocratic, democratic, or laissez-faire.
- Culture is a set of learned values, beliefs, and customs that are shared by a family.
- Advances in technology and the use of electronic media have allowed for research of information and achievement of educational degrees in the home setting.
- Interactive video games and television viewing involving violence can have negative effects on the growth and development of children.
- Posttraumatic stress disorder can occur after viewing a live disaster scene on television and can affect growth and development.
- Parents must be guided to monitor the social networking sites used by children to assure positive outcomes.
- The family plays a crucial role in the development of healthy lifestyle habits.
- Community members, such as teachers, coaches, clubs, and peers, influence growth and development and place demands on the family unit.

Critical Thinking

A newly divorced mother moves with her three children, ages 4, 7, and 15, into a new neighborhood. What interventions could a school nurse or health-care worker use to help the family make a healthy adjustment to their new life?

REVIEW QUESTIONS

1. A family is defined as:
   a. a structure consisting of two parents and at least one child.
   b. a social system involving commitment and interaction.
   c. genetically related groups of people.
   d. a group of people living together.

2. A theory is:
   a. a logical, consistent concept based on research findings.
   b. concepts and thoughts accepted by most people.
   c. an unproven concept based on an individual's observations.
   d. a technique or intervention used to treat others.

3. A family Apgar is:
   a. a tool to assess family function.
   b. the financial status of a family.
   c. a family systems theory.
   d. a process of family therapy.

4. A dysfunctional family includes:
   a. stable family members.
   b. changing family memberships and rules.
   c. parents who manage the care of children.
   d. parents who use effective coping skills.

5. The Children's Television Act of 1990 was designed to:
   a. control programs aired when children may be watching.
   b. provide cartoons for young viewers.
   c. limit the number of hours children can watch TV.
   d. provide educational programs for preschool children.

CHAPTER 5

Theories of Development

http://evolve.elsevier.com/Leifer/growth

OBJECTIVES

1. List theories of personality development.
2. Discuss one behavioral theory of development.
3. Discuss one psychosocial theory of development.
4. Discuss one environmental theory of development.
5. Discuss one cognitive theory of development.
6. Discuss the major forces that influence an adult learner.
7. Discuss how understanding developmental theories can enhance the ability to teach an individual who may be in a specific stage of development.
8. List physiological, cognitive, personality, social, and emotional changes that occur over the lifespan.
9. Discuss the uniqueness of individual personality and behavior at each stage of the life cycle.
10. Practice a deeper understanding of self and family.

KEY TERMS

behavioral theories
behaviorist theory
classical conditioning
cognitive theories
Electra anxiety
extrovert
humanist theories
information-processing theory
introvert
looking-glass self
moral reasoning
Oedipus complex
operant conditioning
psychodynamic theories
social-learning theory
sociocultural theories

DEFINITION

A theory is a statement based on scientific research that helps to make observations and facts meaningful. Behavioral theories are designed to explain the development of specific behaviors and suggest their relationships to other developing social skills. Psychodynamic theories focus on personality-trait development and psychological challenges at different ages; cognitive theories focus on advancement of the development of thinking; humanist theories describe the influence of human experiences such as love and attachment on behavior and personality development; and sociocultural theories describe how culture influences behavior. There is no single theory of development. Each theory provides important insights into different life stages, and human development is most accurately understood by integrating these theories.

IMPORTANCE OF UNDERSTANDING DEVELOPMENTAL THEORIES

Developmental theories focus on changes in physiology, psychology, and behavior that occur normally at different stages in the lifespan. Behaviors at different stages within the life cycle are influenced by culture, environment, past experiences, family, health status, and the reaction of the individual to all these events.

The study of growth and development starts with conception and extends throughout the lifespan. Understanding what affects growth and development, positively and negatively, helps nurses, health-care workers, and educators predict behaviors and responses at each stage and understand why people behave in certain ways. We now know that adults pass through predictable stages of development just as children do. Therefore studying growth and development in a continuum from birth to the geriatric adult provides a comprehensive understanding of how various life experiences affect growth and development at each stage of the life cycle. This understanding of behavior and personality enables health-care workers and educators to intervene effectively and to foster positive physical and mental health-care practices that will improve the lives of those they serve and teach.

Lifespan Considerations

Specific changes occur in each phase of the life cycle (Figure 5-1). Therefore interventions at the appropriate time within each stage can effectively influence health practices and contribute to the achievement of the goals of *Healthy People 2020.* Anticipation of needs can help in the development of an effective health-teaching plan.

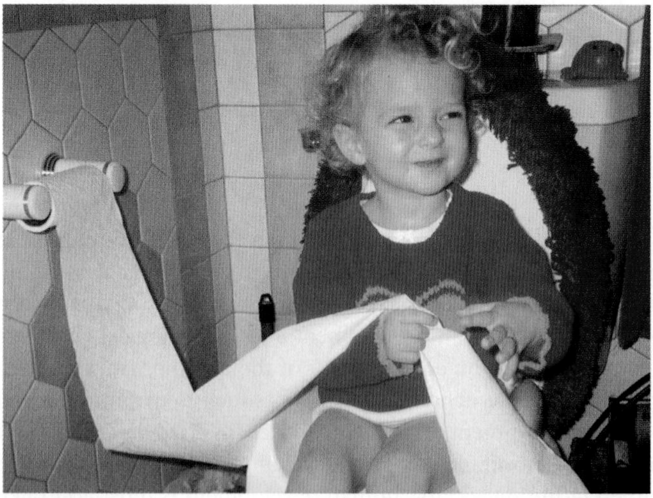

Figure 5–1 **Toilet training.** Learning self-control of the bowel and bladder is a developmental task of the toddler. There are many child-sized potties available, and eventually the child prefers adult facilities.

SELECTED THEORIES OF DEVELOPMENT

Psychoanalytic Theory (Freud)

Sigmund Freud was a psychoanalytic theorist who identified three interacting parts of a person's psychological functioning. They are as follows:

- *Id* (the unconscious) is present at birth and generates impulses that seek immediate pleasure and satisfaction.
- *Ego* is a view of the self or image a person wants to convey to others.
- *Superego* emerges between 3 and 5 years of age, delays immediate gratification for socially appropriate reasons, and represents recognition of good and bad. It is also known as a moral guide or a conscience.

Freud believed that conflict occurs when society provides mixed messages, causing the unconscious (id) to produce anxiety, which rises to the surface (conscious or ego) and becomes evident to the individual in his or her feelings and behavior. Freud described defense mechanisms that protect the ego by hiding unpleasant feelings from a person's conscious awareness thus serving as a defense against anxiety (Box 5-1).

Freud believed that personality grows, develops, and changes during the lifespan, but experiences in the early phases of development have a strong impact on the formation of the adult personality. Freud defined sexuality as any expressed bodily stimulation that is perceived to be pleasurable (Gormly et al, 1989). Freud described specific stages of psychosexual development (Table 5-1).

Freud believed that the Oedipus complex arises during the phallic stage of development and suggested that little boys compete with their fathers for the mother's love and attention. During this stage, the boy prefers attention from the opposite-sex parent. As this stage ends, the boy decides to identify with his father, and attention is desired from both parents again. The Electra anxiety occurs when little girls compete with their mothers for the love and attention of their fathers. At the end of this stage, the little girl stops competing and reidentifies with the mother, again desiring attention from both parents. This occurs at about 5 years of age. Successful resolution of the Oedipus complex and Electra anxiety were thought to be the basis of the development of a mature sexual role and identity. Freud believed that the experiences of children play a role in forming adult personality, but Freud did not view the adult as a developing being. Thus Freud's theory has no identified stages beyond puberty.

BOX 5-1 Defense Mechanisms for Coping

Rationalization – Developing a plausible excuse for unacceptable behavior
Repression – "Forgetting" an unpleasant experience
Projection – Attributing one's thoughts or feelings to another person
Displacement – Expressing feelings (often anger) one has about a person toward another innocent person
Reaction formation – Acting just the opposite of what one feels (e.g., acting sure of oneself when one is really feeling insecure)
Regression – Reverting to immature behavior
Identification – Joining a group so that its positive identity will be reflected on oneself
Sublimation – Rechanneling unacceptable impulses into socially acceptable ones (e.g., channeling aggression into playing football)

TABLE 5-1 Freud's Stages of Psychosexual Development

Stage	Age	Description
Oral	First year of life	Focus is on mouth and the need to suck.
Anal	Toddler age	Focus is on learning self-control of bowels (see Figure 5-1).
Phallic	Preschool age	Attention is self-centered during this stage. Some type of masturbation often occurs at this stage. Child identifies with parent of opposite sex. Superego develops at this time.
Latency	School age	Learns to suppress sexual urges and focuses on industry, achievement, and skills.
Genital	Puberty	Deals with sexual urges involving the opposite sex (mature compared with phallic stage). Seeks mutual pleasure with a partner.

Data from Haith M, Benson J: Encyclopedia of infant and early childhood development, Waltham, MA, 2008, Elsevier; Kleigman R, Stanton B, Geme I, Shor N, Behrman R: Nelson's textbook of pediatrics, Philadelphia, 2011, W.B. Saunders; Carey W, Crocker A, Elias E, Feldon H, Coleman W: Developmental-behavioral pediatrics, ed 4, Philadelphia, 2008, W.B. Saunders.

Psychodynamic Theory (Jung)

Carl Jung, a Swiss doctor, studied with Freud but did not believe sexuality was the basis of behavior development. He believed development extended into adulthood and that age 40 was the "noon of life." Jung believed the roots of personality were a reflection of the past culture of the family, which unconsciously molds the way a person perceives experiences as an adult. He was most recognized for describing personality traits, including the introvert (a quiet person who focuses inwardly on self) and the extrovert (an outgoing person who focuses on others in the environment). Jung believed that the personality could be changed in the middle-adulthood phase, when repressed feelings are recognized and coping mechanisms mature. Jung defined the process of recognizing one's own talent and abilities as self-actualization.

Stages of the Life Cycle: A Psychosocial Theory (Erikson)

Erik Erikson's theory describes the parts of personality development that are dependent on the social environment and social interactions. Each stage involves a social crisis or task that must be positively resolved to pass successfully to the next stage. For example, failure to establish trust with caregivers in the infant stage of development may affect the stage of intimacy later in life, which is based on the ability to establish trust with another person. Successfully passing through each of these stages is thought to contribute to the overall development of the individual personality and its unique strengths and weaknesses (Table 5-2).

The stage of adulthood also proceeds through phases, which include occupation, marriage and family, friends, culture and religion, and leisure. Each phase has a period of stability, which could last several years, where values are pursued and choices are made. The phases are bridged by a transitional period of change, when reassessment occurs and

TABLE 5-2 Erikson's Stages of the Life Cycle

Stage	Age	Positive Achievement
Trust vs. mistrust	Infant	Develops trust of others to meet personal needs of self and, as a result, begins to trust others and himself/herself.
Autonomy vs. shame and doubt	Toddler	Ability to act independently is equated with trusting oneself to be good.
Initiative vs. guilt	Preschool	Imitates role models and follows rules. Experiences self-control in social interactions.
Industry vs. inferiority	School age	Develops ability to make friends and independently achieve school tasks.
Identity vs. role confusion	Adolescent	Learns to know oneself and what one believes and develops a career goal.
Intimacy vs. isolation	Young adult	Develops an ability to share all aspects of life with others.
Generativity vs. self absorption	Middle adult	Can contribute to society in a meaningful way.
Integrity vs. despair	Older adult (geriatric)	Maintains a sense of life achievement and absence of deep regret.

Data adapted from Haith M, Benson J: Encyclopedia of infant and early childhood development, Waltham, MA, 2008, Elsevier; Kleigman R, Stanton B, Geme I, Shor N, Behrman R: Nelson's textbook of pediatrics, Philadelphia, 2011, W.B. Saunders; Carey W, Crocker A, Elias E, Feldon H, Coleman W: Developmental-behavioral pediatrics, ed 4, Philadelphia, 2008, W.B. Saunders.

TABLE 5-3 Stages of Parenting Behaviors

Stage	Parenting Behavior
Stage 1: Parental image	Picturing oneself as a parent
Stage 2: Authority	Questioning parental skills as the child becomes autonomous
Stage 3: Integrative	Feeling responsible to motivate child as the child becomes more independent
Stage 4: Independent teen	Learning how to support teen while maintaining the authority role
Stage 5: Departure	Relating to the child as an adult as child prepares for the future and leaves home

modifications are made. For example, if a marriage occurred in one phase, divorce can occur in a transitional phase. Choices and changes are discussed in detail in the chapters concerning growth and development during the adult years.

Erikson's theory involves generativity. Erikson believed that parents grow as their children develop and are influenced by parent–child interactions at each stage. He described specific stages of parenting (Table 5-3).

Psychosocial Theory (Levinson)

Daniel J. Levinson was a theorist who elaborated on Erik Erikson's theories. Levinson believed that an interaction among environment, culture, and the individual was the "fabric of life." Levinson believed that each person enters an orderly sequence of events or structures in life. The tasks of each structure are specific and identifiable. For example, Levinson defined the pre-adult as being between 17 and 22 years of age. The pre-adult first leaves the protection of the family, and that period serves as a bridge between adolescence and independent adulthood. He described the early adult (age 22 to 45 years) as being at the height of vigor and vitality and making important choices such as marriage, career, and lifestyle. He described the middle adult, age 45 to 65 years, as being in a transition phase with a gradual decrease of mental and physical functioning. He described the late adult, age 65 to 80 years, as the grandparent generation whose task is to define new goals and levels of involvement with family, friends, and community. The late-late adult (geriatric) stage he described as beginning at 80 years of age and involves the task of facing death, although the individual often continues to be socially interactive. Details of these stages, with more current definitions, are reviewed in later chapters.

Cognitive Theory (Piaget)

Jean Piaget was a Swiss psychologist who emphasized cognitive milestones in development. Piaget described four stages of development related to learning to understand and relate logically to the world (Table 5-4).

TABLE 5-4 Piaget's Four Stages of Development

Stage	Age	Cognitive Milestones
Sensorimotor	Birth to 2 years	Gains developmental understanding of object permanence. Understands cause and effect. Understands differences in time of day.
Preoperational	2 to 7 years	Attributes life to inanimate objects. Child believes he or she is the center of world. Sees only the obvious. Understands only one bit of information at a time without seeing abstract relationships. Develops language skills. Uses pretend play. Begins to use logic to understand rules.
Concrete operations	7 to 11 years	Can understand more than one piece of information simultaneously. Has a realistic understanding of the world. Focuses on the present, not the future.
Formal operations	Adolescent	Can think abstractly and understands symbols. Can think in hypothetical terms. Is future oriented. Understands scientific bases of theories. Cultural practices play a role in helping the adolescent understand "rules" and develop the moral sense of what is right.

Data from Haith M, Benson J: Encyclopedia of infant and early childhood development, Waltham, MA, 2008, Elsevier; Kleigman R, Stanton B, Geme I, Shor N, Behrman R: Nelson's textbook of pediatrics, Philadelphia, 2011, W.B. Saunders; Carey W, Crocker A, Elias E, Feldon H, Coleman W: Developmental-behavioral pediatrics, ed 4, Philadelphia, 2008, W.B. Saunders; Piaget J: The language of the child, Philadelphia, 1926, Harcourt Brace.

Piaget's theory involved sensory and motor interactions with the environment. An infant learns how to grasp a block and learns the relationship it has to the infant's body. The infant then learns when he or she drops the block that it will fall down and be out of reach. Gradually the infant learns that he or she can stack the blocks on top of one another, and eventually the infant can use the blocks to build something that represents a house or other object in the environment.

This interaction involves the child's thinking or processing of information at different ages and stages of development. The information-processing theory states that information is input, is processed mentally, and is then followed by an output of judgment and decision making. This is believed to be the basis of problem-solving and critical-thinking abilities. The basic technique of information processing does not change with age. Only the speed and efficiency of the processing improves with age to adulthood. Piaget's stages involve qualitative, not just quantitative, changes in thought.

Cognitive Theory (Loevinger)

Jane Loevinger stretched Piaget's model of development into the stages of adulthood. She believed that the ego adapts to demands and is an important basis for critical thinking. Loevinger believed ego development was progressive, with observable milestones throughout adult life.

Constructive Theory (Kegan)

Robert Kegan expressed a constructive developmental theory similar to Piaget's. Kegan believed that there was a lifelong interaction with the environment, in which the individual moved through periods of changes in stability that provided meaning for living. The core of Kegan's theory was the need to be included in reciprocal relationships with others and the need to maintain independence.

Theory of Language and Culture (Vygotsky)

Lev Vygotsky believed social and cultural experiences were necessary for optimal growth and development. Physiological maturation of the brain enables language development, which influences how a child thinks and behaves. His theory suggested that language was a major force in the growth and development of the personality. Table 5-5 shows how language skills and social interaction affect each other and contribute to learning. People learn what they can achieve for themselves, and, through social interaction, what they can do with the help of others. This has implications for health education.

Social and Economic Influences (Bronfenbrenner)

Urie Bronfenbrenner presented a combination of social and economic factors that influence growth and development (Table 5-6). This theory offers insight into how children may be treated differently in different environments and the effect that those differences may have on a child's understanding of himself or herself.

TABLE 5-5 Vygotsky's Language and Development Theory

Age	Verbal Ability	Adult Response
Infant	Cries and coos	Parents respond to cries by cuddling infant and providing toys to stimulate responses.
Toddler	Points to objects	Adults give names and definitions to the objects at which the child is pointing.
Preschool		
3 years old	Speaks to self during play or movement	Parents may or may not listen to all the words.
4 years old	Uses inner speech to guide behavior	Parents praise the child for demonstrating delayed gratification or self-control.
School age	Engages in speech and social interactions	Parents who listen to their child understand the child's interpretation of events and experiences. Parents allow child to discover what he or she can do independently and with the help of others.

Data from Haith M, Benson J: Encyclopedia of infant and early childhood development, Waltham, MA, 2008, Elsevier; Kleigman R, Stanton B, Geme I, Shor N, Behrman R: Nelson's textbook of pediatrics, Philadelphia, 2011, W.B. Saunders; Carey W, Crocker A, Elias E, Feldon H, Coleman W: Developmental-behavioral pediatrics, ed 4, Philadelphia, 2008, W.B. Saunders; Vygotsky L: Thoughts and language, Cambridge, MA, 1962, MIT Press.

TABLE 5-6 Bronfenbrenner's Social Theory of Growth and Development

Social Contacts	Influence on Personality Development
Parents, siblings	Gender of child influences how others treat child, which influences child's behavior. Parental expectations of child influence child's perception of self-worth.
Teachers, babysitters	Teachers' and babysitters' perceptions of the child influence child's sense of self. The active or aggressive child can frustrate teachers and babysitters, and the quiet child is often more appreciated.
School, neighborhood, community	Coach may value an athletically talented child. The academically talented child may not achieve similar recognition.
Political community	Funding for school community centers and programs influences ability of child to experience these social opportunities. Some energy and behaviors, if not appropriately channeled, may become antisocial; poverty can result in poor nutrition that can decrease the ability to learn and develop.

Data from Haith M, Benson J: Encyclopedia of infant and early childhood development, Waltham, MA, 2008, Elsevier; Kleigman R, Stanton B, Geme I, Shor N, Behrman R: Nelson's textbook of pediatrics, Philadelphia, 2011, W.B. Saunders; Carey W, Crocker A, Elias E, Feldon H, Coleman W: Developmental-behavioral pediatrics, ed 4, Philadelphia, 2008, W.B. Saunders; Brofenbrenner U: The ecology of human development, Harvard University Press, 1979, Cambridge, MA.

Hierarchy of Needs (Maslow)

Abraham Maslow described a hierarchy of needs. According to Maslow, if basic needs are met, then the individual can move to higher levels of thought and self fulfillment. These needs are described using a triangle. The base of the triangle represents the basic physiological needs of survival. As the sides of the triangle narrow, achievement of needs at each level allows movement toward a higher level (Figure 5-2). After basic needs are met, a person can move toward self actualization. Self actualization is the realization of one's own talent and abilities and the achievement of satisfaction in life's goals and desires. It is reaching the peak of one's potential. For example, in severe poverty, basic physiological needs for food and shelter may be unmet. The person cannot think beyond meeting these basic needs of survival and so will not proceed to higher goals and ultimate self actualization. Some characteristics of self actualization include the accurate understanding of reality, judgments based on evidence, and the acceptance of self as independent and creative.

Environmental Theory (Rogers)

Carl Rogers believed people naturally form their own positive destiny, based on the concept of the self, if obstacles are removed. He theorized that mastery over the environment and positive relationships helped form the self concept. A person has an idea of the type of person he or she would like to be. Sometimes there are differences between this idealized self and the actual self. If the ideal self shares a lot in common with the actual self, then that person discovers his or her full potential and achieves happiness. According to Rogers, self actualization happens as a person realizes he or she can do many things to be like the ideal self.

Behaviorist Theory (Watson)

John Watson was known as the father of behaviorism. He believed the environment and experiences molded the personality. Inborn traits or drives are not the basis of his theory. Watson's theories are related to Pavlov's conditioning theory of personality development and Skinner's operant theory.

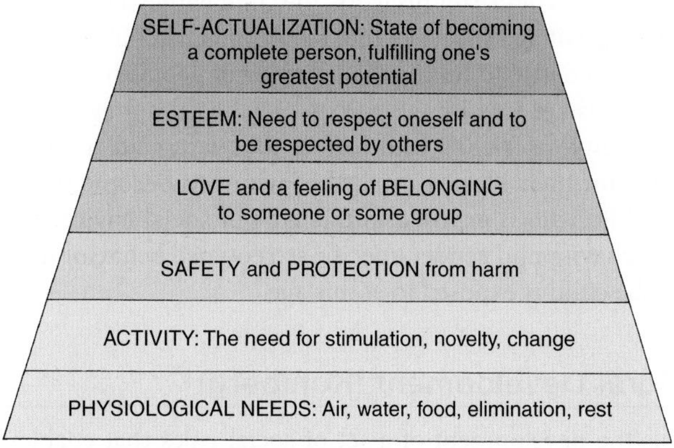

Figure 5–2 Modified version of Maslow's hierarchy of needs. (From Leifer G: *Introduction to maternity and pediatric nursing*, ed 6, Philadelphia, 2011, WB Saunders.)

Behaviorist Theory of Personality (Pavlov and Skinner)

Ivan Pavlov and B.F. Skinner's theories describe learning and interaction with the environment as the center of development. This is known as the behaviorist theory of development. Behaviorists believe that personality and behavior are learned. Therefore they believe that there are no identifiable stages. Each experience helps to mold the adult personality.

These theorists believed that the environment and the way people respond to it influence personality development. Pavlov developed the theory of classical conditioning. Conditioning has to do with associating (pairing) things in the environment. For example, when an individual eats a food that causes the unpleasant symptoms of food poisoning, that individual may develop an aversion to that food. The food poisoning was paired with that food, because they were experienced together. Because of this, that particular food is associated with negative feelings even without food poisoning occurring again.

Skinner attributed learning to operant conditioning, which involves behavioral consequences such as reward or punishment. For example, reinforcing positive behavior with a reward will eventually develop a regular practice of that behavior. Reward can be praise, special privileges, or material rewards such as toys, money, or candy.

These theories are useful in health education, because positive reinforcement of learned information can result in positive health practices. The opposite is also true. If a coach uses exercise as a punishment, by making the student run around a course or do 15 pushups after bad behavior, then exercise can become perceived as a negative activity and not considered as a pleasurable experience. This can lead to a sedentary lifestyle and obesity later in life. Rewarding healthy behaviors, such as exercise or medical compliance, can increase the occurrence of these behaviors.

Social-Learning Theories of Personality (Bandura and Mischel)

Albert Bandura and Walter Mischel were theorists who believed that social learning formed the basis for personality development (Bandura, 1977). Social-learning theory involves exposure to and imitation of a behavior. Children often imitate what they see. If a father mows the lawn and receives praise for his work, the child witnesses the scenario and receives reinforcement for the positive aspects of that behavior. The child may copy that behavior because of curiosity or a desire to mimic the behavior of people he or she admires. In early childhood, these models are usually the parents. In the school-age child, models may be peers or teachers. Therefore friends who belong to a gang and receive high praise from other gang members for their illegal or risky behavior can become the behavioral models for the school-age child who is exposed to this type of social environment. The development of aggressive behavior and gender-specific stereotyped behavior may be intensified by the gangs or clubs the child is exposed to at this age.

Theory of Moral Development (Kohlberg)

Moral reasoning is the development of a set of social rules that enables a person to differentiate right from wrong, and moral behavior is based on perception and integration of these rules. Lawrence Kohlberg's theory of moral development consists of three levels

TABLE 5-7 Kohlberg's Stages of Moral Development

Stage	Age	Behavior
Preconventional	Toddler Early childhood	Obeys rules to avoid punishments. Seeks to avoid punishment.
Conventional	School age	Conforms to rules to gain recognition or reward.
Postconventional	Adolescent and adult	Follows rules that lead others to perceive person as "good." Develops a sense of responsibility.
	Older adult	Develops own set of principles that may overrule social laws or customs. Is independent.

Data from Haith M, Benson J: Encyclopedia of infant and early childhood development, 2008, Elsevier; Kleigman R, Stanton B, Geme I, Shor N, Behrman R: Nelson's textbook of pediatrics, Philadelphia, 2011, W.B. Saunders; Carey W, Crocker A, Elias E, Feldon H, Coleman W: Developmental-behavioral pediatrics, ed 4, Philadelphia, 2008, W.B. Saunders; Kohlberg L: Development of moral character and moral ideology. In Hoffman H, Hoffman L, editors, Review of child development research, Troy, NY, 1964, Russell Sage.

that are closely related to Piaget's views (see Table 5-4). Kohlberg's stages of moral development (Table 5-7) remain a respected theory today, although modification of level three (the postconventional stage) has been suggested as a result of research findings. Carol Gilligan's work challenged the description of postconventional moral thought, and Gilligan also believed that Kohlberg's research excluded women.

Moral behavior is generally considered to be learned. Parents and teachers provide rewards when children demonstrate desired morally sound behaviors. Teaching a child right from wrong in a firm, loving way will result in the development of moral behavior.

Health Promotion

Helping a child understand how someone else feels in reaction to his or her behavior (empathy) is a preferred method for encouraging the development of moral behavior. Punishment often results in resistance and denial and can turn the focus away from learning, and thus punishment may not be an effective tool for teaching moral behavior.

Development of Self-Image (Cooley and Mead)

Charles Horton Cooley created the theory of the looking-glass self, which states that the self-image is formed through three steps: (1) imagining how we portray ourselves to others; (2) imagining how others evaluate us; (3) combining these impressions to formulate a self concept or idea of what we are like. For example, if a teacher criticizes a child, the child may think the teacher believes the child is stupid; therefore, the child's self-image may incorporate the thought that he or she is stupid.

George Herbert Mead furthered Cooley's theory by presenting three stages in the development of the self. In the first stage, children imitate those around them. The child uses a toy broom to imitate the mother sweeping or a toy lawn mower to imitate the father mowing the lawn. The

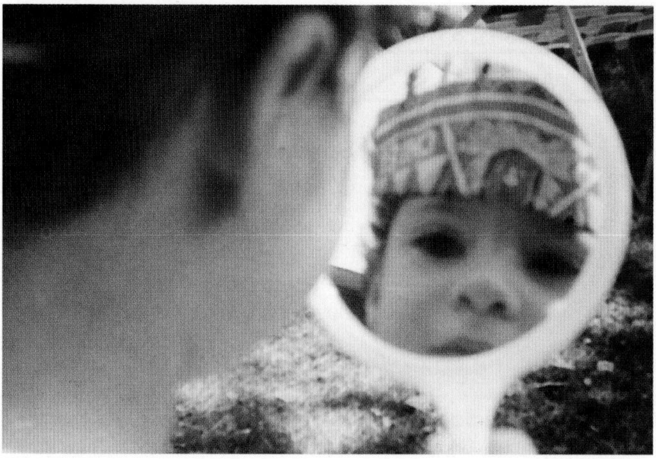

Figure 5–3 A self-image begins to develop with imaginative play during the preschool years.

child may vicariously feel proud of the clean floor or manicured lawn. When children are ready to experience the world of language, television (TV), and books, they are ready for stage two, which involves the use of language or other symbols during interaction with others, such as making a sad, pouting face; a happy face; and so on. In the third stage, the child pretends to be other people—for instance, a superhero such as Spiderman—and may play the role of the pretend person. In middle childhood, the child understands his or her own role and the way it affects the role of others (Figure 5-3). A child learns about others' expectations and appreciates that each person assumes multiple roles in life, such as daughter, sister, mother, grandmother, and teacher.

Developmental Tasks of the Older Adult (Peck)

Robert Peck's theory is based on the developmental tasks of the older adult, which include coping with retirement from work; adapting to the normal physiological decline because of aging; and facing the inevitability of death. Peck's theory involved the need to positively meet these challenges so as to maintain generativity (as described by Erikson) and to avoid despair. Maintaining a positive self-image and feelings of self-worth, despite changing abilities and increasing limitations, is essential to making a healthy transition during this stage.

Developmental Tasks of the Older Adult (Havighurst)

Robert Havighurst (1974) was a theorist who also described the developmental tasks of late adulthood, which involve accepting oneself and maintaining meaning in life. The older adult's developmental tasks include adjusting to a decreasing health status, adjusting to decreased income, adjusting to the death of a spouse, adapting to changing social roles with peer groups, and adapting to changing living arrangements.

Developmental Stages of Retirement (Atchley)

Robert Atchley described five developmental stages in the older adult related to retirement, as described in Table 5-8.

TABLE 5-8 Developmental Stages of Retirement

Stage	Focus
Preretirement	Dreams of retirement
Honeymoon	Enjoys freedom of retirement
Disenchantment	Designs new priorities as a result of boredom
Stability	Begins to feel needed and respected
Terminal	Changes occur because of need for reemployment or decline in health

Additional Influences on Growth and Development

In addition to the theories described above, there are other influences on growth and development. *Cultural beliefs and practices* (discussed in Chapter 3) and *gender differences* affect development according to how the child is treated by others. At birth a girl is often dressed in pink frilly clothes and a boy in blue or brown. Toys selected by parents also enhance gender differences.

Poverty can decrease experiences available to the child, and it can also deprive the child of nutrition needed for brain and body development. The homeless child often does not have access to health care, and homeless adolescents may be exposed to drugs, sexual abuse, and other problems that affect growth and development.

There are *developmental tasks* to be achieved and challenges to be met in each phase of development through the lifespan. Psychological growth occurs through all stages of the life cycle and can modify a person's personality, behavior, and health.

KEY POINTS

- Personal development is influenced by many factors, including genetics, birth order, gender, and environment.
- A theory is designed to explain the development of specific behaviors and is based on research findings.
- Developmental theories can aid health-care workers, nurses, and educators in understanding needs, learning styles, and behaviors at various stages of the life cycle.
- Understanding needs, learning styles, and behaviors at each stage of development enables the nurse, health-care worker, or educator to plan teaching interventions that will contribute to the goals of *Healthy People 2020*.
- Understanding growth and development can help in the designing of teaching styles that will foster positive health-care practices.
- Freud was a psychoanalyst who identified the id, ego, and superego and described stages of psychosexual development.
- Carl Jung believed that development extended into adulthood, with age 40 as the "noon of life."
- Erik Erikson expressed a psychosocial theory that defined stages of life from infancy through the older-adult phase.
- Jean Piaget developed the cognitive theory of development that centered around understanding and relating to the world environment.
- June Loevinger stretched Piaget's theory of development into adulthood.

(*Continued*)

KEY POINTS—cont'd

- Robert Kegan expressed a constructive developmental theory similar to Piaget's, which involved lifelong periods of change and stability.
- Lev Vygotsky presented a theory of language and culture related to the developmental process.
- Urie Bronfenbrenner believed social and economic pressures influenced growth and development.
- Abraham Maslow described a hierarchy-of-needs theory leading to self actualization.
- Carl Rogers believed people form their own destinies based on mastery of the environment.
- Ivan Pavlov and B.F. Skinner developed the behaviorist theory of personality development. They described how classical and operant conditioning influence behavior in response to the environment.
- John Watson was known as the father of behaviorism.
- K. Bandura and W. Mischel researched social-learning theory as the basis for personality development.
- Lawrence Kohlberg described personality development based on moral reasoning. He believed moral behavior was a learned behavior.
- Charles Horton Cooley proposed the looking-glass self theory of personality development, and George Herbert Mead expanded the theory by presenting three stages in the development of the self.
- Robert Peck described developmental tasks of the older adult.
- Robert Havighurst described developmental tasks of late adulthood.
- Robert Atchley described developmental stages in the older adult related to the retirement phase of life.

Critical Thinking

Using information from established theories of growth and development, explain why the diagnosis listed on the left might have the greatest influence on the development process of the age group listed on the right.

Diagnosis	*Age Group*
Fractured jaw	Infant
Fractured leg	Toddler
Fractured arm	School-age child

REVIEW QUESTIONS

1. Which theorist described a hierarchy of needs that leads to self actualization?
   a. Ivan Pavlov
   b. Abraham Maslow
   c. Lawrence Kohlberg
   d. Robert Peck

2. Health-care workers need to understand developmental theories because this understanding will help them:
   a. pass the licensing examination
   b. intervene effectively to promote positive, healthy practices
   c. design effective discipline for young children
   d. analyze the goals of *Healthy People 2020*

3. Which psychoanalytic theorist first described defense mechanisms?
   a. Abraham Maslow
   b. Sigmund Freud
   c. Jean Piaget
   d. Lawrence Kohlberg

4. An understanding of object permanence is part of the stages of development described by:
   a. Jean Piaget
   b. Abraham Maslow
   c. Lawrence Kohlberg
   d. Sigmund Freud

5. Ivan Pavlov was a behaviorist who believed that personality and behavior develop under the influence of:
   a. conditioning responses
   b. genetic control
   c. close parental guidance
   d. chronological age

CHAPTER

6 Prenatal Influences on Healthy Development

http://evolve.elsevier.com/Leifer/growth

OBJECTIVES

1. State the goals of the Human Genome Project.
2. Trace the steps of human fertilization and implantation.
3. Discuss the critical periods of fetal development.
4. Describe the role of exercise during and after pregnancy.
5. Describe the modifications required for exercise during pregnancy.
6. Compare the similarities and differences among two types of twins.
7. Discuss the importance of prenatal health and nutrition as related to the health and life expectancy of the newborn.
8. Discuss the emotional changes that occur during transition to motherhood.
9. Discuss the importance of understanding culture as it affects the care of parents and newborns.
10. Discuss bonding and attachment between parents and newborns.
11. Describe the techniques for calming a newborn infant.
12. List the types of toys and activities that foster the growth and development of the neonate.

KEY TERMS

allele
Apgar score
attachment
bonding
chromosome
dizygotic
dominant gene
ectopic pregnancy
en face
engrossment
fetal alcohol syndrome
fetus
gene therapy
genetic code
genetic counseling
genome
gestation
gestational diabetes
monozygotic
multifetal
mutated
neonatal
sibling rivalry
syndrome
viable
virus vector

THE HUMAN GENOME PROJECT

Growth and development are influenced by biology and by the environment. Research concerning the maternal–fetal origins of adult disease contributed to the development of the Human Genome Project. The National Institutes of Health (NIH) and the U.S. Department of Energy (DOE) assumed leadership of the many scientists who probed the secrets of human genetic makeup for this project. The Human Genome Project involved gene mapping, which determined the makeup of human genes, and the completion of the project in 2001 resulted in the identification of all human genes. Various grants were awarded to finance the research. The project officially began in 1990, and a draft of the findings was published in 2001. The original goals of the project involved the following:

- Identifying the more than 30,000 genes contained in human DNA
- Determining the sequence of the billions of chemicals that are contained in DNA
- Developing tools for analysis of the findings
- Addressing the **e**thical, **l**egal, and **s**ocial **i**mplications involved (ELSI)
- Transferring the technology for use by the public in the private sector

HEREDITY

Cells are the basic working units of all living systems, and a genome is a complete set of DNA that is contained in all cells. The DNA in the genome is the genetic code of a cell that is carried on the chromosomes. A chromosome is a thread of protein and DNA that is contained in the nucleus of every cell. Each chromosome contains genes, and there are approximately 30,000 genes in a genome. The genes or genetic code within these cells carry information about all the proteins within the cell that will determine the characteristics that will be inherited by the newborn (Figure 6-1).

Heredity is controlled by pairs of genes from both the mother and father. This pairing of genes is called an allele. Genes can be dominant or recessive. A dominant gene will overpower a recessive gene most of the time, so that its characteristic will be inherited in about three of four offspring. The fourth offspring may exhibit characteristics of the recessive trait (Figure 6-2).

Studying the characteristics and roles of mutated (variations that may be abnormal) and normal genes enables genetic therapy to be used to correct mutated genes and to replace missing genes that cause specific syndromes. A syndrome is a group of symptoms or signs of an abnormal condition. It is known that specific genetic syndromes contribute to specific behavior patterns. Behavior patterns can result in a response from the environment, which can then affect a child's self-image, as well as growth and development. For example, a genetic abnormality that causes Down syndrome, or an uncontrolled glucose (sugar) level in a diabetic mother, or poor nutrition during pregnancy, can each cause cognitive damage in the newborn infant that will impact the child's growth and development.

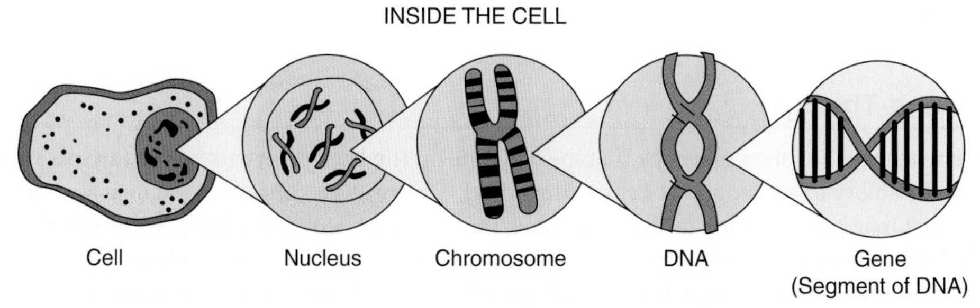

Figure 6-1 The cell contains the nucleus, chromosomes, DNA, and genes. (From Leifer G: *Maternity nursing: an introductory text*, ed 11, Philadelphia, 2012, Saunders.)

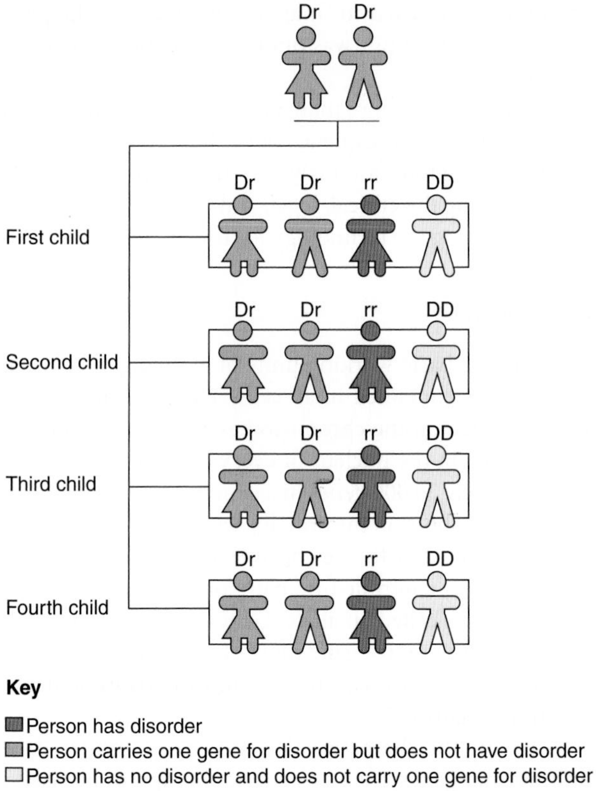

Figure 6-2 Transmission of dominant and recessive traits. Each parent has one dominant gene (D) and one recessive gene (r) for a disease. This figure shows the chances of each offspring being affected by the disease. (From Leifer G: *Maternity nursing: an introductory text*, ed 11, Philadelphia, 2012, Saunders.)

Genetic Counseling

Genetic counseling is the communication between a geneticist (a specialist in inherited conditions) and the parents to discuss the risk of their infant inheriting genes that could result in an abnormality. It is known that behavior is molded by the influence of genes as well as environmental factors. The success of the Human Genome Project allows more detailed research concerning genetic problems and resulting behaviors. Researchers have developed therapeutic genes that repair defective DNA, suicide genes that can be programmed to destroy defective genes, and pure genes that can replace a missing gene.

Gene Therapy

Gene therapy involves placing a therapeutic gene on the back of a virus vector (a virus that has the ability to enter specific cells in the body). The virus vector carries the new gene into the cell that has a missing or defective gene. Gene therapy is in its infancy. Some problems and side effects must be controlled before gene therapy is available for widespread clinical use. However, gene therapy holds much promise. The ethical, social, and legal aspects of gene therapy will need to be clarified in the near future, and standardized policies will need to be developed.

Screening Procedures and Therapies

In the past it has been possible to screen individual patients for the existence of some specific genetic problems without looking at DNA, such as using hemoglobin electrophoresis for types of anemia or the Guthrie test for phenylketonuria (PKU) (a condition in which phenylalanine accumulates in the body and causes mental retardation). However, DNA-based genetic tests can detect carriers, identify susceptibility, and enable diagnosis before symptoms occur. Carrier testing is possible, and genetic counseling can be initiated for sickle-cell and thalassemia disease (a genetic trait that causes an abnormal shape or type of red blood cells), Tay-Sachs disease (a destruction of nerve cells that causes mental and motor deterioration and death during early childhood), and cystic fibrosis (a malfunction of the exocrine glands that results in lung and digestive dysfunctions).

Some adult-onset diseases can be diagnosed before symptoms appear, such as kidney disease, Huntington's chorea, and Lou Gehrig's disease (amyotrophic lateral sclerosis). However, genetic specialists are needed to ensure accurate interpretation of test results. This type of testing requires a team of professionals who can determine the psychological impact of this knowledge on the patient and perhaps the impact on the patient's employment eligibility, now and in the future. Genetic testing is available but may not always be affordable, appropriate, or relevant to optimal medical management.

ELSI

The **ELSI** program has been developed to study the **e**thical, **l**egal, and **s**ocial **i**mplications of gene therapy. Techniques of gene therapy still need to be refined to ensure that inserting a gene on a vector virus to repair DNA does not damage the DNA in a way that could potentially cause a new illness. The refinement of a suicide gene might be used to stop the gene therapy process if genetic damage is noticed. Research is ongoing and is very promising.

FETAL DEVELOPMENT

Fertilization occurs when the sperm penetrates the ovum as it enters the upper portion of the woman's fallopian tube. The time in which fertilization can occur is brief. The sperm lives for up to 5 days, but the ovum lives for only 24 hours after ovulation (see Chapter 10). The ovum always contributes an X chromosome, and the sperm contributes either an X or a Y chromosome. The combination of XX chromosomes produces a female fetus, whereas an XY combination creates a male fetus. Because it is only the sperm that carries the Y chromosome, the male partner determines the sex of the infant. However, the female has some influence on which sperm fertilizes the ovum, because estrogen levels and the pH of the reproductive tract affect the survival rate of the X- or Y-bearing sperm and the speed of their movement to the fallopian tube.

The *zygote* is the cell formed by the union of the sperm and ovum. The cell rapidly multiplies and develops. Within 1 week it enters the uterus and attaches to the upper posterior portion of the uterine wall. (If the zygote does not move freely through the fallopian tube, its increasing size will rupture the fallopian tube, and this condition is known as an ectopic pregnancy.) After implantation into the wall of the uterus, the cells differentiate into layers called the endoderm, mesoderm, and ectoderm. Each layer develops into different organs of the body. After 2 weeks of growth and development, the zygote is called an embryo. From the ninth week of life to birth, the developing baby is called a fetus. Fetal development is shown in Table 6-1.

TABLE 6-1 Embryonic and Fetal Development

Age	Length and Weight	Development
Week 3 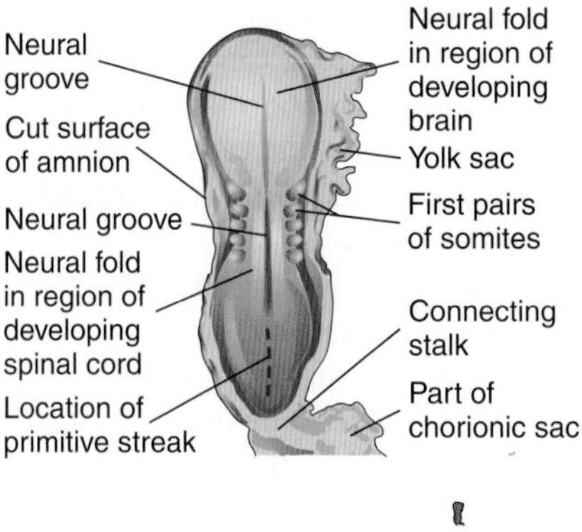 Actual size 2.5 mm	1.5–2.5 mm	Single tubular heart is formed. Neural tube forms; primitive spinal cord and brain appear.
Week 4 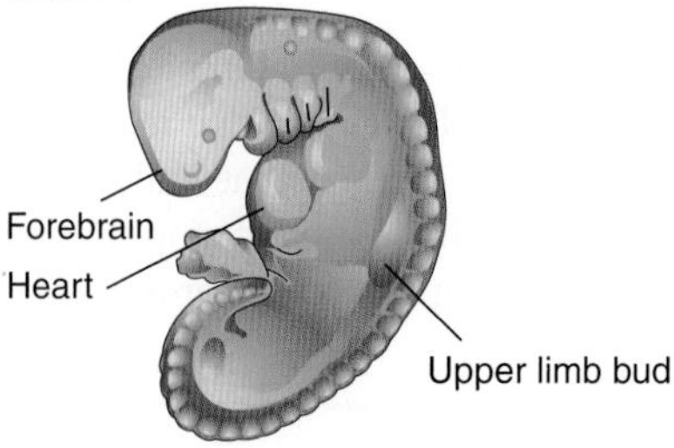	3.5–4 mm	Heart pumps blood. Esophagus and trachea separate; stomach forms. Neural tube closes; forebrain forms. Upper and lower limb buds appear. Ears and eyes begin to form.
Week 6 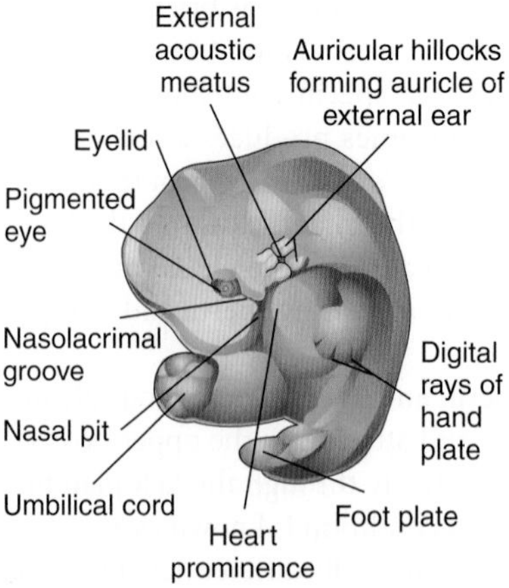 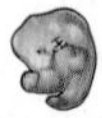 Actual size 11.0 mm	11–13 mm	Skull and jaw ossify; hands and elbows differentiate. Auditory canal forms; eye is obvious. Heart has all four chambers. Nasal cavity and upper lip form.

Age	Length and Weight	Development
Week 8 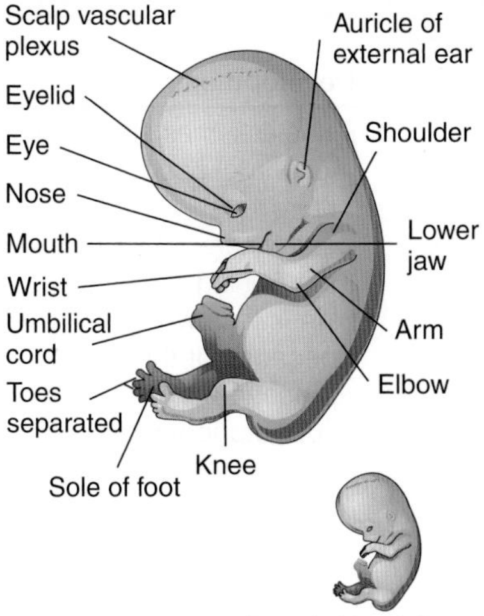 Actual size 30.0 mm	30 mm crown-rump 6 g	Embryo has distinct human appearance. Purposeful movements occur. Tail has disappeared. Sex organs form. Beginnings of most external and internal structures are formed. Enters Fetal Period.
Week 17 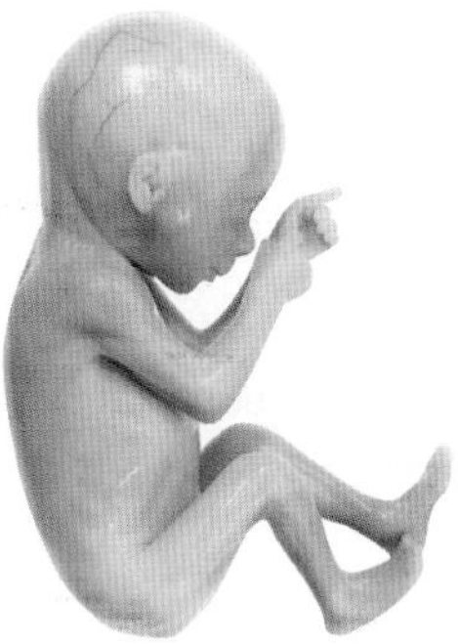	150 mm crown-rump 260 g	Genitalia and leg movements are visible on ultrasound; movement may be felt by the mother. Bones are ossified. Eye movements occur. Fetus sucks and swallows amniotic fluid. Ovaries contain ovum. No subcutaneous fat is present. Thin skin allows blood vessels of scalp to be visible.
Week 25 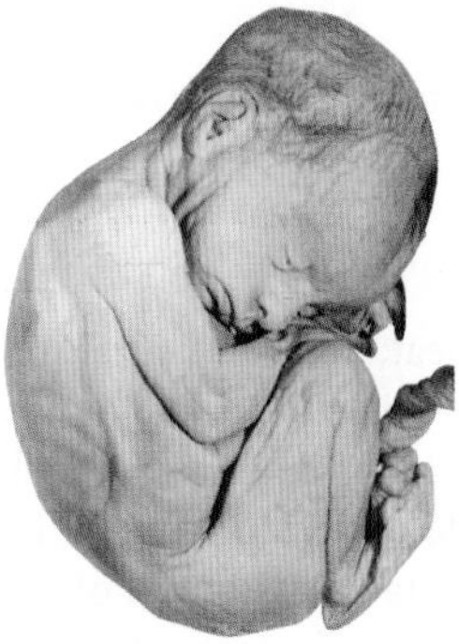	28 cm (11.2 inches) crown-heel 780 g (1 lb, 10 oz)	Wrinkled skin, lean body results from lack of subcutaneous fat. Eyes are open. Fetus is now viable. Mother feels stronger movement (quickening). Fetus has schedule of sleeping and moving. Vernix caseosa is present on skin. Lanugo covers body. Brown fat is formed. Lungs begin to secrete surfactant. Fingernails are present. Respiratory Movements Begin.

(Continued)

TABLE 6-1 Embryonic and Fetal Development—cont'd

Age	Length and Weight	Development
Week 29 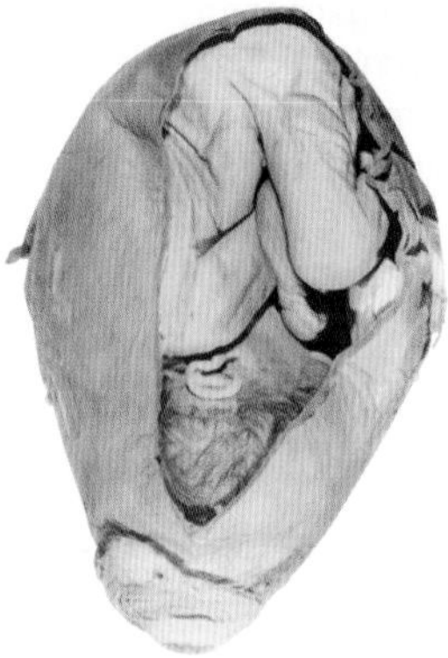	38 cm (15 inches) crown-heel 1260 g (2 lb, 10 oz)	Fetus assumes stable (cephalic) position in utero. Central nervous system is functioning. Skin is less wrinkled because of the presence of subcutaneous fat. Spleen stops forming blood cells, and bone marrow starts to form blood cells. Increased surfactant is present in lungs.
Week 36 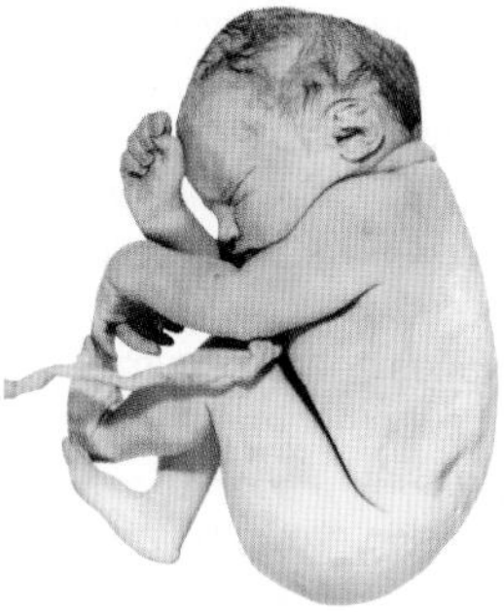	48 cm (19 inches) crown-heel 2500 g (5 lb, 12 oz)	Subcutaneous fat is present. Skin is smooth. Grasp reflex is present. Circumferences of head and abdomen are equal. Surge of lung surfactant is produced.

NOTE: Full-term is considered 38-40 weeks. The crown-heel length is 48–52 cm (18–21 inches), and the weight is 3000–3600 g (6 lb, 10 oz, to 7 lb, 15 oz).
Unnumbered figures 6-1, 6-2, 6-3, 6-4 from Moore KL, Persaud TVN: *The developing human: clinically oriented embryology*, ed 8, Philadelphia, 2008, Saunders.
Unnumbered figures 6-5, 6-6, 6-7, 6-8 from Moore KL, Persaud TVN, Shiota K: *Color atlas of clinical embryology*, ed 2, Philadelphia, 2000, Saunders.

During the third week after fertilization, the heart begins to beat, and the neural tube (the beginning portion of the central nervous system) forms. For this reason, the mother should take prenatal vitamins to ensure adequate intake of folic acid, which is essential for normal neural-tube development. Conditions such as spina bifida can occur if there is a deficiency of folic acid when the neural tube is forming. The placenta takes control of fetal circulation at the end of the third month of pregnancy. The umbilical cord attaches the fetus to the placenta, and a thin membrane separates the maternal and fetal blood, because the two blood supplies do not normally mix.

By 20 weeks of gestation (fetal life), the fetus is considered viable (able to survive outside the uterus). However, the lack of a substance called surfactant in the lungs at this stage of fetal development would require that special neonatal intensive care be provided. Some surfactant is produced by 28 weeks' gestation, and another spurt of surfactant is deposited into the fetal lungs at 32 weeks' gestation. After 38 weeks of gestation, the fetus is considered to be full term and is ready to be born.

A woman should start prenatal care as early as possible. Adequate nutrition and exercise during pregnancy are beneficial, and monthly visits to the health-care provider enable monitoring of the pregnancy to ensure a healthy outcome for both mother and baby.

Twins

Twins or other multifetal births (e.g., triplets, quadruplets, and so on) can occur. Dizygotic twins, also called fraternal twins, occur when two ova are released at ovulation, and each ovum is fertilized by a separate sperm. The twins may or may not be of the same sex, and they are as alike as any siblings. Monozygotic twins, also called identical twins, occur when one single fertilized ovum separates into two separate embryos. These twins will be of the same sex and will be genetically identical (i.e., they will look alike). Many twins are born prematurely because the uterus becomes overdistended or the placenta is unable to supply the nourishment required to carry the pregnancy to term.

THE PRENATAL PHASE

Critical Periods

Many of the critical periods during fetal growth occur during the first trimester of pregnancy (first 3 months) when basic structures are developing. Many of these factors can affect growth and development throughout fetal life, such as undernutrition, which can cause a reduction in the number of cells produced, resulting in health problems after birth.

Inadequate nutrition during fetal development can change the structure, physiology, and metabolism in the body and can predispose the fetus to the development of coronary artery disease or stroke in adult life (Rines, 2009). There are strong indications that coronary disease in adulthood originates in utero. A newborn who has low birth weight with a small head circumference may be at risk for coronary disease. Low placental weight may be associated with predisposition for stroke in later life (Burton, 2011). Every system in the body has a critical period in which nutrition, drugs, and other environmental factors influence its development and function. Illness, lack of nutrition, or exposure to toxins during this critical period can cause a maldevelopment or malfunction of a specific organ or system that may not manifest until adult life.

Lower respiratory tract infections in infancy may be an indicator of impaired lung growth that can increase the risk for chronic bronchitis in adulthood. Exposure to environmental factors such as smoking can increase vulnerability to serious bronchitis and respiratory problems in adulthood. The balance of maternal protein and cholesterol levels in late pregnancy and the amount of fat in the mother's diet can influence the development of diseases in the child later in life even though the infant may appear normal at birth.

Exercise During Pregnancy

It is important to maintain levels of health and fitness during pregnancy, benefits of which include improved energy level, mood, sleep, and muscle tone, as well as decreased

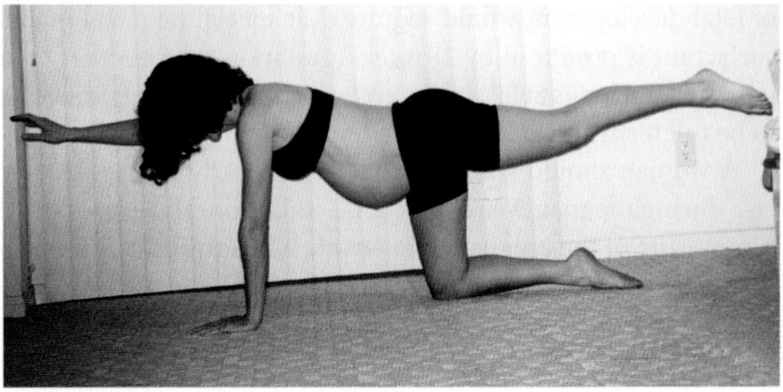

Figure 6-3 Stretch exercises at home are appropriate and healthy for the pregnant woman. Other appropriate activities are step aerobics, swimming, and prenatal yoga, among others.

risk of gestational diabetes. Diabetes that occurs during pregnancy can negatively affect pregnancy outcome but often disappears after pregnancy. Exercise programs also play a significant role in managing glucose levels in women who have type 2 diabetes mellitus when becoming pregnant. A fitness program can also improve the mother's ability to cope with labor as well as enhance recovery and decrease the risk of postpartum depression. At least 30 minutes per day of regular exercise also helps prevent excessive weight gain during pregnancy (Figure 6-3).

A pregnant woman who was previously sedentary can slowly begin a light exercise program that includes walking or swimming. A previously active woman can, in most cases, safely continue her exercise program with a few simple modifications, such as avoiding becoming overheated (since heat is transmitted to the fetus, causing an increase in oxygen needs). There are several safety issues to consider while exercising during pregnancy. Hormones released during pregnancy cause increased joint laxity, which could lead to injury if range of motion is exaggerated. Also, a shift in center of gravity can create balance challenges, thus increasing the risk of falls. The pregnant woman should avoid the supine position during exercises after the first trimester to ensure uninterrupted blood flow to the fetus. Pregnant women should also stay well hydrated.

A pregnant woman should stop exercising if she experiences vaginal bleeding or other discharge, uterine contractions, or decreased fetal movement. Food intake must be adequate for appropriate weight gain during pregnancy.

Health Promotion

The well-being of the mother and fetus can influence the life expectancy of the newborn. In accordance with the goals of *Healthy People 2020,* to prevent disease in the next generation we need to improve the nutrition of mothers and babies and reduce exposure to infection in early childhood.

Toxins

Teratogens (toxins) are harmful influences on fetal growth. Exposure to toxins during fetal development can cause abnormalities, illness, or miscarriage. Maternal ingestion of substances such as alcohol can interfere with cell growth in the developing fetus. For example, fetal alcohol syndrome is characterized by mental retardation and abnormal facial features. Recreational drug exposure during pregnancy can cause prematurity, seizure disorders, and learning disabilities in the newborn infant. Maternal cigarette smoking can cause decreased birth weight in the newborn. Mothers are cautioned to avoid contact with cat-litter boxes during pregnancy because of the risk of developing a condition called toxoplasmosis, which can be devastating to the newborn. Radiation exposure during X-rays and lead contamination in the environment are examples of other environmental toxins that are harmful to growing fetuses.

Health Promotion

Maternal illness must be prevented and certain teratogens should be avoided during pregnancy to prevent untoward effects in the fetus.

Maternal Adaptations During the Prenatal Phase

The changing patterns of childrearing, the increasing number of dual-career households, and the increasing distances among extended family members, influence the social support systems available for parents-to-be. Dependency on physicians is decreased, because the large health maintenance organizations (HMOs) or health-care facilities may not guarantee a regular personal physician to follow each pregnant woman throughout her pregnancy.

Health Promotion

Parents need to be well informed to make healthy decisions about pregnancy, delivery, and child care. Parents need to be involved in developmental issues concerning their parental roles and impending changes in their lifestyles.

If the pregnancy is planned and wanted, attitudes will most likely be positive. If the pregnancy is unplanned or unwanted, interventions and referrals may be necessary to help the parents develop a positive attitude or to help parents select alternatives such as adoption or abortion. The timing of the pregnancy in the life of the parents is also an important consideration. Adolescent parents may not have completed the transition to adulthood, may still be in the protective environment of their parents' homes, and so may need a more intensive adjustment period to establish their independence.

The initial phase of establishing a family after marriage (see Chapters 4 and 11) involves adjusting to a marital adult affiliation with the establishment of mutual goals, housing, financial responsibilities, educational pursuits, and lifestyle choices. Entering into the role of a parent who is responsible for a dependent child is, according to Erikson, the beginning of the stage of generativity. The mother is motivated to prepare psychologically for the arrival of the infant as she feels the fetus move in her womb (uterus). A state of attachment occurs, and rapport with the fetus develops. The partner may attend parenting classes with the pregnant woman and may be included in the attachment process as the fetus grows and develops (Figure 6-4).

The first period of parental development includes three distinct phases, each with specific tasks (see Table 6-2 on p. 85). The first phase is the response to discovering that conception has occurred. The parents may be elated or disappointed. Lifestyle changes will be discussed. The second phase occurs in the second trimester (months 4 to 6 of the

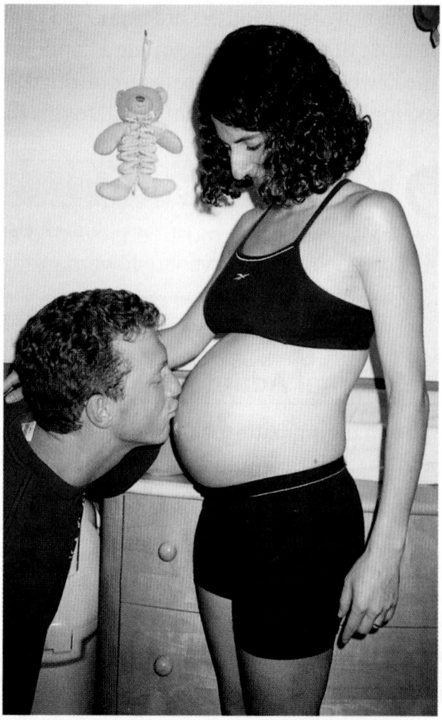

Figure 6-4 The father begins to bond with the fetus as the fetal heart and fetal movement can be felt.

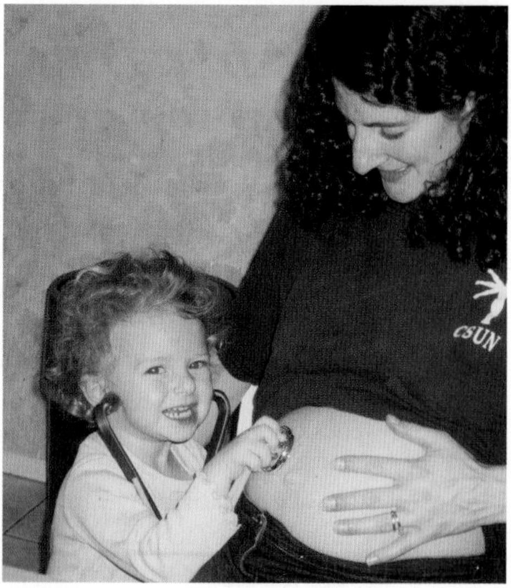

Figure 6-5 A sibling begins to anticipte the birth of her brother.

pregnancy), during which time fetal movement is felt, an ultrasound picture of the fetus is often seen, and the reality of the pregnancy becomes evident. Parents may worry about the health of the infant and plan for its place in the home and family (Figure 6-5). The third phase occurs in the third trimester (months 7 to 9), when plans for the actual birth of the baby become the focus. The father may worry about competing for attention and may feel left out. Old conflicts may resurface. Parents may feel inadequately prepared for the responsibility of caring for the newborn. Parents can be referred to parenting classes that are available in most communities.

THE BIRTH PROCESS

Childbirth is a normal physiological process that affects the health of the mother and fetus. Labor and delivery are often a family affair with fathers or significant others participating and grandmothers closely involved. Attendance at preparation classes during pregnancy and the cultural background of the parents usually dictate the extent to which the partner or grandmother play supportive roles in the labor and delivery unit. A woman can choose to deliver the baby in a traditional hospital setting, in a freestanding private birthing center, or at home. *Obstetricians* (doctors with special education in women's health), *nurse practitioners* (registered nurses with advanced practice education), or *nurse midwives* (registered nurses with advanced labor and delivery education) may be in attendance to monitor the process. A *doula* is a specially trained labor and delivery coach who may stay with the mother during labor and birth. The birth process occurs in four stages. The first stage is the dilation (opening) and effacement (shortening) of the uterine cervix. The second stage is the descent and birth of the baby, and the third stage is the birth of the placenta (afterbirth). The fetal heart rate and the contractions of the uterus are monitored closely during the birth process. The fourth stage is the recovery stage, when bonding takes place and the family is united and monitored.

THE NEWBORN INFANT

After the infant is born and the umbilical cord is cut, many physiological changes occur in the infant's body to enable it to adjust to life outside of the uterus. The lungs expand and the circulation pattern that allowed bypass of the lungs during fetal life changes so that all blood circulates to the infant's lungs to receive oxygen. The cyanotic (blue) color of the skin quickly changes to its natural color as the infant cries and oxygenation is established. The infant is dried and placed in a prewarmed bed, and the head is covered to minimize heat loss until the infant can stabilize its own body temperature.

The newborn's vital signs are monitored, and an Apgar score is assessed at 1 minute and 5 minutes after birth. The Apgar score is a rating of heart, respiration, muscle tone, color, and reflex irritability (not to be confused with the *family* Apgar described in Chapter 4). A score from 1 to 10 provides an estimate of the condition of the infant and determines the need for further resuscitation efforts. The infant receives vitamin K to aid in blood clotting in the umbilical cord, and an antibiotic ointment is placed in the infant's eyes to prevent ophthalmia neonatorum and chlamydia infection, which if left untreated could lead to blindness in the neonate. An identification band with a special number is placed on the wrist of the infant, mother, and significant other, and the newborn's footprints may be taken.

It is important for the nurse to promote bonding and attachment between parents and newborns as soon as possible after birth (Figure 6-6). Bonding refers to a strong emotional tie between parents and the newborn. Attachment refers to an affectionate tie that occurs over time as a result of parent–infant interaction. Bonding begins during pregnancy, but it is most important that touch and visual interaction occur as soon as possible after birth. The newborn should be placed in the mother's arms, and put to breast for breastfeeding. The *en face* (face-to-face) position facilitates eye contact between infant and parent (Figure 6-7).

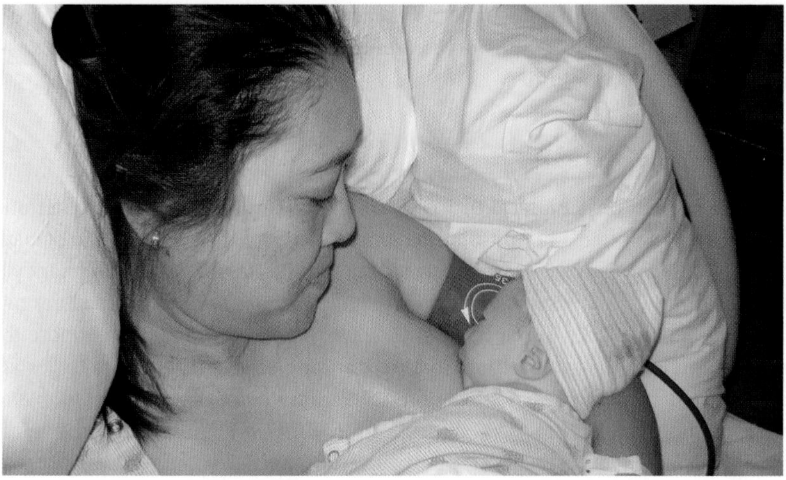

Figure 6-6 A new mother bonds with her newborn infant using skin-to-skin contact during breastfeeding.

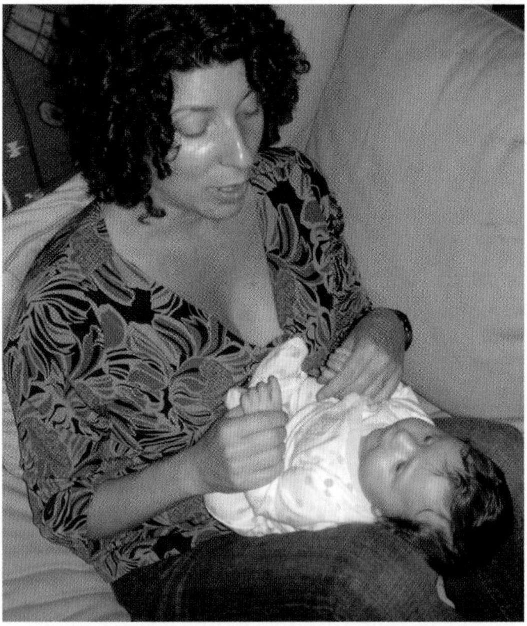

Figure 6-7 The en face position between mother and infant. The mother positions her baby to provide close face-to-face interaction to promote bonding. The newborn gazes at the mother and responds to her voice and touch.

The infant can see a short distance at birth and responds to close face-to-face encounters. The infant is most alert in the first hour after birth, and then several hours of sleep and decreased motor activity will follow. Parent–infant bonding should be the focus of care during this first hour of life outside the womb.

TABLE 6-2 Rubin's Psychological Changes After Birth

Phase 1	"*Taking in.*" The woman is passive, lets others care for her and her infant, and talks about the delivery experience. The mother usually requests food and opportunity to sleep.
Phase 2	"*Taking hold.*" The woman begins to initiate care of the infant and assumes responsibility for self care. The woman is most receptive to teaching at this stage.
Phase 3	"*Letting go.*" The parents recognize the reality of the new lifestyle and responsibilities they face and accept the gender and unique appearance of the new child.

Data from Rubin R: Attainment of the maternal role: part 1 processes. *Nursing Research* 16, 237-245, 1967; Rubin R. Maternal tasks in pregnancy, *J Maternal-Child Nursing* 4(3):143, 1975; Rubin, R. Maternal behavior, *Nursing Outlook* 9:692, 1961; Rubin, R. Maternal identity and the maternal experience, Springer, New York, 1984; Rubin, R. Puerperal Change, *Nursing Outlook* 9(12);743-755, 1961; Rubin, R. Binding-in in the postpartum period. *American Journal of Maternal Child Nursing* 6(1);65-75, 1977.

THE TRANSITION TO MOTHERHOOD

The transition to motherhood involves hormonal changes, changes in self-image, and reorganization of tasks. Mood swings are common. Irritability and fatigue may peak by the fifth day after delivery. Conflicting feelings of joy and depression are called the *postpartum blues,* and the symptoms are typically self-limiting. Discharge teaching concerning self care and infant care, support, and reassurance should be offered. Rubin's descriptions of the psychological changes that occur after birth have been a framework for the care of new mothers for more than 45 years. The described behavioral changes help health-care workers understand the new mother as she progresses through these stages (Table 6-2).

Postnatal Exercise

Exercise can also be an important part of postpartum recovery. In addition to assisting with weight loss, exercise can increase energy levels, restore muscle strength, and decrease the risk of postpartum depression. Exercise in the early postpartum period can include modified sit-ups and kegel exercise to strengthen abdominal muscles and perineum. Abdominal breathing, head lifts, and modified sit-ups are good beginning exercises.

If there were no complications during labor and delivery, gentle exercises such as walking can begin when the woman feels ready. More vigorous exercises can begin following doctor's approval, usually after about 6 weeks of recovery. Caesarean sections and other complicated births may require a longer recovery period before exercise.

FATHERS OR SIGNIFICANT OTHERS

Fathers or significant others often develop an intense focus on the newborn, which is called engrossment (Figure 6-8). A realignment of relationships with his own parents, past experience with children, and relationship to his wife or partner are factors that will affect his bonding experience. When a new infant is added to the family, some of the father's or partner's roles and responsibilities may also change. The partner may be expected to take

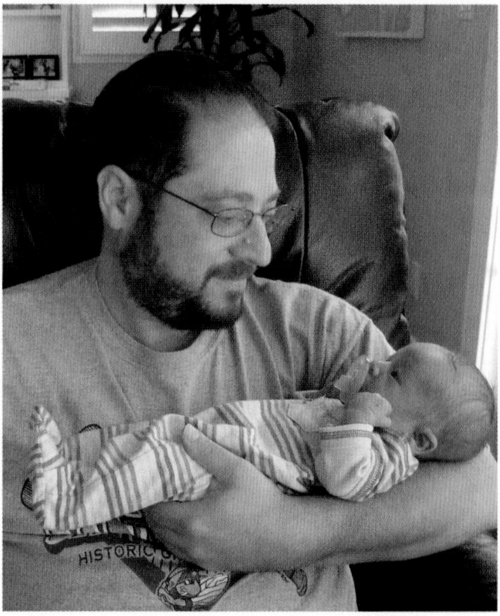

Figure 6-8 The en face position between father and infant. The intense fascination that fathers exhibit is called *engrossment*.

more time and responsibility for the older sibling or siblings, who will need repeated reassurances and validation of continued love. A change in sleep patterns, new financial stresses, and changes in routines can be stressful for some fathers or partners. Plans for child care for other children, while both parents are focused on the birth of the newborn, need to be in place well before the occasion arises.

SIBLINGS

The influence of the new child's birth on siblings depends on their age and developmental level. Toddlers may regress and be angry. Older children may enjoy helping with the newborn, and adolescents may feel embarrassed about their mother giving birth. A sibling relationship is lifelong and can be characterized by both close friendship and intense rivalry. Sibling rivalry is the competition between siblings, usually for parental attention and love.

The initial relationship between a newborn and a sibling is established by the parent's interaction with each child (Figure 6-9). When the newborn is presented to the sibling as being a person with feelings, the sibling is likely to develop positive attitudes and experience good interactions. The birth of a baby is a positive and exciting event for the family, but often a sibling views the event as a loss of the sibling's place in the family. Relationships in the family change, expectations are different, and the parents may become somewhat less accessible, because the parent must focus on the feeding and physical care of the new infant. A 2-year-old may have a low tolerance to change in the relationship with parents, and a 4-year-old may be still struggling to maintain impulse control.

A sibling in the egocentric stage of development cannot be expected to understand clearly the needs of the new baby. Allowing the sibling to participate in the anticipation of the birth may help in the adjustment and transition tasks. Providing an opportunity for the sibling to

Figure 6-9 Remaining nearby her older children, a mother makes the initial introduction between a newborn and its siblings.

help with the care of the baby, under the supervision of the parents, can help the sibling feel involved rather than displaced. Major changes in child-care arrangements, routines, or location of residence should be avoided during the first 6 months after a baby arrives.

Twins often have the opportunity to share experiences early, which can be positive, but when adults compare their achievements with one another, sibling rivalry can intensify. Sibling rivalry may also intensify when a baby is born into a blended family, where a stepchild may foster resentment toward the new arrival.

Siblings are reliable and available playmates in the home and later may become role models and confidants for one another; therefore sibling relationships generally include long-term benefits.

GRANDPARENTS

Culture and physical distance in living arrangements influence the role of grandparents in the lives of this new family. Some grandparents seek an interactive role, and some grandparents prefer minimal involvement. When parents and grandparents agree on their roles, they can avoid conflict. Because the process of bonding and attachment between parents and the newborn involves learning the cues of newborn behavior, it is essential that parents have the opportunity to spend time with the newborn in the first few weeks or months of life. Grandparents therefore can be most helpful if they assume the role of home manager by preparing meals, shopping, and helping with household tasks. When grandparents take on the care of the newborn, or when a nanny is employed to care for the newborn, the critical time for bonding between parents and the newborn is interrupted and may never be recaptured. This may affect the lifelong relationship between parent and child.

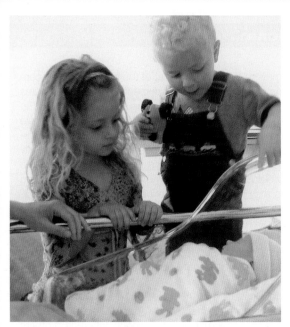

Cultural Considerations

The Influence of Culture

The family's cultural background may be different from that of the nurse or health-care worker, but different practices must be understood and respected. In some cultures the husband or partner is expected to be present during the birth process, and in others the presence of the husband or partner is discouraged. In some cases a male practitioner in attendance at birth may be forbidden. Some parents practice the hot-and-cold theory related to diet, and any diet prescription needs to be carefully designed to ensure compliance. The postpartum phase may last 30 days or longer in some cultures, with the woman forbidden to leave the home. Bathing may be delayed by cultural regulations; cold packs may be refused for perineal comfort. In some cultures women believe that the colostrum portion of breast milk is unhealthy and therefore do not breastfeed immediately after delivery. Ritual circumcision of the newborn is practiced in the Jewish religion and is avoided in some other religions. Some Asian women do not praise the newborn to protect the infant from evil influences. This behavior may be misinterpreted as a noncaring attitude or a failure to bond.

Culture may also influence the accuracy of pain assessment. Nurses and health-care workers often use a horizontal illustration of the score of 1 to 10 to assess the level of pain. Certain cultures read downward rather than left to right and may need a vertical chart for accuracy. In some cultures women suffer in silence, whereas in others women chant or moan loudly. Understanding pain and the influence of culture on the expression of pain is essential to providing comprehensive care. Interpreters should be used whenever possible for patients who speak little English. Family members should not serve as the interpreters when sensitive information is discussed, because a family member may interpret selectively (see Chapter 3).

DEVELOPMENTAL TASKS AND RESPONSES OF THE NEONATE

The main task after birth is the establishment of feeding patterns and habits. The infant learns how to latch on to the breast and suck to obtain nourishment, which will last for 2 to 3 hours. Parents who plan to bottle feed their infants are taught about techniques and the types of formulas available. The mother must learn to recognize cues that indicate the infant is hungry even before crying occurs. This is the first *trust* experience. The mother learns to recognize the different cries of the infant and knows whether they mean that feeding, cuddling, or diaper changing is necessary. Various organized behavioral states of the newborn can be observed. They include (1) quiet sleep, (2) active sleep, (3) quiet alert, (4) active alert, and (5) cry.

The neonate sleeps 15 to 20 hours daily and is most responsive to interaction during the quiet-alert stage of responsiveness. Rocking an infant in a vertical fashion (upright) is likely to maintain alertness, whereas gentle rocking in a horizontal position (lying flat) while wrapped snugly will promote sleep. Each newborn infant has a unique temperament that will influence the intensity of responses to environmental stimuli. The neonatal period (first 30 days of life) serves to solidify parent–infant expectations and relationships. The newborn initiates environmental support by crying or turning away from excess stimulation and learns to self-console and eventually to interact socially by smiling. Nurses and health-care workers can help cement a positive parent–infant relationship by observing parent–infant responses, educating parents concerning the abilities and behaviors of the newborn, and using opportunities to promote bonding and attachment. Newborns who exhibit frequent startles or tremors, gaze away from the face of the caregiver, and appear irritable when stimulated require further professional assessment. Distressed parents who feel inadequate and who believe their infant to be highly vulnerable need special guidance and support to assist the infant to achieve trust and to grow toward autonomy.

Parent Teaching

The alert neonate has predictable responses to environmental stimuli that parents learn to understand and anticipate. This interaction fosters effective parenting and infant growth and development.

During the neonatal period, the infant develops *conditioned responses,* or unconscious responses to external stimuli. For example, the hungry infant who stops crying at the sound of a caregiver's presence, even though food is not yet offered, is exhibiting a conditioned response.

The neonate can hear clearly after the first sneeze clears the eustachian tubes. The newborn's sucking response is increased when stimuli are introduced, and sucking stops when attention is focused elsewhere. The newborn is capable of feeling pain, and pain relief should be offered before any painful procedures are undertaken. Swaddling, cuddling, wrapping, rocking, *nonnutritive sucking* (use of a pacifier), and a quiet environment provide comfort for the neonate. Oral sucrose (sugar) placed on a pacifier often serves as a mild pain reliever. The behavior and appearance of the newborn are influenced by reflexes that are present at birth and gradually disappear (Table 6-3). These reflexes help the neonate adapt to the environment and gradually disappear as voluntary motor ability develops. Assessment of the neurological system is achieved by testing for the presence of these reflexes.

Development of Intelligence

Intelligence is difficult to define because it includes so many aspects and different types of abilities. Intelligence involves the ability to learn from experience and to adapt to the environment and its challenges. It includes the ability to reason, solve problems, and learn. Researchers have classified the study of intelligence to include *psychometric* variables such as reasoning, memory, perception, and abstract thinking; *computational* variables such as the ability to process information; *biological* variables such as neural (brain) functioning; and *complex system* variables that involve language intelligence, spatial intelligence, musical intelligence, interpersonal intelligence, and so on. Each of these areas of intelligence may be studied separately, but they interact to form an individual's intelligence potential.

Molecular technology has enabled research into genetic influences on intelligence (Gale, 2006). Both genetics and environment influence the intelligence potential of a newborn infant. Poor nutrition, environmental toxins, or oxygen deprivation can inhibit optimal brain development. Family, schooling, and availability of preschool programs also will influence

TABLE 6-3 Ages of Appearance and Disappearance of Neurological Reflexes of Infancy

Response	Age at Time of Appearance	Age at Time of Disappearance
REFLEXES OF POSITION AND MOVEMENT		
Moro Reflex 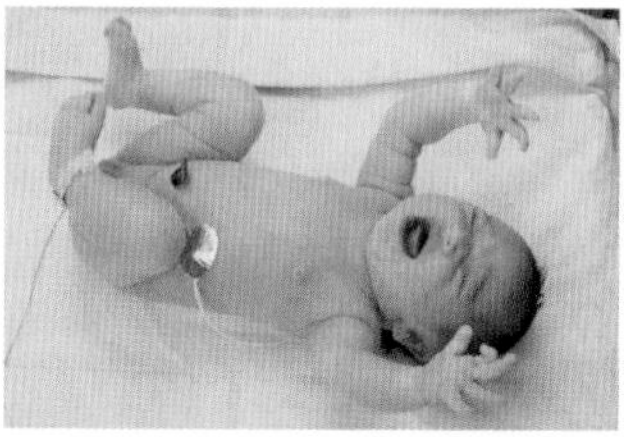	Birth	1-3 months
Tonic neck reflex 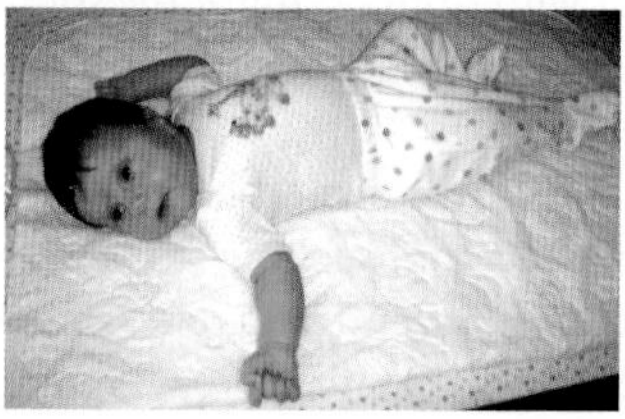	Birth	5-7 months
Palmar grasp reflex 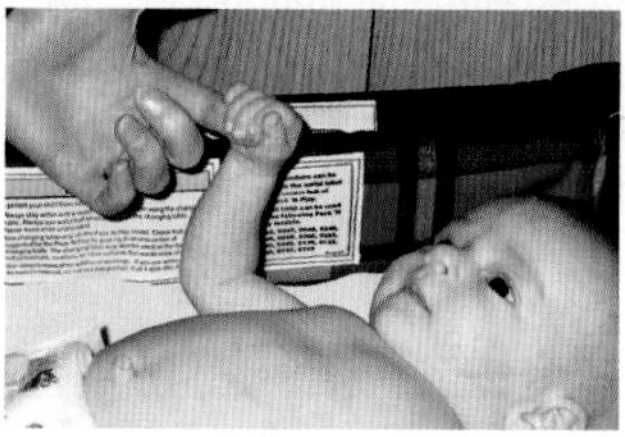	Birth	4 months
Babinski reflex	Birth	Variable*
RESPONSES TO SOUND		
Blinking response	Birth	NA
Turning response	Birth	NA
REFLEXES OF VISION†		
Blinking to threat	6-7 months	NA
Horizontal following	4-6 weeks	NA
Vertical following	2-3 months	NA
Postrotational nystagmus	Birth	NA

*Usually of no diagnostic significance until after age 2 years.

†Holding the newborn infant upright under the arms will induce eye opening.

TABLE 6-3 Ages of Appearance and Disappearance of Neurological Reflexes of Infancy—cont'd

Response	Age at Time of Appearance	Age at Time of Disappearance
FOOD REFLEXES		
Rooting response (awake)	Birth	3-4 months
Rooting response (asleep)	Birth	7-8 months
Sucking response	Birth	12 months
OTHER SIGNS		
Handedness	2-3 years	NA
Spontaneous stepping	Birth	4-5 months
Straight-line walking	5-6 years	NA

NA, Not applicable.
Unnumbered Figure 6-9 from Leifer G: *Maternity nursing*, ed 11, Philadelphia, 2012, Saunders.
Unnumbered Figures 6-10, 6-11 from Leifer G: *Introduction to maternity & pediatric nursing*, ed 6, Philadelphia, 2011, Saunders.

the infant's ability to reach the full potential of his or her intelligence. Environmental influences affect the potential and rate of development (see Chapter 7). The environment can influence temperament and motivation that then influence the development of intelligence. Intelligence quotient (IQ) scores remain the valid measure of intelligence in research settings. Intelligence testing began with Binet intelligence tests in 1905 and is used for routinely identifying mental retardation, gifted children, school placement, vocational assessment, learning disabilities, neuropsychological exams, and military placement. Several IQ exams are validated as reliable by the American Psychological Association, but commercially marketed, web-based tests have questionable validity (Boake, 2002). Intelligence tests can measure potential, but they may not be a measure of future capabilities (Nio Leon, 2005).

Play Activities and Neonatal Development

Because hearing and vision are present in the newborn, an appropriate toy would include a musical mobile that is placed above the crib within the infant's sight. Music can capture the attention of the newborn. A developmental task of the neonate is to learn how to focus on and follow objects as they move across the field of vision. An overhanging mobile with sharply contrasting colors will foster this development.

The neonate can detect the smell of mother's milk by 6 days of age and prefers sweet tastes. The sense of touch is well developed, and stroking the cheek will cause the infant to turn toward the person stroking his or her face. An infant can be quieted and bonding promoted by placing the infant in skin-to-skin contact with the parent. A nude infant placed on the nude chest of the parent will quiet and snuggle.

The neonate is in Piaget's sensorimotor stage of cognitive growth (see Chapter 5). Infants can learn and repeat behavioral responses. Looking, listening, and touching the environment help the infant master the tasks of this stage. Close contact with the infant will help parents recognize cues to specific needs so that cry time is minimized. The best time to interact with the neonate is during the quiet-alert state of responsiveness. The infant will quickly halt physical activity and become very still when approached and talked to, eyes will focus on the parent's face, and beginning communication will be evident.

KEY POINTS

- A genome is a complete set of DNA contained in all human cells.
- The goal of the Genome Project was to identify the 30,000 or more genes in the DNA; develop tools for analysis; and address the ethical, legal, and social implications of this knowledge and ability.
- The Genome Project may enable gene therapy to correct or replace abnormal genes.
- One of the critical periods during fetal growth occurs during the first 3 months of pregnancy, when basic structures are developing.
- The well-being of the mother and fetus can influence life expectancy of the newborn.
- Exercise during pregnancy contributes to a healthy outcome.
- Improvement in the nutrition and health of mothers and babies may prevent disease in the next generation.
- Exposure to toxins such as drugs and alcohol during fetal development can cause abnormalities in the newborn.
- According to Erikson, parenting a dependent child is the beginning of the stage of generativity.
- A combination of an XX chromosome from the mother and father will produce a girl, and an XY combination will produce a boy fetus.
- Only the sperm carries the Y chromosome, so the male partner determines the sex of the infant. However, the female has some influence on which sperm may survive to fertilize the ovum.
- An adequate intake of folic acid early in the maternal diet is essential to prevent neural-tube defects in the newborn infant.
- Fraternal twins are the result of two ova released at ovulation, each fertilized by a separate sperm. Identical twins are the result of one fertilized ovum separating into two embryos.
- Bonding refers to a strong emotional tie between the parents and the newborn.
- Attachment refers to the affectionate tie that occurs over time because of parent–infant interaction.
- The influence of the new child's birth on siblings depends on their ages and developmental levels.
- Breastfeeding, bonding, and attachment are developmental tasks of parents and the newborn.
- The neonatal period encompasses the first 30 days of life.
- Swaddling, cuddling, rocking, and use of a pacifier calm the newborn infant.
- Newborn reflexes help the neonate adjust to the environment, and reflexes disappear as voluntary motor abilities develop.
- An overhanging mobile with sharply contrasting colors will foster the growth and development of the neonate.

Critical Thinking

A woman has just confirmed that she is pregnant. List at least five ways she can reduce the risk of exposing her developing fetus to dangerous teratogens that may produce negative effects on fetal growth and development.

REVIEW QUESTIONS

1. **Neural tube defects such as spina bifida can be prevented by:**
   a. eating a well-balanced diet during pregnancy.
   b. taking folic acid supplements early in pregnancy.
   c. avoiding alcohol and smoking during pregnancy.
   d. engaging in early antibiotic therapy for infections during pregnancy.

2. **The neonatal period refers to the:**
   a. first 30 days after birth.
   b. period between birth and 1 year of age.
   c. period immediately before birth.
   d. moment of birth.

3. **To promote growth and development in an infant, an overhead mobile should have *(select all that apply)*:**
   a. contrasting colors.
   b. bright colors.
   c. animated characters.
   d. sound integrated with movement.

4. **Fraternal twins are the result of:**
   a. two ova fertilized by two separate sperm.
   b. one ovum fertilized by one sperm.
   c. two ova fertilized by one sperm.
   d. one ovum fertilized by two sperm.

5. **A complete set of DNA that is contained in all human cells is known as a(n):**
   a. chromosome.
   b. nucleus.
   c. genome.
   d. allele.

CHAPTER

7 The Infant

http://evolve.elsevier.com/Leifer/growth

OBJECTIVES

1. Define the term *infant*.
2. State the developmental tasks of infancy.
3. Describe the physical development of infants from 1 month to 1 year of age.
4. Discuss milestones of motor development.
5. Understand five basic guidelines for physical activity for infants.
6. Discuss the development of language.
7. Describe the theories of Piaget, Freud, and Erikson concerning infant development.
8. Define separation anxiety.
9. Discuss the development of attachment.
10. Describe the basic nutritional needs of infants from 1 month to 1 year of age.
11. List the immunization schedule for infants under 1 year of age.
12. State four safety precautions essential in infant care.

KEY TERMS

autonomy
cephalocaudal
coping skill
defense mechanism
development
expressive
growth
infant
length
nonverbal language
norms
nursing caries
object permanence
ordinal position
personality
pincer action
preverbal
receptive
separation anxiety
sudden infant death syndrome (SIDS)

DEFINITION

The infant stage of development is the period between ages 4 weeks and 1 year. Growth indicates an increase in size, measured by inches (centimeters) and pounds (kilograms). Development indicates an increase in function and mastery of tasks for the specific phase in the lifespan.

The process of growth and development is orderly and proceeds from simple to complex in an expected pattern but at a variable pace. Growth spurts are common. Norms (averages) are only guidelines concerning the ages at which specific abilities or skills are achieved. Cephalocaudal growth refers to the progression of the growth pattern that proceeds from head to toe. For example, infants are able to lift their heads before they can sit, and they are able to sit before they can stand. Proximodistal growth refers to growth from the center of the body to the periphery. Height refers to a standing measurement, whereas length is measured while the infant is lying down. The average height of a person is generally a result of family traits, although nutrition and other factors may alter the attainment of the specific individual's adult height. A general estimation for infants of potential adult height can be determined by the following formulas:

$$\text{Boys} = \frac{\text{Father's height} + \text{mother's height in inches} + 2.5\,\text{inches}}{2}$$

$$\text{Girls} = \frac{\text{Father's height} + \text{mother's height in inches} - 2.5\,\text{inches}}{2}$$

The length of the newborn is normally about 20 inches (50 cm), and by 1 year of age, the birth length increases by almost 50%. A normal newborn weighs approximately 7.5 pounds (3.4 kg). The infant's birth weight doubles by 6 months of age and can be expected to triple within 1 year.

Many factors influence the growth and development of the infant. Development is a process that continues throughout the life cycle, with mastery of specific tasks occurring in each phase. Successful mastery of the tasks in one phase of the life cycle enables the person to proceed more easily to the next phase. Development is an interaction among the child, the parent, and the environment. If there is a problem with the parents or environment, the child responds by developing *defense mechanisms* or *coping skills.* A defense mechanism is a reaction that is protective to the individual or helps conceal conflicts or anxieties. Denial and projection of blame are examples of defense mechanisms. For example, if an infant is hurt, he or she may blame the caregiver for causing the pain and may react by hitting or thrashing (an infant cannot yet understand the concept of an accident).

A coping skill is a behavior that helps an individual adapt to or manage a stressful situation. If a goal is obstructed, the infant may find a way around the obstacle to reach the unachievable goal; modify the goal to an achievable level; or perhaps develop an alternative goal. For example, an infant may learn how to climb over a crib rail to reach a toy.

Infants thrive with parental support and praise. This interaction fosters an attachment between child and parent that provides a sense of security, enabling the infant to try to master developmental tasks. Mutual attachment involves not only a close feeling between the infant and parent but also a responsiveness to needs presented. If the needs of the infant are not met, the development of attachment may not be achieved as easily if at all.

Cultural Considerations

Ethnic and cultural practices influence nutrition and behavior development.

The ordinal position in the family—that is, whether the infant is an only child, an oldest child, a youngest child, or a middle child—may influence the age and rapidity of mastering developmental tasks.

Both the prenatal environment and the home environment influence the growth and development of the infant. The development of personality is an interaction between biological and environmental factors. Personality is most often defined as a unique combination of characteristics that result in the individual's recurrent pattern of behavior. The influences of the family and family interactions on growth and development are discussed in Chapter 4. Theories of behavioral development abound, and a summary of popular theories is presented in Chapter 5. The roles of heredity and prenatal influences are discussed in Chapter 6.

DEVELOPMENTAL TASKS

Trust Versus Mistrust

The functioning of all humans is goal directed and involves the tasks of developing social competence and the mastery of skills necessary for functioning in their environments. Some tasks of infancy include weaning, self feeding, walking, and acquiring language and communications skills.

Trust versus mistrust is the first psychosocial crisis in infancy that must be resolved (Erikson, 1994) (see Chapter 5). In the first year of life, trust develops when infants learn that their basic needs will be met. Crying infants who are left alone cry more at 1 year than infants who are picked up and comforted or who are fed promptly when they evidence hunger. Infants fed on a rigid schedule rather than as a response to hunger signs generally show more spitting up and gastrointestinal disturbances as well as later behavioral problems (Kleigman, 2011). By 2 months of age, parents react positively to the infant's responsive smile, and a mutual bond (attachment) is secured.

Intelligence

Understanding Cause and Effect

Infants discover at an early age that there is a relationship between cause and effect, and experiences at each stage of the life cycle build on this discovery. Newborns suck their thumbs to feel secure and will seek out the thumb or pacifier to achieve this feeling of comfort. A cry usually elicits a response from adults, and so the cry becomes a means of communication.

From 1 to 4 months of age, the infant is focused on the parent and, when held, prefers the ***en face*** (face-to-face) position. After 4 months of age, the infant begins to become more aware of the surroundings and may prefer to be held outwardly or away from the parent, facing the activity happening in the room. By 4 months, infants discover their hands and feet. If a mobile gym is placed above them, infants discover there are predictable sounds and tactile responses that occur when reaching out to touch the mobile. The infant strives to recognize behavior patterns that elicit special responses from the environment. When infants feel secure, they will explore the world around them. Infants who have not developed an attachment to the parental figure do not explore as readily.

At 4 months, the infant drops a spoon from the highchair and believes it is gone. By 7 months, the infant will continue to look for it. This is called object permanence, or knowing the object is there even though one cannot see it. Playing peek-a-boo with the infant at this age helps to develop the concept of object permanence.

Memory

Studies have shown that infants can retain memory of a traumatic experience (Paley, 2003). General comforting may not be enough to achieve full emotional recovery. Newborns demonstrate a physiological response to pain, and so a stress response can develop and influence later behavior. For example, a choking episode (anoxia) early in breastfeeding may cause an infant to reject further attempts at breastfeeding. One study showed that a 10-week-old infant, repeatedly abused by the father and placed in a foster home, showed an aversion to male caretakers for many months afterward (Gaensbauer, 2002). This evidence has led psychologists to advise parents to talk about stressful events that may have occurred early in the lives of their children, so that the child does not have to deal with those memories alone.

Emotional Development

When placed face-to-face *(en face)* with an adult, an infant will mimic the facial expression of the adult. For example, if the adult's tongue is thrust out, the infant will eventually thrust out his or her tongue also. Smiling, eye widening, and puckering of the lips occur when the infant focuses on the adult or activity that the infant can see. When stimulation reaches a high level, the infant will turn away to rest and then return to the view when ready for further stimulation. If the adult turns away before the infant is ready, the infant will lean forward and attempt to get the adult's attention with sound and movement and will eventually cry with frustration if unsuccessful. When adult stimulation is not available, the infant will eventually lose energy and stop efforts at communication. Interaction between parent and infant is necessary in the first months of life and is important for later social development.

Attachment

The process of attachment begins long before the infant is born, when the mother feels the fetus moving in the womb. The father or partner feels the fetal movement by touching the mother's abdomen and feeling the fetus kick. Both parents can hear the heartbeat with the aid of a stethoscope or a Doppler device. A relationship with an imagined child starts to develop. At birth, the real child emerges, and if he or she is not too different from the imagined child, attachment easily intensifies. However, the infant must respond positively in this mutual interaction. An infant who is sleepy, does not focus on the face of the parent, has difficulty latching on to the breast for breastfeeding, or spits up or vomits during feedings cannot contribute to the attachment process as readily, and the nurse or health-care worker may need to help the process along.

Parents slowly develop an instinctive response to infants' cues. The way infants cry, and the pitch or intensity of the cry, may indicate to the parent whether the infant is expressing a cry of pain, discomfort, hunger, or boredom. If the parent's response is prompt, attachment becomes secure. Providing time for *en face* interactions is important. The infant from birth to age 3 months can respond with varied facial expressions. After age 2 or 3 months, a responsive smile by the infant brings joy to the parent's efforts at interaction. By 5 or 6 months of age, the infant clearly recognizes and prefers the parent to other casual caregivers. The infant also looks to the facial expression and body language of the parent in new situations and responds accordingly. For example, if a relative from out of town visits, and the mother, while holding the infant, smiles and embraces the relative, the infant will likely smile and coo and respond calmly. However, if the person entering the room is a health-care provider for a well-child visit, and the mother is concerned about the pain of the immunizations to be administered, her facial expression and nonverbal behavior or body language (e.g., a stiffened posture) will be communicated to the child, who may then cry as the health-care provider approaches.

Separation anxiety begins at 6 months of age. The infant cries or protests when the parent leaves the room. Stranger anxiety peaks at 9 months of age when the infant is approached by a stranger, babysitter, or substitute caregiver in the absence of the parent. The mastery of object permanence will enable the infant to understand that the parent is still available even though he or she is not visible at the moment.

By 18 months, memory development helps the child remember the parent's image and to trust that the parent will return after an absence. Affectionate, responsive parents who respond to the child's needs help develop a secure attachment and bonding. The process of attachment is a gradual one, but attachment abilities stretch across the lifespan. Mastery of this task is essential for the child to be successful in later attachments to school friends or partners in the adult phase of the life cycle. The infant's temperament can influence the success of the attachment process, because parents usually have expectations concerning temperament of the child. Parents may say, "he is a difficult child," or "she is an easy child." This usually means that the parents' expectations do not exactly fit the infant's temperament, and the health-care worker may need to guide the parent's response (Table 7-1).

Parents who have psychiatric problems or marital stress or who both work long hours may not have the energy to respond to a demanding infant. Infants who receive inconsistent responses to their needs may withdraw from the risks of exploring the world around them, even when the parent is present. These infants or toddlers may become clingy, angry, and rebellious or become nonresponsive to the soothing and care they do receive. Child abuse becomes a risk at this time. The nurse should be alert to signs and symptoms of child abuse (Figure 7-1).

This understanding of attachment behavior is one of the reasons for providing one consistent core teacher in the elementary-school setting, whereas in high school the student usually interacts with multiple teachers in one day, because the typical adolescent has achieved independence, trust, and autonomy. It is also the basis of the rooming-in concept, where the parent is encouraged to stay in the room with the infant or child day and night when the child is hospitalized.

Observation of the parents' ability to comfort the infant, distract the infant, and respond to the emotional cues of the infant's behavior can be observed at each well-child visit, and appropriate guidance should be offered as needed. For example, following a clinic immunization, the mother can be encouraged to hold, rock, or breastfeed her infant to calm the infant before leaving the room.

Parents often need help with the separation experience. Sometimes it is not the child who cannot accept separation, but the parent who has the difficulty. Step 1 of separation starts with the placement of infants in their own beds, perhaps in their own rooms. Cosleeping can prolong this first step in separation. Step 2 involves leaving the infant with a relative or babysitter. Parents often do not realize that such short separations help infants develop independence and enable them to prepare for the next stage of autonomy. Coping skills are developed, and trust is strengthened when the infant learns from many small experiences with short separations. Protest at the initial separation is to be expected but will diminish as the child learns to trust the caregiver and to trust that the parents will return.

Hospitalization is a unique experience of separation that is filled with strangers, pain, and fear of the unknown. For this separation experience, it is strongly recommended that a parent room-in with the child, and most hospitals have facilities to accommodate parents.

Parents who perceive their child as especially vulnerable and who therefore avoid most separation experiences are exhibiting overprotective parenting, which can stifle the normal

TABLE 7-1 Temperament

Factors	Characteristics	Interventions
Activity level	Activity level of the infant can be high, medium, or low. It can be assessed by watching activity during feeding, bathing, or playing.	High activity: Provide opportunity for high activity. Low activity: Provide enough time for tasks.
Regularity	Regularity can be assessed by predictability of the infant's sleep–wake cycle, hunger, or elimination schedule.	Make provision for regularity by bringing food and diapers on trips.
Approach/withdrawal	The infant may respond to a stimulus with gusto and exploration or with caution and avoidance. Stimuli include people, foods, and toys.	Use a time-limited trial and praise.
Adaptability	How easily an infant can tolerate and respond to new stimuli.	Provide multiple short exposures to events.
Threshold	The level of stimulation response. Can also indicate hyperreactivity to minor stimuli.	Limit stimuli before bedtime.
Intensity of response	Involves the energy.	Do not yield to the child's will to buy peace.
Distractibility	Easily changes focus of interest.	Calmly redirect wandering attention.
Attention span	Loses interest rapidly.	Plan brief periods of activity; monitor completion of task. Warn if task must be interrupted for meal or sleep.

Modified from Carey W, Crocker A, Elias E, Feldman H, Coleman W: *Developmental-behavioral pediatrics*, ed 4, Philadelphia, 2010, Saunders.

process of child development. Crises in separation experiences can recur later in life when the school-age child must leave the home environment to attend elementary school or when the teenage child leaves home to enter college. Leaving home may precipitate a recurrence of the separation anxiety.

Language Development

Language development consists of verbal language that is both expressive (can say it) and receptive (can understand it) and body language that follows a predictable course of development. Body language, also known as nonverbal language, is the language of the motions, postures, and gestures of the body and is learned as part of communication. There appears to be an innate ability to develop language skills.

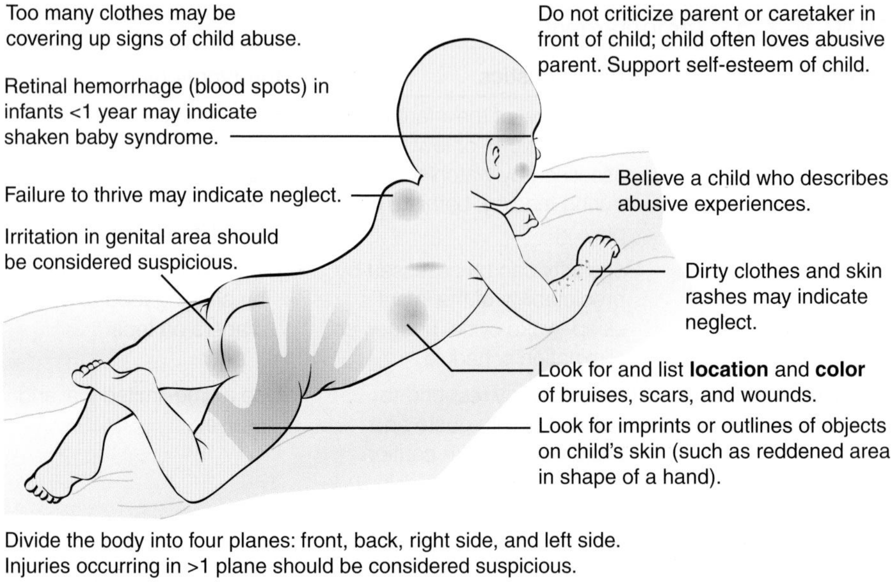
Too many clothes may be covering up signs of child abuse.
Retinal hemorrhage (blood spots) in infants <1 year may indicate shaken baby syndrome.
Failure to thrive may indicate neglect.
Irritation in genital area should be considered suspicious.
Do not criticize parent or caretaker in front of child; child often loves abusive parent. Support self-esteem of child.
Believe a child who describes abusive experiences.
Dirty clothes and skin rashes may indicate neglect.
Look for and list **location** and **color** of bruises, scars, and wounds.
Look for imprints or outlines of objects on child's skin (such as reddened area in shape of a hand).
Divide the body into four planes: front, back, right side, and left side. Injuries occurring in >1 plane should be considered suspicious.

Figure 7-1 Assessing for child abuse. The nurse should be alert for inconsistent statements about injuries, bruises at various stages of healing, or delay in seeking care. (From Leifer G: *Introduction to maternity & pediatric nursing*, ed 6, Philadelphia, 2011, Saunders.)

The first year of life, before the infant can express understandable speech, is called the preverbal stage of language development. In the early months, the infant initially communicates needs by crying or smiling. The infant will stop all random motor activity when listening to a voice, and the baby learns the rhythms and speech patterns of what will be his or her native or primary language. At 3 or 4 months of age, the infant will utter repetitive sounds, which develops into babbling, using combinations of vowels with some consonants. By 7 to 8 months, syllables using the D, P, and B sounds appear, and parents are gleeful when they hear "ma" or "da." By 9 or 10 months of age, specific sounds are used consistently to refer to objects or events. At this age, infants share their emotions by showing a favorite toy to an adult, because they are sure it will bring joy to the adult also.

The first words may occur between 10 and 13 months of age. Body language, such as pointing, leaning, or staring, assists the infant to make desires or needs understood. The first single words used often have multiple meanings. For example, "ball" can mean "that is a ball" or "give me the ball." Nonverbal behavior often assists the parent to understand what the infant means.

By the time infants are 1 year old, their brain is committed to the language that is used regularly in the environment around them. Initially, at birth, the infant was able to tune in to the covert sounds that often separate language with different sounds, such as English and Japanese. By the time the infant is a year old, the rhythm and pattern of the language is set, and the ability to distinguish sounds from other languages wanes. Infants soon learn combinations of syllables that separate words by hearing them often and separating them according to the frequency heard. For example, in the phrase "pretty girl," babies learn that "ty" goes with "pret," not "girl." It is not "pret-tygirl," it is "pretty-girl." This is a learned skill and is an important reason parents should talk to their infants in a natural language and should not use slang or baby talk (Figure 7-2).

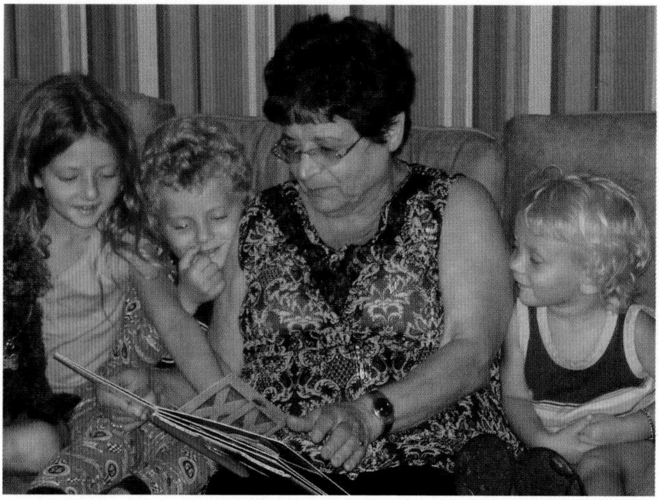

Figure 7-2 Reading to infants and children promotes language development. Infants enjoy books that provide colorful pictures and varied textures.

Motor Development

The development of motor skills is closely related to the development of perception, emotion, and cognition. Reaching out and touching what they see enable infants to establish visual-motor skills. Many motor skills are dependent on the disappearance of newborn reflexes (see Chapter 6). With the disappearance of the tonic neck reflex (the arm extends when the head turns to the side), the infant is able to bring both hands to the midline of the body into prayer position. At 3 months, the infant attempts to grasp whatever he or she touches. At 6 months, the infant shapes the hand to prepare to touch and grasp an observed object. By 9 months, the pincer action enables the infant to grasp with the thumb and forefinger. By 2 years, wrist action enables the use of spoons during feeding.

As posture and balance develop, infants first learn to lift their heads, then to sit and stand, and then to take their first steps around 1 year of age. Infants start to walk about 4 to 5 months after they are able to pull themselves up to a standing position (Table 7-2).

Physical Activity

The acquisition of motor skills in infancy lays the foundation for a lifetime of physical activity. In order to develop fine and gross motor skills, an infant must be provided with a safe and stimulating environment to move and explore. Early motor competence and confidence can contribute to the enjoyment of physical activity throughout childhood and beyond (Figure 7-3 on p. 105). The National Association for Sport and Physical Education (NASPE) (2009) recommends five basic guidelines for physical activity during infancy (Box 7-1 on p. 105).

Autonomy

Autonomy refers to independence. Striving for independence starts early in infancy. Self-consoling behavior is an early form of independence. Infants learns to bring their hands

(Text continued on p. 105)

TABLE 7-2 The Development of Locomotion, Prehension, and Perception

	Locomotion	Prehension	Perception
1 Month	Chin up. 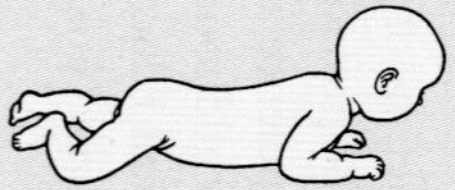	Hand held closed. Fingers move without coordination from mind. 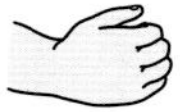	Able to focus on sharply contrasted, angled mobile above.
2 Months	Chest up. Elevates self with arms. 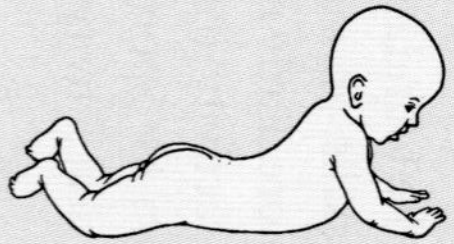	Hand held open most of the time. 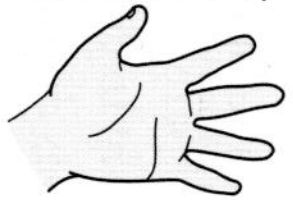	Selectively responds to patterns, colors. Imitates expressions. Is self-centered. Prefers to look at familiar sights.
4 Months	Rolls over at will. 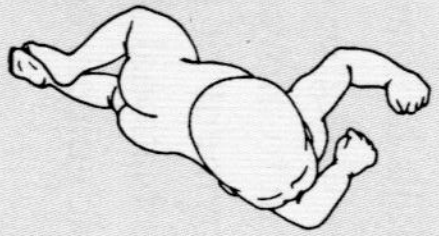	Reaches for overhead objects with fingers, with hit-and-miss action. 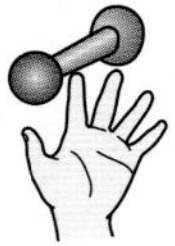	Perceives differences in facial expressions.
5 Months	Sits alone momentarily. 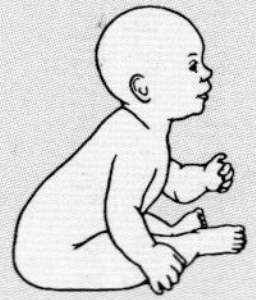	Picks up toy with squeeze action. 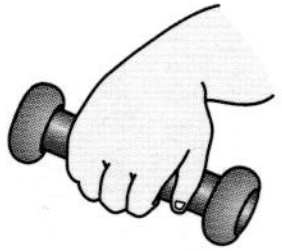	

6 Months	Sits alone steadily with hands forward for support. 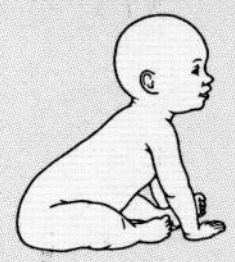	Grasps with thumb on one side and 3 fingers on other. 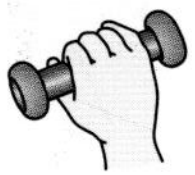	Can distinguish between familiar and unfamiliar sights. Separation anxiety begins. Sees self and parent as one.
8 Months	Sits with support. Pulls to standing position. 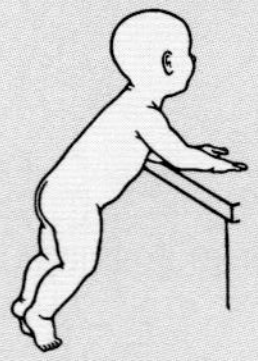	Thumb and index finger can hold object without pressing it into palm. Can transfer from one hand to the other. 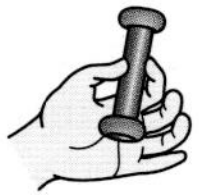	Can distinguish happy from fearful face.
9 Months	Creeps. 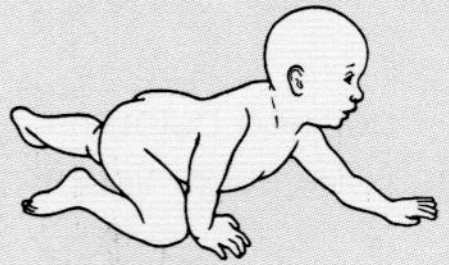	Uses finger to explore what eye sees. Has hand–mouth coordination. 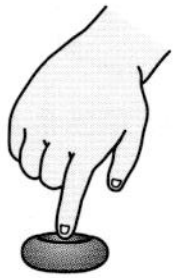	Fears strangers. Recognizes self as separate from parent.

(*Continued*)

TABLE 7-2 The Development of Locomotion, Prehension, and Perception—cont'd

	Locomotion	Prehension	Perception
10 Months	Walks when led. 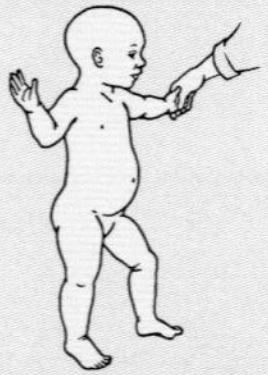	Can release from grasp one toy at a time. 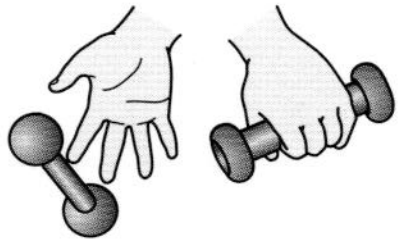	Separation anxiety peaks.
11 Months	Stands alone and can sit from standing position. 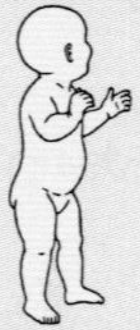	Pincer action enables infant to pick up small objects. 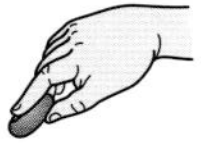	
12 Months	Walks 3 steps. 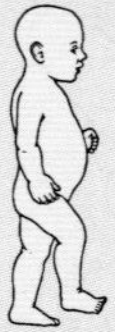	Hand obeys direction from mind. Aim is poor but can place toy in pan. Can attempt to feed self. 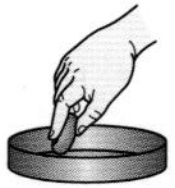	"Goal corrected partnership" enables infant to grasp onto parent because he or she anticipates being left with stranger.
15 Months	Can walk up stairs with support. 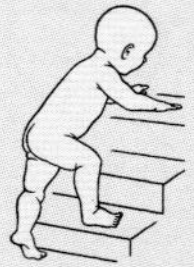	Mind is 100% in control of hands. Places round peg in round hole. Builds tower of 2 cubes. 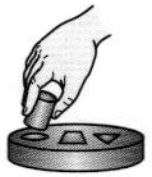	

From Leifer G: *Introduction to maternity & pediatric nursing*, ed 6, Philadelphia, 2011, Saunders.

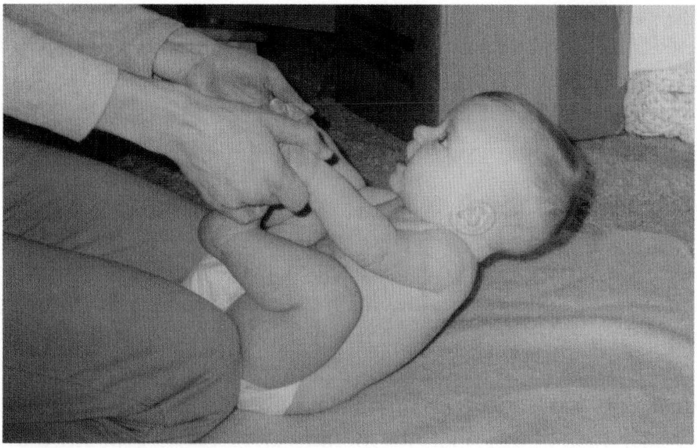

Figure 7-3 Age-appropriate exercise for the infant. The infant learns head control by gentle lifting. The infant will soon assist in pulling up by using her arm muscles.

BOX 7-1 Physical Activity Guidelines for Infants

1. Infants should interact with caregivers in daily physical activities that are dedicated to exploring movement and the environment.
2. Caregivers should place infants in settings that encourage and stimulate movement experiences and active play for short periods several times daily.
3. Infants' physical activity should promote skill development in movement.
4. Infants should be placed in an environment that meets or exceeds recommended safety standards for performing large-muscle activities.
5. Those in charge of infants' well-being are responsible for understanding the importance of physical activity and should promote movement skills by providing opportunities for structured and unstructured physical activity.

Adapted from National Association for Sport and Physical Education (2009). *Active Start: A Statement of Physical Activity Guidelines for Children Birth to Age 5*, ed 2. Accessed November 11, 2011, from www.aahperd.org/naspe/standards/nationalguidelines/activestart.cfm.

to their mouths and to suck their fingers to bring comfort or to relieve boredom. At 6 to 10 months of age, body rocking is used to achieve self-comforting. Nine-month-old babies with newly developed pincer ability will insist on self–finger feeding and will resist the attempts of parents to feed them at mealtime.

Sleep Patterns

A maturing central nervous system combined with parental responses aids in the development of sleep patterns. By 3 months, most infants develop a pattern of sustained sleep between midnight and 5:00 a.m., but a few do not develop this pattern before 1 year of age. In the first year, waking at night is considered normal. The goal is to help infants develop self-regulatory skills so that they return to sleep without prompting. This can occur more quickly if parents wait until there is evidence that infants are fully awake before picking them up. In a semiwakened state, gentle body patting or use of a pacifier should be enough consolation to help the infant return to sleep. The establishment of a prebedtime routine of quiet activity (e.g., rocking or reading to the infant) helps with the acceptance of bedtime during the first years of life.

Health Promotion

The establishment of an appropriate sleep pattern is important, because adequate sleep is related to memory, attention, learning, and general behavior.

Role of Play in Fostering Growth and Development

Piaget's sensorimotor theory of development (see Chapter 5) is evident in the infant's play activities, which are activated by sensations and relate to the infant directly. Play is the work of a child, and age-appropriate play activities can effectively foster growth and development. For example, a newborn must learn to focus and follow with the eyes. Hanging a bright mobile with contrasting colors (such as black and white) above the crib within sight of the infant can promote the development of this skill. At 3 months, an interactive mobile that is activated by kicking helps develop the cause–effect understanding. At 6 to 7 months of age, playing peek-a-boo helps solidify the object permanence concept. Dropping food from the highchair when someone is there to pick it up is also part of the learning process, although the messiness involved often tries the patience of parents. In the young infant, all toys are explored for taste and touch, but by 1 year, the infant typically understands the function of the toy. A car will be pushed; a telephone will be put to the ear. All toys and activities are related to the child's body. Egocentric behavior is evident in 1-year-olds who drink from a toy cup or place a toy telephone to their ear, but a toddler at 18 months of age will offer the drink to a doll. The 1-year-old enjoys push toys that foster the newly mastered walking abilities.

According to Freud's theory of development, the infant is in an oral phase, which involves exploring with the mouth (see Chapter 5). Oral sucking, biting, and chewing toys are appropriate activities for this stage of development.

By applying learned skills to environmental experiences, children learn about the world around them. Often the health-care worker must reassure parents that a child picking up everything from the floor and placing it in the mouth, or a child intentionally dropping food from the highchair tray onto the floor, are developmentally normal behaviors and are definitely not signs of a child who is behaving badly.

HEALTH MAINTENANCE

Nutrition

In the first year of life, the brain and the body grow and develop rapidly. Proper nutritional intake is essential to support optimum development. The newborn has a rooting reflex that seeks out the nipple and a sucking reflex that is elicited when the nipple touches the lips. A tongue extrusion reflex prevents ingestion of solid foods in the first few months of life.

Health Promotion

The best nutrition for the newborn is breast milk, which contains antibodies and easy-to-digest fats. For mothers who cannot breastfeed, most commercial formulas provide adequate nutrition, although they do not have the extra benefits of the antibodies and other protective ingredients in breastmilk.

Cultural Considerations

Breastfeeding

Cultural factors influence breastfeeding choices. Some mothers from North American or European backgrounds are uncomfortable with the body contact and exposure required for breastfeeding. In American cultures, returning to the workplace soon after delivery may influence the mother's choice to bottle-feed her newborn, although many current workplace environments provide accomodations for breastfeeding mothers, and user-friendly breastpumps and milk storage containers are available and inexpensive. In many cultures, breast pumping is not accepted as a relief for engorgement or as a convenience for working mothers.

In cultures such as the Cambodian, Mexican-American, and Filipino, colostrum is discarded, and in some Asian cultures, sterile water may be provided for the newborn to drink until maternal milk flow is well established. In African-American cultures, solid food may be added to the formula bottle in the early months of life. Breastfeeding may be medically contraindicated in most women with human immunodeficiency virus/acquired immunodeficiency syndrome (HIV/AIDS) and in women receiving medications that may pass into the breast milk and cause adverse effects in the newborn.

Newborns are usually fed on demand at 2- to 3-hour intervals, and by 4 to 6 months of age infants may skip a nighttime feeding. If the newborn is lethargic, efforts to maintain a state of alertness will aid nutritional intake. Infants should be fed formula or breast milk for 1 full year. At 1 year of age, the infant can be placed on cow's milk. Low-fat milk should not be given to children under age 2, because the fats are necessary for development of the nervous system. At 6 months of age, the tongue extrusion reflex has disappeared. The infant will no longer spit out solid foods and is ready for strained rice cereal. Gradually, vegetables and fruits are added to the diet, but only one at a time to allow identification of foods that may upset the infant's stomach or result in a food allergy response. By 11 months of age, meat and eggs can be added to the diet. By 1 year, the infant typically eats table food three times a day and can join the family meal schedule.

Introduction of foods before 6 months of age is not recommended, because the infant does not have the digestive enzymes necessary for complete digestion and utilization of the nutrients. Foods such as nuts, jellied candy, and large pieces of solid foods should not be offered to the infant, because these items present a choking hazard. Honey should not be given to children under 2 years of age because of the risk of botulism poisoning. Commercially prepared foods such as beets, turnips, spinach, celery, and collard greens are high in nitrates and should be used sparingly for infants under 1 year of age. Commercially prepared baby food in jars are vacuum packed, and parents should check the safety seals and expiration dates before purchase. When a jar is first opened, a pop should be heard as the vacuum is broken. Foods should not be fed directly from the jar, and leftovers should not be returned to the jar, because saliva contamination can alter the foods. Parents should avoid tasting the food from the same spoon used to feed the infant, because organisms from their mouth will be passed to the baby.

The development of autonomy dictates the need for finger foods by 9 or 10 months, when the infant can be expected to prefer self feeding. The temperament of the infant will influence the development of mealtime challenges. For example, infants with a high activity level should not be expected to sit for a long period at the family meal table. Infants who are highly distractible may not even finish a meal. Infants who are slow to adapt may not easily try new foods.

Health Promotion

The health-care worker can help the parent develop strategies to accommodate temperament as it relates to feeding, so that conflicts will not arise. The prevention of obesity is a *Healthy People 2020* goal, and overfeeding during infancy is thought to be a contributing factor to obesity later in life. The health-care worker can provide parents with information regarding feeding concerns during the first years.

Teeth

The eruption of the first 20 deciduous teeth, which are also known as *primary* or *baby teeth*, usually begins at 5 to 7 months of age (Box 7-2). The upper and lower central incisors are usually the first to emerge. At this time the infant enjoys holding toys that can be chewed. The primary teeth serve the purpose of helping the intake of nutrition by allowing the chewing of foods, and they also help in the formation of the jaw. If an infant or child loses a primary tooth because of an accident, a spacer is usually inserted by the dentist to preserve the space for the later eruption of the permanent tooth, thus avoiding expensive orthodontic care. Nursing caries (cavities) occur when the infant is put to bed while sucking on milk or juice from a bottle. The sugars in the milk or juice coat the teeth and promote tooth decay. If the infant insists on a bottle at bedtime, it should be a bottle of water to prevent the development of nursing caries.

Immunizations

Well-child visits should be scheduled after birth before the newborn is discharged from the hospital. Community resources should be assessed and the parents informed about available help for breastfeeding problems, such as the La Leche League or Healthy Starts programs offered by some health-insurance companies. Home visits are often available through the Visiting Nurse Association, the local health department or through the home-health services of a hospital for new mothers of high-risk newborns. The growth, development, health, and nutrition of the infant should be checked every 2 months and appropriate immunizations scheduled (see Appendix A).

Parent Teaching

Well-child checkups are the best time to answer questions the parents may have and to provide anticipatory guidance concerning the developmental stages and needs of the growing infant.

BOX 7-2 Estimating the Number of Erupted Primary Teeth

The number of primary teeth that should be present in an infant or toddler can be anticipated using the following formula: Age in months – 6

Accident Prevention

Accidents are a major cause of morbidity (illness) and mortality (death). The first injury prevention activity for the newborn, now required by law in most states, is the use of car seats. When held in the lap of a parent instead of in a car seat, the infant becomes a high-speed missile in the event of a motor vehicle accident. Also, front-seat airbags in cars can be lifesaving for adults but can be lethal to infants or young children during accidents (see Chapter 8).

Safety Alert

A safe or "childproof" home is essential for the prevention of accidents. There are private agencies in many communities that will come to the home to evaluate safety and offer childproofing suggestions for parents. Local police stations or highway patrol stations offer assistance in assessing car-seat installations. Falls are common causes of injury to infants younger than 1 year.

- Keeping the crib's side rails secured in the raised position prevents the infant from rolling out of the crib.
- The use of safety straps when infants are placed in highchairs or strollers prevents falls.
- Gates are needed at the top and bottom of stairs to prevent the infant from falling.
- Placing the infant supine, to sleep on their back, and not using pillows in the crib can aid in preventing accidental suffocation and **sudden infant death syndrome (SIDS).**
- When the infant masters the pincer action of the thumb and forefinger, choking becomes a high risk, because small objects picked up from the floor are typically placed in the mouth.
- Infants can drown in a shallow tub bath if left unattended even for a minute.
- Burns can be a risk for infants who pull on the cord of a hot iron, reach for the handle of a pot on the stove, or stick fingers into an exposed and inviting electrical outlet.

KEY POINTS

- Infancy includes the period between 4 weeks and 1 year of age.
- Developmental tasks involve the goals of developing social competence and mastery of skills necessary for functioning in an environment.
- Some developmental tasks of infancy include weaning, locomotion, self-feeding, and acquiring language.
- The development of a sense of trust begins in infancy.
- The infant's birth weight doubles by 6 months and triples by 1 year of age.
- The infant is in Piaget's sensorimotor stage of development.
- Object permanence involves knowing an object is there even though it is not in sight.
- The infant is in Freud's oral stage of development. Sucking and exploring textures with the mouth are normal behaviors.
- Separation anxiety begins at 6 months of age, when the infant protests if the parent leaves the room.
- Language development involves both verbal language and body language.
- Verbal language involves expression and receiving (understanding) communication from others.

(Continued)

KEY POINTS—cont'd

- Egocentric behavior is evidenced by the 1 year old, who relates all toys to his or her own body.
- Major risk factors for heart disease begin developing in early childhood. Regular physical activity can help slow the development of these risk factors.
- Infants should be placed in environments that stimulate movements and exercise.
- A natural pattern of intermittent play is age appropriate physical activity for infants.
- Breast milk is the best food for infants under 6 months of age, and mothers should be encouraged to continue to provide breast milk until 1 year of age.
- To prevent SIDS, infants should be placed on their backs to sleep.
- By 1 year of age, the infant eats table food three times a day.
- At 1 year of age, whole milk can be introduced, but low-fat milk should not be provided to children under 2 years of age.
- The most common type of dental caries in infants is nursing caries, which are preventable.
- By 9 months of age, the pincer action enables the infant to grasp small objects with the thumb and forefinger.
- A childproof home is essential for preventing accidents.

Critical Thinking

Accidents are the major cause of illness and death in children. List three types of accidents that commonly occur in the first year of life, and discuss how they can be prevented.

REVIEW QUESTIONS

1. **The period of infancy occurs between:**
   a. birth and 1 month.
   b. 4 weeks and 1 year.
   c. 1 and 3 years.
   d. 1 and 12 years.

2. **A 1-year-old who regards all toys in relation to his or her own body is exhibiting which type of behavior?**
   a. Dysfunctional
   b. Selfish
   c. Sexual
   d. Egocentric

3. **Separation anxiety typically begins at what age?**
   a. 3 months
   b. 6 months
   c. 1 year
   d. 2 years

4. **By 9 months of age, a pincer action is well developed, enabling the infant to:**
   a. increase locomotion.
   b. grasp small objects with the thumb and forefinger.
   c. scoop up toys within reach.
   d. achieve increased depth perception.

5. **By 1 year of age, the normal infant should weigh approximately:**
   a. twice the birth weight.
   b. quadruple the birth weight.
   c. triple the birth weight.
   d. 30 pounds.

CHAPTER

8

Early Childhood

http://evolve.elsevier.com/Leifer/growth

OBJECTIVES

1. Define early childhood.
2. Describe characteristics common to toddlers.
3. Describe characteristics common to preschool children.
4. Discuss the developmental tasks of early childhood.
5. List three factors that aid in the development of language skills.
6. List at least three guidelines for selecting a preschool or day care center.
7. Describe the role of physical activity in maintaining health.
8. Describe the characteristic play and appropriate toys for a toddler and preschool child.
9. List three safety risks common to the early childhood years.
10. Discuss the principles of guidance and discipline for children during the early childhood years.

KEY TERMS

age-appropriate toys
cooperative play
corporal punishment
dental caries
discipline
early childhood
immunity
oropharynx
parallel play
pincer grasp
preschool phase
time-out
toddler phase

DEFINITION

The early childhood period includes children from 1 to 6 years of age. Early childhood is typically separated into two phases; 1 to 2 years of age is the toddler phase, and 2 to 6 years is the preschool phase. During early childhood, physical growth slows and stabilizes.

DEVELOPMENTAL TASKS

Tasks to be mastered include acquiring *receptive language* and *expressive language* (understanding and speaking words); developing social interaction skills; mastering self-control in such areas as toilet training); and beginning to develop a self-image and sense of autonomy. The toddler, between 1 and 4 years of age, is in Erikson's stage of autonomy versus shame or doubt. The preschooler, between 4 and 6 years of age, is in Erikson's stage of initiative versus guilt.

Increased motor ability allows expanded exploration in the family and within the community. The willingness to separate from the mother and to explore enhances the development of autonomy and communication skills.

PHYSIOLOGICAL CHANGES

Most children learn to walk steadily between 12 and 15 months of age. By age 2, an exaggerated lumbar curve of the spine causes the abdomen to protrude. By age 3, the posture is more erect. The legs appear bowed between 12 and 18 months of age, and the feet strike the floor flat when walking. A knock-knee appearance develops between 18 months and 2 years. The gait gradually becomes steadier, and by age 2 the knees and toes appear more in alignment. At age 2, the child can run. By age 2 ½ the child can climb stairs gracefully; by age 3 the child can alternate feet when climbing stairs and can ride a tricycle. By age 4 the child can hop and by age 5 can skip.

The anterior fontanel of the skull closes at 18 months. By age 2, twenty primary teeth have erupted. Continued myelinization of neurons within the brain increases brain function. Although complete myelinization of the brain does not occur before 6 to 7 years of age, the rate of brain and body development during the preschool years influences behavior and motor coordination. The neocortex of the brain is responsible for thought, emotion, and higher-level brain functions. The frontal lobes are responsible for memory, attention, behavior, and emotions. For example, the skill of bike riding involves vision, hearing, sensation, balance, and using the thalamus and neocortex brain functions (Figure 8-1). A school-age child can ride a two-wheel bicycle, whereas a toddler struggles to learn skills involved in controlling a tricycle. The left hemisphere of the brain has been implicated in language disorders, cerebral palsy, and deafness (Guyton, 2011). Language-rich interactive play helps to enhance language development. Children who have difficulty in one area of brain development may be predisposed to other areas of developmental delay. Developmental screening should be part of every well-child visit.

The preschooler gains about 5 to 7 pounds (2.7 to 3.2 kg) and grows about 2 ½ to 3 inches (6.25 to 7.5 cm) per year. Approximately half of the adult height is achieved by age 2 (Kleigman, 2011), and the birth weight is quadrupled.

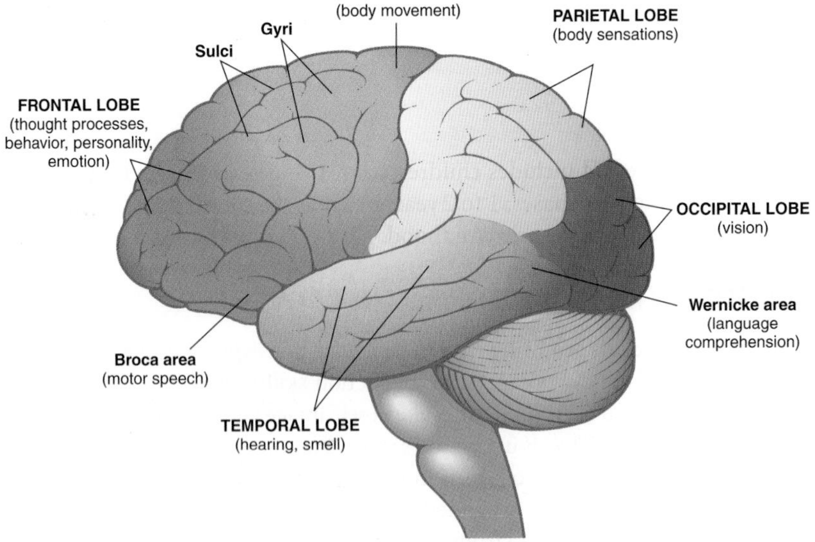

Figure 8-1 Anatomy of brain function.

The toddler has a well-developed pincer grasp (the ability to pick up small objects with the thumb and forefinger) by age 1 and can touch the thumb to each finger sequentially by age 5. A 2-year-old can copy a straight line on paper; a 3-year-old can copy a circle and can use scissors. A 4-year-old can draw a person with three body parts, and most 5-year-olds can print their names. Between 18 months and 5 years, the child shows a preference for using one hand or the other and so becomes left-handed or right-handed. Attempts to change hand preference are often met with frustration and are rarely successful. The eye muscles strengthen, depth perception increases during the preschool period, and 20/20 vision is usually achieved by age 4. When asked to find a specific picture on a page while reading a book, the toddler will examine the page in a random pattern to find the specific picture. However, in the same situation with a preschool-age child, the child will examine the page in an organized fashion (up and down or side to side), indicating reading readiness has occurred. Successful reading requires examining the page in an organized pattern.

Hearing is fully developed in the toddler and is necessary for speech development to occur. The eustachian tube connects the middle ear to the oropharynx (back of the throat). The eustachian tube is short and straight; therefore bacteria can easily travel from the throat to the middle ear causing an ear infection. A child who is put to bed while drinking milk or juice from a bottle may have a pooling of the sugary fluid in the back of the throat that enables bacteria to grow. These bacteria then have easy access to the ear through the eustachian tube and can cause a middle-ear infection. If a child must be put to bed with a bottle, only water should be in the bottle to prevent development of frequent ear infections, as well as dental caries (cavities).

During early childhood, fine motor skills develop, which include self feeding, dressing, and undressing. Toddlers are able to eat with a fork and spoon but often prefer finger foods. At age 2, the appetite decreases.

Toilet (potty) training occurs as sphincter control develops and the child masters some form of communication to indicate the need to use the toilet. Modeling behavior, using specially equipped dolls and celebrating successes aids in achieving toilet training, but the process cannot be hurried and may not be complete before 3 ½ years. Bowel control occurs before full-bladder control, and nighttime or stress accidents are common. Accidents should not result in scolding or punishment, because mastering sphincter control is related to the development of the self concept.

During toilet training, a child's refusal to sit on a toilet may stem from the fear of falling in or being flushed away. The child's fear is real, and the parents cannot dismiss it and expect to gain cooperation.

Nutrition

During the early childhood years, the dependent child is fed by adults whose eating habits may be based on ethnic, cultural, folklore, or fad concepts. Some families are poor, some need guidance on how to select nutritious foods, some need guidance on how to cook foods to preserve the nutritious qualities, and many families do not consider food a priority in the home. However, adequate nutrition is essential for optimal physical and mental development in young children. The U.S. Department of Agriculture (USDA) and The U.S. Department of Health and Human Services (USDHHS) offer guidelines for healthy eating. The private company beBetter Health has created the The Portion Plate to help kids make conscious food choices (Figure 8-2).

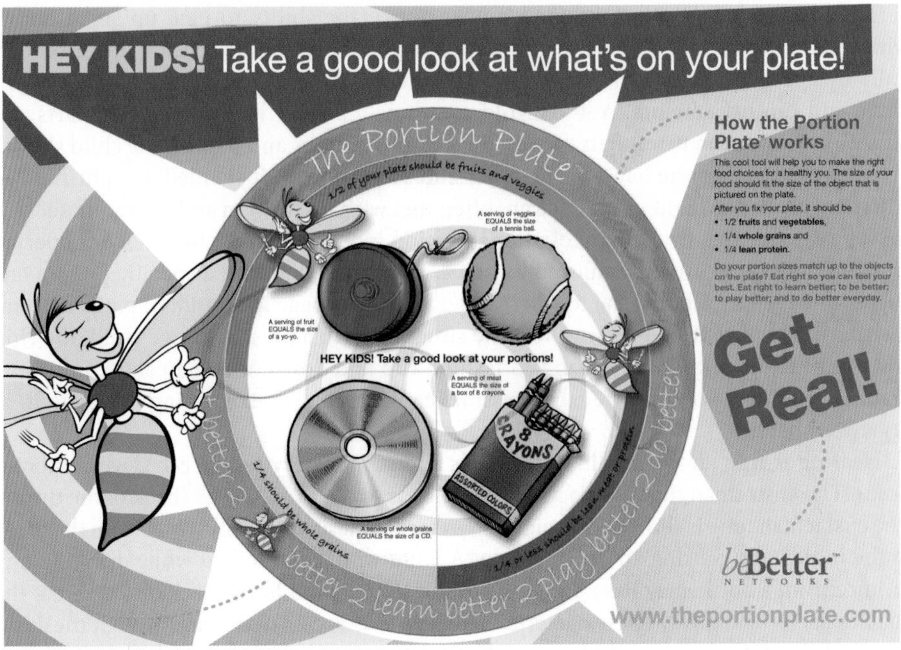

Figure 8-2 The Portion Plate for Kids is an educational placemat that can be used to guide portion amounts in terms children can understand, such as making the serving portion of vegetables in one meal about the size of a tennis ball. The reverse side of the mat offers tips on food selection. Preventing the supersizing of portions is an important step in preventing obesity. *(Courtesy beBetter Health, Inc., Poca, WV.)*

High-fiber diets are not adequate for children, because the foods are filling but do not provide the essential nutrients for growth and development. Children 1 to 6 years old are susceptible to nutritional deficiencies, because growth is rapid and energy output is high. There are no known advantages in consuming excess nutrients or vitamins. Obesity should be prevented and support for growth and development provided through a varied and nutritious diet. Eating habits are developed during the early childhood years, and children may carry these healthy (or unhealthy) habits with them into adulthood. The effect of childhood nutrition on adult health and illness has been well established.

PSYCHOSOCIAL DEVELOPMENT

Language Development and Communication Skills

The Toddler

Children develop *receptive* language before *expressive* language. That is, they are able to understand words before they can express them. Communication is evidenced in the neonatal period by the cry, coo, or smile. The initial purpose is to communicate needs, to regulate another's behavior, to attract attention, and to interact socially.

By 1 year of age, the toddler usually says the first clear word and responds to simple, single demands or statements such as "bye-bye" or "no!" By 15 months, the toddler may speak four to six words and typically uses one finger to point to various parts of the body. By 18 months the toddler speaks about 15 words and by 19 months may speak in two-word sentences. By age 2, the child has a vocabulary exceeding 100 words and can follow two-step commands such as "pick up the toy and put it away." When learning to speak, the toddler can learn more than one language if both languages are used at home. When one language is used at home and a different language is used at school, difficulties tend to arise. By age 5, parents have usually assisted their child to achieve competence in their native language.

The Preschooler

Language development occurs rapidly during the preschool years. A typical 2-year-old has a vocabulary of just over 100 words, whereas a typical 5-year-old has a vocabulary exceeding 2000 words. In a preschool child, the number of words in a typical sentence is equal to the child's age (Kleigman, 2011). By age 2 ½ the child expresses possession, as in "my doll." By age 4, the past tense is expressed, and by age 5 the child can express the future tense. Although speech development is directly influenced by the experiences of others talking to the child and encouraging the child to verbalize, speech development follows a predictable sequence and occurs even without the benefit of encouragement or imitating the words of others, albeit at a much slower pace. Speech development is a reflection of mental and emotional development, and often mental retardation can be detected by age 2, when speech delay is obvious. However, speech can also be delayed under conditions of abuse and neglect.

By age 2, a child can be heard to repeat the commands of others. When tempted to touch a forbidden object, the child can be heard to state, "don't touch." From this observation it is apparent that the child's own internal language plays a part in the child's behavior. When the child's skill at language allows him or her to express basic fears, the need for acting out on the fears or frustrations decreases. For this reason, language-delayed children are apt to experience more frequent behavioral outbursts or temper tantrums.

The language skills acquired during the preschool years set the stage for success for the school-age child in the task of achieving literacy at school. A school-age child is expected to enter the classroom with competency in his or her native language. Literacy milestones can be used to aid in the assessment of the child's development (Table 8-1).

Speech ability may be delayed. For example, a child may use only single words at 18 months, few vocabulary words by age 2, or words that are not clearly understood by age 3. In these cases, a referral for speech and hearing evaluations should be offered (Table 8-2).

Cognitive Development

The sensorimotor stage of cognition ends when the toddler begins to use words to express ideas and to solve problems, which marks the beginning of symbolic thought. By age 1, the toddler can push aside an obstacle to gain access to a toy. By 18 months, the toddler learns that dropping a ball, block, or stuffed toy down a flight of stairs results in different rates of descent and heights of bounce. By age 2, the toddler remembers past experiences and adjusts behavior accordingly. A 1-year-old child may exhibit stranger anxiety when the parent leaves the room. By age 2, the child can anticipate a temporary absence (e.g., a parent going to work) in an accepting manner.

TABLE 8-1 Literacy Milestones

Age	Motor	Cognitive/ Language	Interaction
6-12 months	Reaches for book Puts book to mouth	Looks at pictures Vocalizes, pats picture	Face-to-face gaze Parents follow baby's cues for "more" and "stop"
12-18 months	Holds book with help Turns several pages at a time	Points at pictures with one finger Labels pictures with same sound	May bring book to read Child becomes upset if parent does not let child "control" reading
18-36 months	Turns one page at a time Carries book around house	Names familiar pictures Attention highly variable Demands story over and over	Parent asks "what's happening?" questions Parent shows pleasure when child supplies word

Adapted from Carey W, Crocker A, Elias E, Feldan H, Coleman W: *Developmental-behavioral pediatrics*, ed 4, Philadelphia, 2010, W.B. Saunders.

Preschool thinking involves Piaget's preoperational or prelogical characteristics, such as magical thinking and egocentrism (see Chapter 5). Two-year-olds attribute life qualities to inanimate dolls or toys and typically feel their wishes caused things to happen. They feel their point of view must be the same as everyone else's. Although preschoolers are empathetic, they believe that whatever comforts them will also serve to comfort others.

Through experience, preschoolers gradually learn about cause and effect and how to solve problems. Having one object represent another, such as a box representing a train, evidences symbolism and fantasy play. Pretend play is common at age 2. By age 3, children can understand the motivations of others that may differ from their own, and by age 5 they can role-play scenarios with elaborate plots and characters. During the preschool years, while the child is trying to understand the differing opinions of others, fears and other forces in life may be represented by monsters, bad people, or invisible friends.

One of the major tasks of the child during preschool years is to develop impulse control for behaviors such as biting, kicking, and throwing toys. Impulse control is typically achieved by age 4, with minor relapses in times of stress. By 18 months, the toddler develops a sense of self (Carey, 2008) and by age 3 is able to express complex feelings and ideas through pretend play (Figure 8-3). At age 4, the child can understand the wishes and emotions of others and how they differ from the child's own. Whatever the preschooler cannot understand or express is often acted out in the form of negativism or tantrums. The natural temperament of the child influences the intensity of the emotional responses of joy, anger, or frustration. Many parents need guidance in helping their toddlers manage these challenges in a positive way.

TABLE 8-2 When a Child with a Communication Disorder Needs Help

Age	Behavior Indicating Help Is Needed
0-11 months	Before 6 months the child does not startle, blink, or change immediate activity in response to sudden loud sounds. Before 6 months the child does not attend to the human voice and is not soothed by the mother's voice. By 6 months the child does not babble strings of consonant + vowel syllables or imitate gurgling or cooing sounds. By 10 months the child does not respond to his or her name. At 10 months the child's sound making is limited to shrieks, grunts, or sustained vowel production.
12-23 months	At 12 months the child's babbling or speech is limited to vowel sounds. By 15 months the child does not respond to "no," "bye-bye," or "bottle." By 15 months the child will not imitate sounds or words. By 18 months the child is not consistently using at least six words with appropriate meaning. By 21 months the child does not respond correctly to "give me…," "sit down," or "come here" when spoken without gestural cues. By 23 months two-word phrases have not emerged that are spoken as single units (e.g., "whatzit," "thank you," or "all gone").
24-36 months	By 24 months at least 50% of the child's speech is not understood by familiar listeners. By 24 months the child does not point to body parts without gestural cues. By 24 months the child is not combining words into phrases ("Go bye-bye," "Go car," "Want cookie"). By 30 months the child does not demonstrate understanding of the words "on," "in," "under," "front," or "back." By 30 months the child is not using short sentences ("Daddy went bye-bye"). By 30 months the child has not begun to ask questions using "where," "what," and "why." By 36 months the child's speech is not understood by unfamiliar listeners.
All ages	At any age, the child is consistently dysfluent, exhibiting repetitions and hesitations. Child evidences blocks or struggles in saying words. Struggle may be accompanied by grimaces, eye blinks, or hand gestures.

Adapted from Kleigman R, Stanton B, St. Geme J, Schor N, Behrman R: *Nelson's essentials of pediatrics*, ed 5, Philadelphia, 2011, W.B. Saunders. Originally adapted from Weiss CE, Lillywhite HE: *Communication disorders: a handbook for prevention and early detection*, St Louis, 1976, Mosby.

Figure 8-3 This child engages in pretend play as she feeds her doll.

Moral Development

According to Kohlberg, learning self-control and learning to share with others are moral tasks of early childhood (see Chapter 5). Preschoolers look carefully at parents as models of moral behavior, and this is often acted out in their play. Preschoolers must organize and synthesize what they view at home, in the community, and on television. They constantly test limits either to confirm that a behavior is unacceptable or just to gain attention. A child of 3 becomes ritualistic and aware of rules that he or she feels must be obeyed, and the child will feel guilty if scolded (Figure 8-4). A 2-year-old cannot differentiate between intentional acts and accidents and readily assigns blame. A 3-year-old can understand the difference between intentional acts and accidents but still may extend blame to another. By age 5, the child extends blame for only the intentional act and easily excuses the accident.

Some parents complain that their preschool child lies. Preschoolers do not have the abstract reasoning to lie for the purpose of deceiving others. They tell the truth as they interpret it or wish it to be true. Stealing is a behavior that a preschooler does not feel is wrong because ownership is not completely understood. Respecting the property of others is a learned behavior. A child will learn socially acceptable behavior through consistent, positive reinforcement and discipline.

Discipline

Discipline must have as its basic purpose the guiding, teaching, or correcting of behavior, not punishment. Preschoolers are naturally egocentric and may not understand the rights

Figure 8-4 Children can learn to wash their hands at an early age. Regular handwashing can prevent the spread of infection and can assist in meeting some of the goals of *Healthy People 2020*.

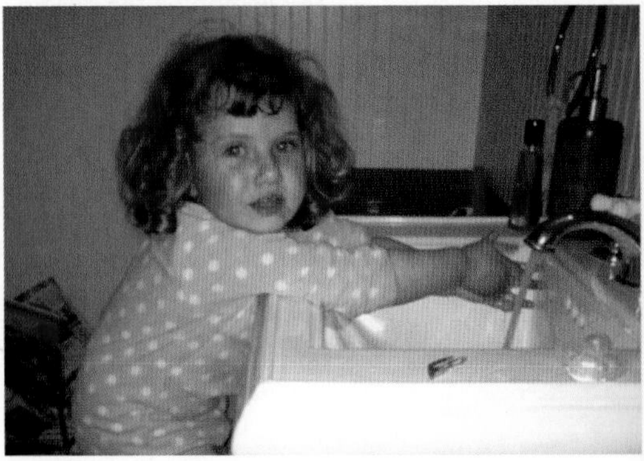

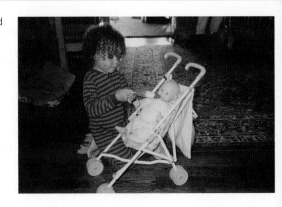

and needs of others. The preschooler may hit the mother in anger yet expect to be loved, hugged, and comforted by the mother in his or her frustration.

The purpose of discipline for toddlers should be to help them develop self-control while maintaining positive self-esteem. Setting limits should include praise for good behavior. A time-out response to unacceptable behavior is effective for children between the ages of 1 and 6 years. This response places the child in a safe place with time for self regulation. The child is removed from the situation, is placed in time-out with just a very brief explanation of why it is happening, and is reminded of the cause at the end of time-out. Time-outs usually are limited to 1 minute per year of age. With consistent use, the child will learn to anticipate this disciplinary response to certain behaviors and will learn to control those behaviors.

Corporal punishment (spanking) focuses on the pain of the punishment, can model aggression, and rarely accomplishes the true goal of discipline. Young children may model the behavior of the parent and may hit the parent. Children can also become accustomed to the spanking, so that the parent has to hit harder, and child abuse can become a risk. Severe physical punishment may affect the psychological health of the child.

Rewarding good behavior is the positive and most effective technique of discipline. A hug, smile, praise, or material reward for good behavior is effective. Consistency in parental response is the key to successful discipline. It is best to ignore the behavior of a child who whines, nags, or has a tantrum and to express frequent praise when the behavior is good. If a behavior receives attention, it will be used again with more intensity to attract attention. Operant conditioning, as described by B.F. Skinner, occurs when the learner repeats behaviors that result in the positive outcome of reaching his or her goals, and the learner stops behaviors that have negative outcomes. The operant theory of discipline is described in Table 8-3. An example of the operant theory during play is the use of an interactive mobile that is activated when the infant kicks or touches a footpad. The infant's kicking will increase if the infant enjoys the resulting sound and movement of the mobile.

When discussing with parents disciplinary techniques for children, the health-care worker should be nonjudgmental and should help parents develop a mutually acceptable plan that will be consistent and safe. Support groups, parenting classes, and counseling should be available for referral as needed.

TABLE 8-3 The Operant Theory of Effective Discipline Techniques

Type of Discipline	Example	Effect
Positive reinforcement	Child receives a lollipop or toy for helping mommy	Increases the "helping mommy" behavior
Negative reinforcement	Restrict privileges for bad behavior Remove restrictions for good behavior	Increases likelihood of desired behavior occurring again (useful in older children as well)
Negative punishment	Take away fun and interaction with others Ignore behavior	Decreases or stops unwanted behavior

Sexuality

In the past, toddlers and preschool-age children were thought to be free of sexuality or in a period of sexual dormancy. Today it is recognized that children in early childhood do have the capacity for sexual pleasure and response, which include penile erection, pelvic thrusting, rhythmic movements, and masturbation. Kinsey (1948) and other researchers have shown that children between the ages of 4 and 7 years experience play activities that involve viewing or touching the genitals, which results from normal curiosity (Table 8-4).

Parents have an impact on the molding of sexuality in their infants and children. The parents' response to the child's urinary and fecal elimination is an early influence related to sexuality. A negative response to a dirty diaper, the label of "stinky" to the soiled underpants of a toddler, or forced toilet training all influence the development of sexuality. Treating the natural process of bodily functions as secret or as dirty promotes embarrassment or discomfort related to the genital area. Modesty appears gradually between 5 and 6 years of age. The acceptance or rejection of hugging and kissing as an expression of emotion by parents can influence sexuality and the ability of the child to establish intimate relationships in later life. Preschool day care centers typically do not separate boys' and girls' bathrooms, and viewing the body is treated as normal and natural. Masturbation or sexual curiosity that interferes with normal play activities, or acting out sexual intercourse with dolls or playmates, may be indications of sexual abuse, and the child should be referred for counseling.

Physical Activity

Current evidence indicates that major risk factors for heart disease begin developing in early childhood (Petra, 2011). Regular physical activity, in combination with healthy eating patterns, can help slow the development of these risk factors as well as establish a foundation of healthy habits for adolescence and adulthood.

TABLE 8-4 Sexual Behavior in Early Childhood

Normal	Requires Referral
When diapers are changed, child may touch own genitals	Prefers touching genitals instead of playing with toys
Plays with feces	Repeatedly uses feces as a toy
Touches genitals, breasts of family and peers	Asks to be touched in genital area
Removes clothes, likes to play nude	Removes clothes in public repeatedly even after correction
Shows interest in watching bathroom functions	Often insists on watching bathroom functions of others
Plays "doctor" to inspect body of others	Forces peers to remove clothes
Places objects against genital area	Insists on placing objects against genital area of self or peers
Plays house, with mommy and daddy roles assigned to peers	Simulates sexual intercourse activities; draws genitals on figures

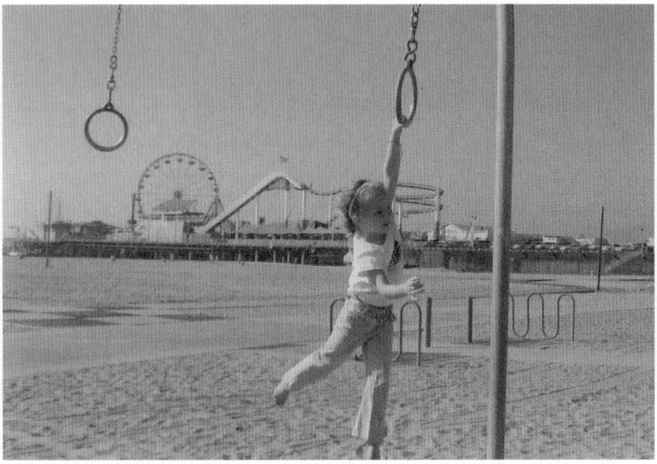

Figure 8-5 Swinging on the rings at the beach or climbing at the playground are age-appropriate activities for the young child.

Children should be physically active for a minimum of 60 minutes every day (NASPE, 2009). Age-appropriate activities should range from moderate to vigorous, often following a natural pattern of intermittent play. Running, jumping, hopping, and climbing are all age-appropriate physical activities for young children (Figure 8-5).

Organized sports can also be good sources of regular physical activity. Caregivers should limit sedentary activities such as television, computers, and video games and should ensure that young children have access to safe, active play.

Caregivers can keep children safe during physical activity by providing appropriate footwear and protective gear for each activity. Shoes should be cushioned and supportive with a good fit. Protective gear may include helmets, pads, mouthguards, shin guards, among others. Equipment and play surfaces should be well maintained to avoid injuries. Children should be kept hydrated by offering water before, during, and after exercise. For details on protective gear for specific physical activities see www.varsityorthopedics.com/specialties/prev.html.

Play

In the toddler period, play is a reflection of the child's experiences. Age-appropriate toys are those that are safe and promote the cognitive and motor development of the specific age-group. The toddler may pretend to put a baby to bed or to shop at a store. The 2-year-old exhibits parallel play, in which he or she plays next to a friend but does not interact with the friend. The 3- to 4-year-old exhibits cooperative play, in which a group of children can cooperate by acting out a scene together or by building a tower of blocks together. By age 5, there is organized group play with assigned roles, such as playing house with one child assigned the mother role, one the father role, and so on.

Play allows the child to imitate adult roles, be the aggressor, assume superpowers, and solve problems. The child's drawings often reflect his or her inner emotional issues or conflicts. According to the preschool child, rules of play are absolute, and fairness means equal treatment regardless of circumstances. Group songs and music are enjoyed by both the

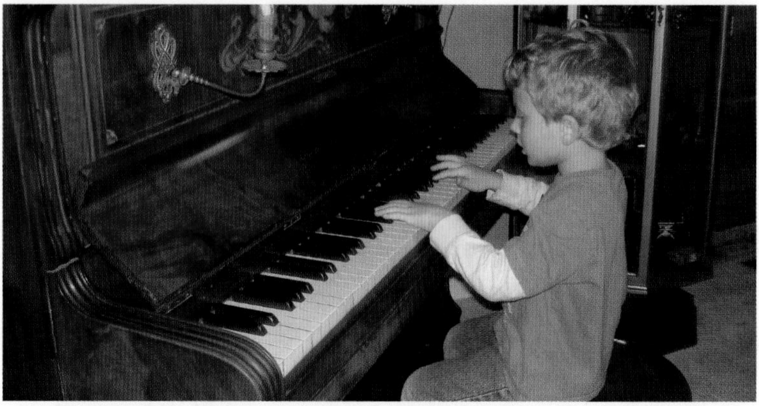

Figure 8-6 Preschoolers share a love of music. This child enjoys playing the piano.

toddler and the preschool child, who respond with unique dancing and random movements (Figure 8-6). Many 2-year-olds enjoy singing along with recorded songs.

Day Care

The experience of spending time in day care or preschool is a big step toward developing independence. The child must accept that the parent will leave and must trust that the parent will return. There are several types of day care settings that may be available in communities for parents who work outside the home.

Parents may choose a private babysitters or nannies to come into their home to offer personal attention to their child. Family day care centers provide child care for small groups of children, and often parents take turns providing child care in this type of setting. *Day care centers* offer structured play and rest activities for groups of children who are supervised by professional staff. Some employers offer day care within the workplace as a service to their employees. *Preschool centers* offer structured activities that foster growth and development and teach coping skills. A good preschool program can help a child gain self-confidence and positive self-esteem. Parents may be offered the following suggestions to help them select a facility that will best meet the needs of their child:

- State licensing agencies offer lists of local day care centers and preschools.
- The school or center should meet accreditation standards set by the National Association for Education of Young Children.
- Staff should have school preparation in early childhood education.
- Student-to-staff ratios should be established with clear limits.
- Techniques of discipline, philosophy of care or education, safety, and sanitary conditions of the environment should be reviewed.
- Facilities for snacks and rest should be reviewed.
- Health history requirements for children should be reviewed.
- Toys and facilities for indoor and outdoor play should be reviewed.
- Parents should visit the school and should observe staff–child interactions.
- Parents can speak to parents of other children in the school to evaluate their input and opinions.

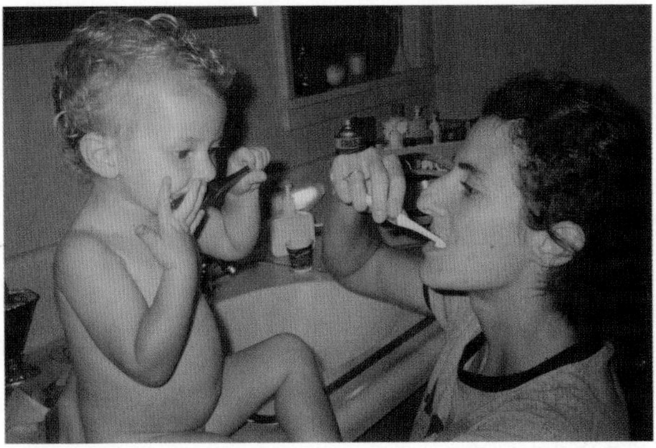

Figure 8-7 The child imitates the mother and brushes her own teeth. The child also "helps" brush the mother's teeth in this nightly ritual.

TEACHING TECHNIQUES

When parents respond to the words of a toddler appropriately, they stimulate the development of positive communication. The use of picture books at regular interactive reading sessions with the toddler also aids in language development. Parents should not demand correct speech of a 2-year-old, and accurate pronunciation should not be a major focus. If speech difficulties are associated with other oral problems, such as the inability to blow a kiss or to eat, medical evaluation should be sought.

Parents can be taught methods for helping the preschooler to express feelings through words such as "You feel angry now, and I understand." Teaching the preschooler how to express feelings verbally rather than by acting out is a key to positive social development. Preschool children who are learning to be autonomous often rapidly shift between dependence and independence, joy and rage, and this changing behavior can cause parents to feel frustrated and inadequate. Parents need to be counseled concerning the normal development and behavior of the toddler and preschool child.

The child should be introduced to the dentist by age 1 (AAPD, 2011), and a soft toothbrush should be used twice daily to maintain oral health. Parents can often model behavior that they wish their child to imitate. For example, regular toothbrushing with toothpaste should be a routine by age 2, and regular professional dental checkups should be initiated (Figure 8-7).

The behaviors of the child and the responses of the parent should be discussed at well-child visits. When a parent does not offer any positive statements about his or her child, and the child misbehaves in preschool and at home, more detailed assessment may be necessary.

Safety and Accident Prevention

Accidents are a major threat during the early childhood years. Young children play hard and have little understanding of the potential dangers around them.

Safety Alert

- Parents may need guidance concerning the need to childproof the house, to keep stairways safe, and to avoid clutter.
- Toys should be sturdy and age appropriate without sharp edges.
- Preschoolers should not be allowed to carry breakable items or sharp objects.
- The appropriate use of car seats is essential (Figure 8-8).
- A child should not sit in the front seat of a car until older than 13 years of age (AAP, 2012).
- Children should not be left inside cars alone.
- Pot handles should not overhang the edge of stovetops, because accidental burns are common dangers in the home.
- Medicines should have childproof bottle caps and should not be left within the sight or reach of a young child.
- Preschool children can be taught the dangers of talking with strangers and should know where to go if a parent or sitter is not in sight.
- Accident prevention techniques should be discussed at every well-child visit (Table 8-5).
- The use of dishes that have a high lead content should be avoided as lead can seep into the food and cause lead toxicity that can impair growth and development.

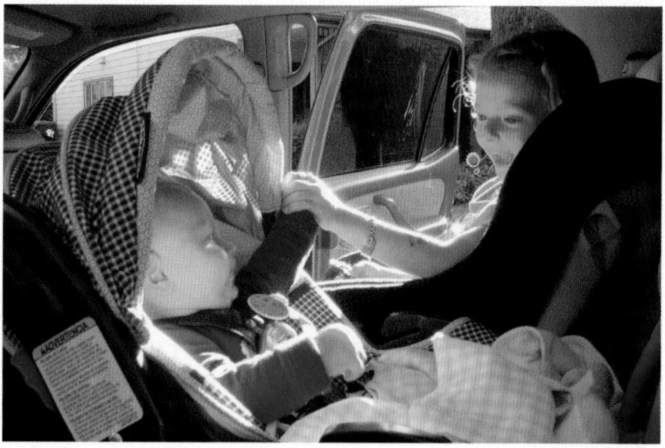

Figure 8-8 An older child, in a front-facing car seat, entertains the infant in a rear-facing car seat. The infant who is less than 2 years of age or weighs less than 35 pounds is secured in a rear-facing car seat behind the driver in the car's back seat to prevent the large and heavy head from falling forward and obstructing the airway when the car stops suddenly or in case of an accident. The driver can look through the car's rearview mirror toward a mirror mounted on the rear window to see the face of the infant. A child of more than 35–40 pounds is secured in a front-facing car seat in the center of the car's back seat. An older child should use a booster seat until (1) the vehicle safety belt fits properly flat across the chest, (2) the lap belt fits low and snug across the thighs, and (3) the child can sit firmly against the seatback with the legs bent at the knees over the seat edge. A child should not sit in the front seat of a car until over 13 years of age.

TABLE 8-5 How to Prevent Hazards Caused by the Behavioral Characteristics of Toddlers

Behavioral Characteristics	Hazard and Prevention Strategies*
AUTOMOBILE	
Impulsive, unable to delay gratification, increased mobility, egocentric	Teach child safety rules of the street. Teach child the meaning of red, yellow, and green traffic lights. Caution child not to run from behind parked cars or snow banks. Use car-seat restraints appropriately. Hold toddler's hand when crossing street. Supervise tricycle riding. Do not allow child to play in car alone. Driver must look carefully in front and behind vehicles before accelerating. Teach child safe areas in and around house. Supervise child younger than 3 years at all times.
BURNS	
Fascination with fire Toddler can reach articles by climbing, pokes fingers in holes and openings; can open doors and drawers; is unaware of cause and effect	Teach child the meaning of "hot" (e.g., allow child to touch sun-warmed beach sand). Put matches, cigarettes, candles, and incense out of reach and sight. Turn handles of cooking pots toward back of stove. Beware of hot coffee; avoid overhanging tablecloths. Keep appliances such as coffee pots, electric frying pans, and food processors and their cords out of reach. Test food and fluids heated in microwave ovens to ensure that center is not too hot. Beware of hot charcoal grills. Use snug fireplace screens. Mark children's room locations to alert firefighters in emergency. Keep a pressure-type fire extinguisher available, and teach all family members who are old enough how to use it. Practice what to do in case of home fire. Install smoke detectors. Cover electrical outlets with protective caps. Check bathwater temperature before placing child in water. Do not allow child to handle water faucets. Protect child from sun with sunscreen and clothing.
FALLS	
Exploring different parts of house; can open doors and lean out open windows; toddlers' depth perception immature	Teach children how to go up and down stairs when they show readiness for these tasks. Fasten crib sides securely and leave them up when child is in crib. Use side rails on large beds when child graduates from crib.

*In every situation, keep first-aid chart and emergency numbers handy. Know location of and how to get to nearest emergency facility.

(Continued)

TABLE 8-5 How to Prevent Hazards Caused by the Behavioral Characteristics of Toddlers—cont'd

Behavioral Characteristics	Hazard and Prevention Strategies*
FALLS (cont'd)	
Capabilities change quickly; may seem grown up at times, but still requires constant supervision at home and on playground	Lock basement doors or use gates at top and bottom of stairs. Mop spilled liquids from floor immediately. Use window guards. Use car-seat restraints appropriately. Keep scissors and other sharp objects away from toddler's reach. Use childproof doorknobs and drawer closures. Secure child in shopping cart at store. Supervise when child is climbing in playground. Clothing and shoelaces should be appropriate to prevent tripping.
SUFFOCATION AND CHOKING	
Explores with senses, likes to bite on and taste things Eats on the run	Do not allow small children to play with deflated balloons, which can be sucked into windpipe. Inspect toys for small or loose parts. Remove small objects such as coins, buttons, and pins from reach. Avoid popcorn, nuts, small hard candies, chewing gum, or large chunks of meat, such as hot dogs. Debone fish, chicken. Learn Heimlich maneuver. Inspect width of crib and playpen slats. Keep plastic bags away from small children; do not use as mattress covers. If child is vomiting, turn him or her on side. Avoid nightclothes with drawstring necks. Discard old refrigerators and appliances or remove doors.
POISONING	
Ingenuity increases, can open most containers Increased mobility provides access to cupboards, medicine cabinets, bedside stands, interiors of closets Looks at and touches everything	Store household detergents and cleaning supplies out of reach in a locked cabinet. Do not put chemicals or other potentially harmful substances into food or beverage containers. Keep medicines in locked cabinets; put them away immediately after use. Use child-resistant caps and packaging. Discard unused/expired medicine appropriately. Follow physician's directions when administering medication. Do not refer to pills as "candy." Explain poison symbols to child and to parents not fluent in English.

TABLE 8-5 How to Prevent Hazards Caused by the Behavioral Characteristics of Toddlers—cont'd

Behavioral Characteristics	Hazard and Prevention Strategies*
Learns by trial and error Puts objects in mouth	Keep telephone number of poison-control center available. When painting, use paint marked "for indoor use" or one that conforms to standards for use on surfaces that may be chewed by children. Wash fruits and vegetables before eating. Obtain and record name of any new plant purchased. Alert family of location and appearance of poisonous plants on or around property or commonly encountered when camping. Use childproof locks on cabinets. Use dishes that do not have high lead content.
DROWNING	
Lacks depth perception Does not realize danger Loves water play	Watch child continuously while at beach or near a pool. Empty wading pools when child has finished playing. Cover wells securely. Wear recommended life jackets in boats. Begin teaching water safety and swimming skills early. Lock fences surrounding swimming pools. Supervise tub baths; be aware that a young child can drown in a small amount of water.
ELECTRIC SHOCK	
Pokes and probes with fingers	Cover electrical outlets. Cap unused sockets with safety plugs. Water conducts electricity; teach child not to touch electrical appliances when wet; keep appliances out of reach. Keep electrical appliances away from tub and sink areas.
ANIMAL BITES	
Immature judgment	Teach child to avoid stray animals. Do not allow toddler to abuse household pets. Supervise closely.
SAFETY	
Easily distracted Trusting of others Falls frequently	Teach toddler safety related to strangers. Do not personalize clothes. Do not allow toddler to eat or suck lollipops while running or playing. Keep sharp-edged objects out of reach. Keep sharp-edged furniture out of play areas.

Modified from Leifer G: *Introduction to maternity & pediatric nursing*, ed 6, Philadelphia, 2011, W.B. Saunders.

Immunizations

Immunity is defined as the body's resistance to disease-causing organisms. Newborns have immunity protection transferred via the placenta from the mother, but this immunity lasts for only a few months. In infants and young children, the immune system is immature and the child is vulnerable to life-threatening infections. After discharge from the hospital nursery, an active immunization program starts at 2 months, when the child is capable of producing his or her own antibodies.

Health Promotion

The recommended American Academy of Pediatrics (AAP) immunization schedule for infants and children is listed in Appendix A.

Sometimes teaching a preschooler about health issues requires the child's' participation, interaction, or cooperation. A preschool child knows that a pin or needle stuck into a balloon will pop the balloon. Therefore it is no surprise that children fear that a pin (or needle) stuck into their arm or leg will cause their body to pop or explode too. One possible approach to relieve this fear is to allow the child to handle the syringe (without the needle) and to administer pretend injections to a doll. The immediate presence of a calm, reassuring parent who is holding the child in a firm hug will assuage fear and anxiety better than any verbal explanation or reassurance.

When teaching parents, it is important to develop a partnership with them and to understand their values so that anticipatory guidance can be provided. The nurse can offer tools to the parents to help them manage their child's behavior, including an explanation of the ongoing developmental process.

KEY POINTS

- The early childhood period is between 1 and 6 years of age and is separated into the toddler phase and the preschool phase.
- Tasks to be mastered during early childhood include understanding and speaking words, social interaction, mastery of self-control in feeding and toileting, and beginning to develop a self concept and a sense of autonomy.
- Toilet training occurs as sphincter control develops and the child masters basic communication skills to indicate the need to use the toilet. Complete bowel and bladder control is typically complete by age 2 ½ to 3 years.
- Adequate nutrition is essential for optimum physical and mental development.
- A 2-year-old child exhibits negativistic behavior and tantrums because of frustrations and struggles for independence.
- Preschool thinking involves Piaget's preoperational or prelogical characteristics.
- A 2-year-old cannot distinguish between intentional acts and mistakes.
- Impulse control is typically achieved by age 4.
- A 3-year-old is ritualistic and feels all rules must be obeyed.

- According to Kohlberg, the preconventional stage of moral development begins during the preschool age. (2 - 6 years)
- Discipline should have as its purpose the guiding, teaching, or correcting of behavior rather than punishment.
- Toddlers and preschoolers do not completely understand the rights of others.
- According to Freud, a conscience begins to develop in the preschool phase, and children begin then to understand how their behavior affects others.
- Age-appropriate, daily, moderate and vigorous physical activities are important to maintain the health of children.
- Children should be kept well hydrated by offering water before, during, and after exercise.
- Sports-appropriate protective equipment should be worn by children to prevent injuries.
- Play is an important part of a child's life. Appropriate toys can promote growth and development.
- Twenty primary teeth erupt by age 2. Half the adult height is reached by age 2, and the birth weight quadruples as well.
- The preschool child can more easily learn more than one language when the different languages are used in the home.
- Language milestones can be used to assess the child's development.
- In a preschool child, the number or words in a typical sentence is equal to the child's age in years.
- A preschool child learns socially acceptable behavior by positive reinforcement.
- Time-outs should last 1 minute per year of age.
- A 2-year-old exhibits parallel play, whereas a 3-year-old engages in cooperative play with groups using a high level of imagination.
- Parents who hold, hug, and rock their children can influence the ability of the child to establish intimate relationships later in life.
- Accident prevention techniques should be discussed with parents.
- An active immunization program schedule starts at 2 months and continues through the preschool years. Many communicable diseases in childhood can be prevented through immunization.

Critical Thinking

When discussing disciplinary techniques for children, the health-care worker can help parents develop a plan that is mutually agreeable. Discuss three appropriate types of disciplinary techniques that can be used consistently and safely for the early childhood years. List examples of how these techniques can be implemented.

REVIEW QUESTIONS

1. Tasks to be mastered during early childhood include:
   a. walking.
   b. bowel control.
   c. abstract thinking.
   d. visual maturity.

2. The toddler-age child is in Erikson's stage of:
   a. trust versus mistrust.
   b. initiative versus guilt.
   c. autonomy versus shame and doubt.
   d. identity versus role confusion.

3. The preschool-age child, between 4 and 6 years of age, is in Erikson's stage of:
   a. trust versus mistrust.
   b. initiative versus guilt.
   c. autonomy versus shame and doubt.
   d. identity versus role confusion.

4. Between 12 and 24 months of age, the child's speech normally includes:
   a. only vowel sounds.
   b. both vowels and consonants.
   c. frequent babbling.
   d. three- to four-word sentences.

5. In early childhood the best disciplinary technique includes:
   a. rewarding good behavior.
   b. punishing bad behavior.
   c. setting rigid, structured rules.
   d. posting rules on the refrigerator door.

CHAPTER 9

Middle Childhood

http://evolve.elsevier.com/Leifer/growth

OBJECTIVES

1. Define middle childhood.
2. Describe the physiological changes that occur in middle childhood.
3. Describe the cognitive development that occurs in middle childhood and its effect on the development of learning styles.
4. Discuss the psychosocial development that occurs in middle childhood.
5. List at least three ways in which Erikson's task of industry can be fostered in middle childhood.
6. Trace the development of moral behavior in the school-age child.
7. Discuss the discipline techniques that are effective in middle childhood.
8. Describe the typical play activities of the school-age child.
9. Discuss the use of intelligence testing for school-age children.
10. Discuss the role of peer groups in the growth and development during middle childhood.
11. Discuss the sexual development of and education appropriate for school-age children.
12. Describe the role of daily physical activity in nurturing growth and development and in preventing illness in later life.
13. List the major health-teaching needs of school-age children.

KEY TERMS

cognitive style
corporal punishment
discipline
latchkey children
middle childhood
mnemonic technique
moral behaviors
moral reasoning
plaque
social cognition

DEFINITION

Middle childhood includes children between the ages of 6 and 12 years. School-age children, between 6 and 12 years, differ from preschoolers, because they focus more on fact rather than fantasy. School-age children interact with teachers and others outside the family who will have a significant impact on their growth, development, and education. One of the major developmental tasks of this age group is forming positive self-esteem from internal sources rather than depending solely on feedback from elders for self-esteem. The ability to develop close peer relationships will affect the development of new ideas, skills, and tools that will enhance the child's advancement toward maturity. Other developmental tasks include changing from concrete thinking to abstract thinking, developing secondary sex characteristics, and accepting more responsibility.

PHYSIOLOGICAL CHANGES

Myelinization of the brain is complete by age 7, and by age 12 the head has reached its adult size. The bones continue to ossify and grow, and the body develops a lower center of gravity than in preschool years, due in part to a shift in posture and an increase in leg length. Physical growth is slow during the school-age years until a growth spurt occurs just before puberty. The average weight gain is 5.5 to 7 pounds (2.5 to 3.2 kg) per year, and the average height increase per year is about 2 inches (5 cm). Children who are taller than their peers may face an extra challenge, because they are likely to be treated as if they are older or more mature. The self concept may suffer if the tall child does not live up to these inflated expectations.

The loss of primary teeth begins at about age 6; the lower central incisor is normally the first tooth to be lost (Figure 9-1). Parents often treat the loss of primary teeth as a sign that the child is growing up, and many parents reward the child whenever a tooth falls out. About four permanent teeth erupt each year in the same order as deciduous teeth (see Chapter 7). Regular dental checkups should be a part of routine health care to screen for dental problems and to have the teeth cleaned. Daily dental care should include tooth brushing with a fluoride toothpaste in the morning, after each meal, and before bedtime (AAPD, 2011). Limiting intake of sticky sweets and chocolates, and encouraging snacks such as apples, raw carrots, and sugarless gum, can reduce plaque formation. Plaque is a sticky, transparent mass of bacteria that grows on the surfaces of teeth and spreads to the roots. Plaque buildup can be prevented by regular tooth brushing and flossing. Flossing between teeth can be modeled by parents and can be quickly learned by the school-age child.

The gastrointestinal tract of the school-age child is more mature than that of the preschooler, and stomach capacity increases. The school-age child requires less caloric intake than the preschooler, and the older child usually snacks less. Preferences for specific foods develop. Sensory organs mature and sharpen the senses of taste, smell, and touch. Large-print books are no longer necessary, because visual maturity is achieved sometime between preschool age and age 6.

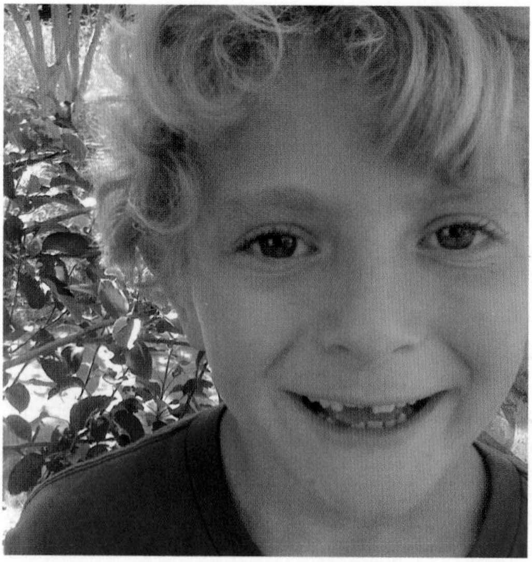

Figure 9-1 One of the most obvious physical changes of middle childhood is the loss of the primary teeth. The loss of primary teeth begins at age 6, and about four permanent teeth erupt each year.

Newly developed fine and gross motor skills enhance school-age children's ability to play independently. Age-appropriate toys include bicycles, skates, swimming gear, and jump ropes. School-age children master coordination and control, allowing them to enjoy team sports such as baseball, play a musical instrument, or tap dance. Excess time spent with computer games and video games may contribute to a sedentary lifestyle and may increase the risk of obesity or health problems in later life. Childhood obesity also carries a risk of negatively affecting the child's self-image and social development.

Exercise and Play

Children between the ages of 5 and 7 engage in rough-and-tumble play. After age 7, children are able to engage in competitive play and use coping strategies to handle team cooperation, conflict, losing, and winning. Competition is often a welcome challenge. Participation in organized sports can develop teamwork and physical fitness (Figure 9-2). High stress and excessive pressure to win are not helpful and should be avoided. In team sports, all children should be encouraged to participate without excluding those who are less physically talented.

School-age children need daily physical activity for the same reasons that young children do: to build strength, endurance, and coordination; to slow the development of coronary risk factors; and to build a foundation of healthy lifestyle habits. Exercise in

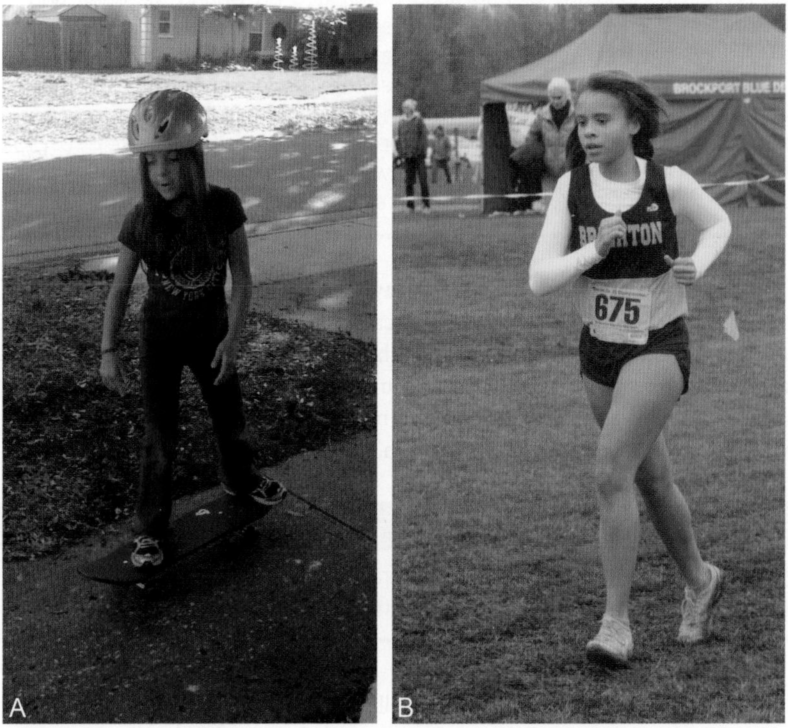

Figure 9-2 Active play **(A)** and competitive play **(B)** are enjoyed by this age group and should be encouraged. Local teams in cross-country running are often partnered with national teams where the child can earn a medal for performance.

childhood also promotes a healthy body composition and bone mass. Additionally, academic achievement has been linked to vigorous physical activity in children.

School-age children should continue to engage in 60 minutes of moderate to vigorous levels of physical activity daily. Organized team sports can contribute to meeting the guidelines as well as contribute to the psychosocial development of the child through increased confidence, focus, and respect for authority. Moderate intensity exercises appropriate for children include hiking, skateboarding, rollerblading, and bicycle riding. Vigorous activities can include running games (such as tag), jumping rope, soccer, basketball, and swimming. Tug-of-war, rope or tree climbing, push-ups, swinging on monkey bars, hopscotch, and jumping rope are all examples of appropriate muscle and bone strengthening exercises for children. A summary of growth and development, nutrition, play, and safety are reviewed in Table 9-1.

Asthma is a common childhood health problem. Symptoms of exercise-induced asthma usually occur 5 to 10 minutes after vigorous exercise that involves rapid mouth breathing of large volumes of cool dry air. Warming the air by breathing through the nose or by covering the mouth with a scarf, and practicing muscle relaxation and diaphragmatic breathing, can decrease hyperventilation and can prevent asthmatic attacks. Swimming, gymnastics, baseball, and weight lifting are preferred sports for asthmatics. Physical activity for asthmatics should not be restricted, because sports and exercise are important for all children.

Health Promotion

The American Academy of Pediatrics Committee on Sports Medicine and School Health recommends teaching motor skills and fitness exercises in the school setting to develop skills and to promote positive attitudes toward exercise, which may lead to a positive lifelong health and fitness philosophy. The focus should be on mastery and enjoyment rather than only on winning. The assignment of the extra running of laps or extra exercise as punishment promotes negative attitudes toward exercise. Protective accessories should be worn by children who engage in high-impact sports, such as football, to prevent injury to the immature skeletal system.

Activities, such as collecting things or playing board games, are often enjoyed by the school-age child. Computer or video games can help develop hand–eye coordination and can challenge intellect. These games are healthy outlets as long as they do not replace daily physical activity. Creativity should be encouraged, because it helps to develop general thinking and problem-solving skills. Art and music lessons, appropriately encouraged, can help to develop lifelong interests, appreciation, and talents in the child.

Health Promotion

Many schools have physical-fitness programs that promote healthy lifestyles consistent with the goals of *Healthy People 2020.*

Eight-year-olds take pride in mastering skills and in showing off their accomplishments. By age 9 or 10, physical strength is greatly increased and interest in specific sports or other activities develops. Increased understanding of rules and teamwork enable these children to

(Text continued on p. 140.)

TABLE 9-1 Summary of Growth and Development and Health Maintenance of School-Age Children

Age (Years)	Physiological Growth	Intellectual Competency	Emotional–Social Competency	Nutrition	Play	Safety
General: 6 to 12 years	Gains an average of 2.5 to 3.2 kg/yr (5.0 to 7.0 lb/yr). Has overall height gains of 5.0 cm/yr (2 in/yr); growth occurs in spurts and mainly in the trunk and extremities. Loses deciduous teeth; most permanent teeth erupt. Progressively more coordinated in both gross and fine motor skills. Caloric needs increase during growth spurts.	Masters concrete operations. Moves from egocentrism; learns that he/she is not always right. Learns grammar and expression of emotions and thoughts. Vocabulary increases to 3000 words or more. Handles complex sentences.	Central crisis; industry vs. inferiority; wants to do and make things. Progressive sex education needed. Wants to be like friends; competition is important. Fears body mutilation, alterations in body image; earlier phobias may recur; nightmares; fear of death. Nervous habits are common.	Fluctuations in appetite because of uneven growth pattern and tendency to become more involved in activities. Tendency to neglect breakfast in rush to get to school. Although lunch is provided in most schools, child does not always eat it.	Plays in groups, mostly of same sex; gang activities predominate. Enjoys reading age-appropriate books. Bicycles important. Sports equipment, cards, board and table games. Most play is active games requiring little or no equipment.	Enforce continued use of seat belts during car travel. Bicycle safety must be taught and enforced. Teach safety related to hobbies, handicrafts, mechanical equipment.

(Continued)

TABLE 9-1 Summary of Growth and Development and Health Maintenance of School-Age Children—cont'd

Age (Years)	Physiological Growth	Intellectual Competency	Emotional–Social Competency	Nutrition	Play	Safety
6 to 7 years	Gross motor skills exceed fine motor coordination. Has good balance and rhythm—runs, skips, jumps, climbs, gallops. Throws and catches ball. Dresses self with little or no help.	Has vocabulary of 2500 words. Learns to read and print. Begins concrete concepts of numbers, general classifications of items. Knows concepts of right and left; morning, afternoon, and evening; coinage. Has intuitive thought process. Is verbally aggressive, bossy, opinionated, argumentative. Likes simple games with basic rules.	Boisterous, outgoing, and a know-it-all. Whiny; parents should sidestep power struggles, offer choices. Becomes quiet and reflective during seventh year; very sensitive. Can use telephone. Likes to make things; starts many projects, finishes few. Adults should give some responsibility for household duties.	Persistence of preschool food dislikes. Tendency for deficiencies in iron, vitamin A, and riboflavin. 100 mL/kg of water per day, 3 g/kg protein daily needed.	Still enjoys dolls, cars, and trucks. Plays well alone but enjoys small groups of both sexes; begins to prefer same-sex peers during seventh year. Ready to learn how to ride a bicycle. Prefers imaginary, dramatic play with real costumes. Begins collecting items for quantity, not quality. Enjoys active games such as hide-and-seek, tag, jumping rope, in-line skating, soccer.	Teach and reinforce traffic safety. Child needs adult supervision of play. Teach child to avoid strangers and never to take anything from strangers. Teach illness prevention and reinforce continued practice of other health habits. Restrict bicycle use to home ground and no traffic areas; teach bicycle safety. Child should wear helmet. Teach and set examples about harmful use of drugs, alcohol, and smoking.

8 to 10 years	Myopia may appear. Secondary sex characteristics begin in girls. Hand–eye coordination and fine motor skills are well established. Movements are graceful, coordinated. Cares for own physical needs completely; is constantly on the move; plays and works hard.	Learning correct grammar and expression of feelings in words. Likes books he/she can read alone; will read funny papers and scan newspaper. Enjoys making detailed drawings. Mastering, classification, serialization, spatial, temporal, and numerical concepts. Uses language as an effective communication tool; likes riddles, jokes, word games. Rules are a guiding force in life now.	Strong preference for same-sex peers. Antagonizes opposite-sex peers. Self-assured and pragmatic at home; questions parental values and ideas. Has a strong sense of humor. Enjoys clubs, group projects, outings, large groups, camp. Modesty about own body increases over time; sex conscious. Works diligently to perfect the skills he/she does best.	Needs about 2100 calories/day; nutritious snacks. Tends to be too busy to bother to eat. Tendency for deficiencies in calcium, iron, and thiamine. Problem of obesity may begin now. Has good table manners. Able to help with food preparation.	Ready for lessons in dancing, gymnastics, music. Restrict television time to 1 to 2 hours daily. Enjoys hiking, sports. Enjoys cooking, woodworking, crafts. Enjoys cards and table games. Likes radio and music. Begins qualitative collecting.	Stress safety with firearms. Keep them out of reach and allow their use only with adult supervision. Know who the child's friends are; parents should still have some control over friend selection. Teach water safety; swimming should be supervised by an adult. Enforce balance in rest and activity.

(Continued)

TABLE 9-1 Summary of Growth and Development and Health Maintenance of School-Age Children—cont'd

Age (Years)	Physiological Growth	Intellectual Competency	Emotional–Social Competency	Nutrition	Play	Safety
8 to 10 years (cont'd)		Very interested in what things are and how they work, such as weather, seasons, and the like.	Happy, cooperative, relaxed, and casual in relationships. Increasingly courteous and well mannered with adults. Gang stage at a peak; secret codes and rituals prevail. Responds better to suggestion than to dictatorial approach.			
11 to 12 years	Vital signs approximate adult norms. Growth spurt for girls.	Able to think about social problems and prejudices; sees others' points of view. Enjoys reading mysteries or love stories.	Intense team loyalty; boys begin teasing girls, and girls flirt with boys.	Male needs 2500 calories/day; female needs 2250 (70 calories/kg/day); both need 75 mL/kg of water/day and 2 g/kg protein daily.	Enjoys projects and working with hands. Likes to do errands and jobs to earn money.	Continue monitoring friends.

	Differences between sexes increasingly noticeable, with boys having greater physical strength. Eruption of permanent teeth complete except for third molars. Secondary sex characteristics begin in boys. Menstruation may begin.	Begins considering abstract ideas. Interested in the reasons for health measures and understands human reproduction. Very moralistic; religious commitment often made during this time.	Wants unreasonable independence; is rebellious about routines; has wide mood swings; needs some time daily for privacy. Very critical of own work. Hero worship prevails. Facts-of-life chats with friends prevail. Masturbation increases. Appears under constant tension.		Very involved in sports, dancing, talking/texting on phone. Enjoys all aspects of acting and drama.	Stress bicycle and in-line skate safety on streets and in traffic and the use of helmets and other protective gear.

Adapted from Betz C, Hunsberger M, Wright S: *Family centered nursing care of children*, ed 2, Philadelphia, 1994, Saunders.

participate in competitive games. School-age children often compare themselves with one another according to their ability to master good grades or to excel at sports. This tendency to compare affects the development of children's self-esteem. Maintaining optimum nutrition and preventing injury are two additional health challenges that exist during the school-age years.

COGNITIVE DEVELOPMENT

According to Piaget, school-age children are concrete thinkers. They think logically and understand rules, although they learn best when they can see and handle objects. Hands-on learning is the most effective educational method for school-age children. Table 9-2 lists

TABLE 9-2 Mastery of Tasks Necessary for School Success

Child's Tasks	Parent's Tasks	Interventions
Adapt to differences in expectations of various teachers.	Communicate with teacher to maintain consistency in expectations and discipline.	School nurse can be contacted to facilitate parent–teacher–child interaction.
Compete with 30 or more peers for adult attention.	Praise child's accomplishments. Avoid comparisons to other children.	Observe parent–teacher interactions and provide guidance and positive support.
Learn to accept criticism from peers and teachers without losing self-esteem.	Supervise peer activities. Facilitate constructive communication.	Provide teacher–parent guidance. Teach constructive and positive feedback.
Assimilate peer values with family values.	Maintain open communication. Encourage peer activity. Introduce and accept other cultures in community.	Provide anticipatory guidance in handling behavior problems. Observe and address signs of prejudice.
Find satisfaction in school achievements.	Help children to achieve. Do not complete tasks for them.	Provide suggestions for identifying strengths and weaknesses. Build on strengths.
Participate in group activities.	Encourage child to join a group or club and actively participate as a member.	Refer to community agencies such as churches, organizations, and club activities as needed.
Learn behavioral self-control. Cope with negative treatment from others in a constructive way.	Encourage participation in activities away from home and with peers. Help build faith in child's problem-solving skills. Discuss coping with prejudices.	Encourage parents to let go and to provide guidance while encouraging independence.

Modified from Leifer G: *Introduction to maternity & pediatric nursing*, ed 6, Philadelphia, 2011, Saunders.

TABLE 9-3 Cognitive Deficits and Their Effect on School Performance

Deficit	Related School Problem
Inability to understand spatial relationships by visual examination.	Repeatedly confuse letters b, d, and g. Difficulty with basic reading and writing.
Difficulty in sensing body position and in programming movements.	Poor handwriting; tight grasp of pencil.
Inability to decipher similar sounding words.	Difficulty following directions, leading to short attention span and behavior problems.
Difficulty with long-term memory and recall.	Delayed mastery of counting and alphabet recital.
Easily distracted.	Difficulty following complex instructions.
Difficulty remembering items in order.	Difficulty in organizing assignments and planning completion.
Difficulty in receptive language.	Difficulty in following directions; attention cannot remain focused.
Impaired expressive language.	Difficulty with recall memory. Difficulty expressing feelings or talking spontaneously in a group setting.

Modified from Kleigman R, Stanton B, St. Geme J, Schor N, Behrmann R: *Nelson's textbook of pediatrics*, ed 19, Philadelphia, 2011, Saunders.

mastery of tasks and behaviors necessary for success in school and also lists the related parental guidance that can be offered. Cognitive deficits must be assessed early so that the child can be successful in school (Table 9-3).

Erikson refers to the school age as the stage of industry. In this stage, the child develops a thirst for knowledge and a desire to master skills and to emulate role models or heroes. If a parent intrudes on children's efforts at achieving a skill—perhaps by helping too much or by doing the task for the child—a sense of inferiority can develop in the child's mind. Even if children receive an excellent grade for a project, they may not attain a sense of industry if *they* know the work was not really the result of their own efforts.

School-age children can group similar items together and can understand that words have more than one meaning. Children may delight in telling jokes to one another, and they may tell jokes to entertain friends or to tease adults.

By age 7, egocentrism decreases. Children realize others may have valid opinions that differ from their own, and they may seek another person's opinion concerning an issue. With a decrease in egocentrism, children become more cooperative and begin to understand how their actions may affect other people. This understanding, called social cognition, enables children to interact better with peers and can enhance their self concept.

The development of moral reasoning happens as the child learns to understand rules and to determine if an action is right or wrong. Moral behaviors are actions based on moral reasoning. In early childhood, rules are important. A 5-year-old child may show intense frustration if a peer breaks a rule. In later childhood, the 10-year-old may enjoy making his or her own rules for a game or bartering to change the rules.

BOX 9-1 Moral Behavior Includes Three Phases

1. Knowledge (logic) – Knowing what is right
2. Emotion – Feeling good or bad about what is right
3. Action (behavior) – Behaving according to the rule of what is right

Culture or an environment such as poverty or war can influence moral behavior. Knowing what is culturally or morally right does not guarantee acting in accordance with that knowledge. Lying, stealing, and cheating behaviors are common in school-age children even as they learn moral behavior. Therefore adult modeling of honesty and fairness is essential as the child is learning moral behavior (Box 9-1).

Lawrence Kohlberg was a theorist who suggested that moral reasoning develops as cognitive function matures (see Chapter 5), so the ability to think logically is related to moral behavior. Other theorists emphasize that moral behavior is learned through positive reinforcement. Parents teach by rewarding desired behavior. Punishment for undesirable behavior is less effective. Punished children may feel less motivated, less capable, or confused, or may focus on the punishment and its emotional consequences rather than the behavior. In addition to using reward or punishment in guiding children's learning, modeling how a child's actions may affect others is also helpful in developing moral behavior.

Cognitive Styles

A school-age child must have an attention span of 45 minutes to process information, encode it into memory, and retrieve or remember it later. Children approach learning and problem solving in various ways. A cognitive style refers to a pattern of thought and reasoning. Some children take a cluster of knowledge and group it in a certain way to better remember the information. Some use mnemonic techniques, such as the rhyme for remembering the number of days in each month of the year.

The elementary-school curriculum is designed to increase cognitive demands gradually for students. The first 2 years of elementary school focus on learning to read, write, and do basic math. By the fourth grade, the volume and complexity of the work increases. If basic skills were not learned well, the child might not progress smoothly. Other factors that affect success in school include the child's desire to please teachers and parents, to compete with other children, to work for delayed rewards, and to take risks by trying new things. Feelings of success encourage the child to continue making efforts. Feelings of failure may lead to avoidance of risks or low self-confidence.

Communication Skills

School-age children are usually able to express themselves verbally, and they often use language as an effective communication tool in their relationships with others. They can tell jokes that tease and express sarcasm. Adults should offer a model of clear and appropriate language use. A child who has a language or other communication problem is at risk for social isolation and underachievement in school.

Cultural Considerations

Bilingual education programs are offered to school-age children who speak English as their second language. However, if the teachers are not proficient in the child's primary language, the child may have to learn English by a total immersion technique, which means the child learns the language by hearing it used every day in the classroom. This may add stress socially, academically, and emotionally. It is important that schools offer support programs for bilingual or language-impaired children to reduce stress and associated behavior problems such as frustration, anger, and rebellion.

Intelligence Tests

The original version of the Stanford-Binet intelligence quotient (IQ) test was published in France in 1905 and was then brought to the United States. This test assesses the mental capabilities of the child and compares set norms or expectations for each age. To determine a score, the mental age is divided by the actual age in years, and the total is then multiplied by 100. For example, if a child performs on tests at a level expected for a 10-year-old, and the actual age in years of the child is 10, the IQ score would be $10/10 \times 100 = 100$.

David Wechsler developed the Wechsler Intelligence Scale for school-age children and adolescents ages 6 to 16 (WISC-III, 1991) and the Wechsler Preschool and Primary Scale of Intelligence (WPPSI-III, 1989) for 3- to 7-year-olds. Both assess verbal and nonverbal intelligence. The tests are not meant to be an overall test of general intelligence, but they can be used to predict school performance and to identify children who may need extra help or additional challenges. The test should be administered to each child by a licensed psychologist.

PSYCHOSOCIAL DEVELOPMENT

Task of Industry

Erikson believed the primary task for school-age children was to develop a sense of industry. A child can gain satisfaction from achieving even small goals. Praise is essential in this stage of development to build motivation to learn and achieve. Seven-year-olds may not have the attention span necessary to complete complex tasks. Nine-year-olds can usually work on a task to completion. By age 11, children are usually able to maintain work and motivation for a delayed reward. A child who does not receive praise for achievements may feel inferior.

Peer Relationships

School-age children begin to compare family values with the values of others. Friendships with same-sex peers are very important for the school-age child. The reliance on and importance of the family can decrease, and sibling rivalry can cause some chaotic episodes. The child may become self-conscious about kisses and hugs from parents in public. Children who have difficulty separating from family and adjusting to school may be responding to the parents' difficulty in letting them go. Divorces, family violence, and other home problems can interfere with a child's achievement of age-appropriate developmental tasks with peers. The school-age child can develop close relationships with friends and share precious toys and innermost thoughts and secrets with them.

School-age children protect their possessions, value privacy, and should be given the responsibility of managing chores and money. However, allowances and family chores work best when kept separate from one another. Regular home chores help children gain a sense of responsibility and achieve a feeling that they are a member of a family group.

The home, the school, and the neighborhood each have an impact on the growth and development of the child. The culture of a school-age child involves memberships in groups of some kind. If parents do not find a socially acceptable group, such as Scouts or a religious group, children may find their own group—for example, a gang—and may be influenced by that group to engage in socially unacceptable behavior to gain acceptance and to achieve a sense of belonging. Conformity to most groups is rewarding and enables social success with peers. When a child is labeled or is outcast by a peer, the identification may remain with the child and may be incorporated into his or her self-image.

Latchkey Children

Latchkey children are those who are left unsupervised after school, because both parents work, and members of the extended family are not available to care for the children. Some children who are left alone at home enjoy the independence and develop maturity and problem-solving skills. Other children are at higher risk for feeling isolated and may be at an increased risk for accidents or getting into trouble. A backup adult should be available in case of an emergency.

After-school programs with supervised activities may be available in some communities, and these programs can help the school-age child maintain contact and interaction with peer groups (Box 9-2).

Sexuality

According to Freud, the child is in a period of sexual latency during the middle childhood years, and children often identify with same-sex parents. Both the family and the school can influence gender identity. Unisex play and clothes are available, but many families tend to dress boys and girls in traditional male or female styles and colors. Toys can also be gender specific. Dolls are often reserved for girls and trucks and tools for boys. Gender-specific toys may guide the development of self-expectations or likes and dislikes.

Between the ages of 4 and 7, children engage in play activities that may involve viewing or touching the genitals. It is the parents who place sexual meaning on the activity, not the children. A negative body image may develop if parents imply that a part of the body is dirty or bad. Children often ask questions related to sexuality and should be given honest and accurate answers. Ten- and eleven-year-olds may be curious and are sensitive about developing secondary sex characteristics, and girls may eagerly await (or dread) signs of breast development. Interest in the opposite sex is often a sensitive topic and may be strongly denied. Ten- to eleven-year-olds appreciate privacy and may be embarrassed to show their bodies.

With the popularity of social media and pop music with sexually explicit lyrics, many 9- to 11-year-old children are now rushed through childhood (Elkind, 2002). They enthusiastically accept adult types of activities and dress. Some preteens wear low-rise pants secured at hip level or very short skirts and halters to school, and some schools have had to adopt strict dress codes or school uniforms to counter this trend.

BOX 9-2 Guidance for Latchkey Families

Teach Child About Safety

Do not enter the house if the door is ajar or if anything looks unusual.
Do not leave the house or yard without permission.
Never admit a stranger into the house.
Never agree to meet with someone you met online.
Never respond to messages on the computer that sound weird.
Do not display keys; keep doors locked.
Teach how to answer the telephone (tell callers that parents are busy, not "out").
Do not take shortcuts to school through alleys or across train tracks.
Walk to and from school with friends.
Never accept rides with strangers.
Know how to contact a trusted adult.
Teach first-aid techniques; know how to call 911.
Review fire-safety rules and the route of escape; walk through the procedure with the child.
Know and obey basic safety rules.

Teach Parents To

List emergency numbers and post them near the telephone.
Designate a neighbor who is usually home for help during emergency situations.
Teach the child his or her own name, telephone number, address, and parents' names.
Leave work number with the child.
Lock up firearms or remove them from the house.
Prepare a first-aid kit and keep it in a designated location.
Address with the child street safety when returning from school; include precautions with strangers.
Consider obtaining a pet for the child.
Be home on time or call the child.
Leave a tape-recorded message to decrease the child's loneliness; recommend specific activities rather than television.
Help the child to feel successful and appreciated.
Assess the home and neighborhood for hazards specific to the locale.

Data from Leifer G: *Introduction to maternity & pediatric nursing*, ed 6, Philadelphia, 2011, Saunders; State of California Office of Criminal Justice Planning, Sacramento, California; and McClellan M: On own: latchkey children, *Pediatric Nursing* 10:2000, 1984.

Sex education is a lifelong process and may begin earlier than many parents believe. Parents convey their attitudes toward sexuality to the growing child, and sometimes parents need guidance in understanding their child's sexual curiosity. School-age children may occasionally masturbate. This behavior is normal and does not cause acne, impotence, mental disease, or blindness as some in the past have claimed. Young boys should be informed about the experience of wet dreams, and young girls should be prepared for menarche.

Facts concerning sex and drugs are an important part of education in the school-age years. Because parents cannot always prevent children's exposure to drug use outside the home, they should educate them about the dangers of drug and alcohol use. Many websites offer age-appropriate tips for parents to teach their children about drugs and alcohol.

Sex education can be introduced in the context of normal anatomy and physiology. Values can be added and influenced by active parental and teacher participation and by

TABLE 9-4 Sex Education of the School-Age Child

Intervention	Observation/Goal
Data collection; history taking Assess readiness to learn.	Readiness to learn is indicated by asking questions concerning sex, menstruation, "wet dreams," and pregnancy.
Analysis	Observe parent–child interactions and determine level of communication.
Assess interactions.	Observe peer interaction to determine the child's self-image, self-confidence, and ability to communicate about sensitive issues.
Assess parents.	Observe parents' knowledge and ability to discuss issues pertaining to sex education.
Assess child.	Determine child's understanding of sexual development and body changes.
Planning/Implementation	Discuss growth and development with the parents and child. Reinforce teaching techniques and opportunities with parents.
Evaluation	With each clinic or home visit, reevaluate parent–child interaction concerning sex education.

Modified from Leifer G: *Introduction to maternity & pediatric nursing*, ed 6, Philadelphia, 2011, Saunders.

encouraging questions and discussion. The Sex Information and Education Council of the United States (SIECUS), located in New York, advocates the idea that sex education programs should be taught from six basic aspects: biological, social, health, personal adjustment, interpersonal relationships, and developing values. Age-appropriate, culturally relevant, written information that treats sexuality as a healthy aspect of life should be included. Table 9-4 reviews the interventions and goals for sex education for the school-age child.

TEACHING TECHNIQUES

Most school-age children have a natural curiosity and are therefore ready and eager to learn. Because the extended attention span of the school-age child is limited to a maximum of 45 minutes, teaching sessions should be planned for no more than this amount of time. All information should be presented to the school-age child in a truthful, factual, and age-appropriate manner. Step-by-step instructions are needed for children who are concrete thinkers. Encouraging verbal feedback from the child will ensure that the information provided was not misinterpreted. During any teaching process, periods of praise and occasional rewards reinforce learning accomplishments. Teaching techniques should encourage the school-age child to accept responsibilities and should provide hands-on reinforcement whenever possible. Group instruction is effective in teaching positive health behaviors, because peer attitudes can influence learning and can enhance the application of values taught.

Patient Teaching

Health teaching needs of healthy school-age children include prevention of injury; maintenance of adequate nutrition; the importance of regular dental care; screening for scoliosis, vision, and hearing deficits; and the need for immunizations (see Appendix A). School nurses can be valuable resources for assisting preadolescents in making positive choices, developing interpersonal relationships, developing positive self-esteem, improving the ability to use problem-solving skills, and accessing community resources. School nurses should be aware that sometimes a school-age child will complain of minor health problems, which have little evidence of pathology, as a way of reaching out for help with psychosocial problems.

School-age children can understand the causes of illness and its consequences in terms of missing school and missing peer activities. Having to live with a long-term, chronic illness can slow cognitive learning. In most cases, illness causes more anxiety related to separation from peers, falling behind in school, and being left out of social activities than anxiety related to the illness itself. An important primary goal in the care of a school-age child is to foster normal growth and development even if some physical or intellectual disabilities are present. Teaching diabetic school-age children to test their own blood sugar and to administer their own insulin is an example of age-appropriate teaching.

DISCIPLINE

The word discipline is derived from the Latin word *disciplinare*, which means "to teach." Discipline should be thought of as providing age-appropriate positive reinforcement of good behavior that plays an important role in the social and emotional development of children.

Punishment is only one aspect of discipline. Reward is another option. If punishment is used, it should be prompt, consistent, and fair. Parents often rely on culturally traditional disciplinary techniques. Some may shy away from asking for help because of the fear that their parenting skills may be criticized. It is through appropriate discipline that children learn self-control and a sense of parental caring. Whenever misbehavior occurs, the motivation should be investigated. Misbehavior often occurs if the child is bored or needs attention, or misbehavior may be a reflection of a larger problem at home. Physical punishment can increase or reinforce misbehavior if it is the only way the child receives attention (Rowe et al., 2010). Negative attention is better than none in the minds of many children.

Certain temperaments may predispose the child to misbehavior. Children with attention deficit hyperactivity disorders (ADHD) are likely to misbehave unintentionally.

Discipline should combine reward and punishment, be based on age-appropriate behavior expectations, offer the child information on alternative choices of behavior, and teach respect for others. Because the school-age child understands cause-and-effect relationships, discipline and rewards need to be immediate and consistent with the action so that the child understands that the behavior resulted in the reward or punishment. The school-age child can understand and respect rules. Therefore behavior standards and social interactions can be guided and reinforced according to rules. Involving the child in designing an appropriate mode of punishment can help develop moral judgment and autonomy.

Including positive reinforcement in disciplinary efforts is crucial to the development of good behavior. Attention or praise from parents or teachers is an example of positive reinforcement. If misbehavior results in extra attention from the parent or teacher, this may reinforce bad behavior. That means that in order to implement effective discipline, attention should be focused on behavior that is good. Rewards for good behavior can be in the form of extra attention, a smile, a hug, a word of praise, extra privileges, or a token reward such as a sticker or a star, and these token rewards can be collected and cashed in later for a material reward. As punishment, a child's stars can be removed as a response to bad behavior.

Discipline should be used only for teaching and not for revenge, to vent anger, or to demand behavior that is beyond the child's ability. Time-outs (discussed in Chapter 8) are appropriate for the 18-month to 6-year-old age group. Removal of privileges such as television, texting, or computer use can be an effective punishment for the school-age child. Verbal reprimands in the form of scolding can provide the needed correction for the child, but scolding can escalate into shouting matches or can result in frustration or increased noncompliance.

Corporal punishment is spanking, hitting, or inflicting pain to stop or alter behavior. Acceptable spanking has been defined as "the use of an open hand on the buttocks with the intention of modifying behavior without causing injury" (American Academy of Pediatrics, 1998). There is a fine line between corporal punishment and child abuse. For this reason, many child experts discourage the use of corporal punishment. Spanking may be initially effective to stop a dangerous situation because of its shock value, but spanking may not be effective as a long-term disciplinary tool. Frequent spanking can teach violent behavior and can lead to decreased self-esteem, depression, and low educational achievement. Positive reinforcement (reward), removing privileges, or adding chores are other effective forms of discipline that clearly are nonabusive (American Acadamy of Pediatrics, 2009).

Parent Teaching

Parents benefit from guidance in formulating effective disciplinary techniques. Every well-child visit should include a discussion of behavior management and discipline in the home. Teacher education programs also should include discipline techniques for classroom management. Discussion should include alternatives to corporal punishment, anger-control skills, and discipline that matches the developmental and educational needs of the school-age children. Community resources may include referral to parenting classes, support groups, or professional counselors.

KEY POINTS

- Middle childhood includes school-age children between the ages of 6 and 12.
- In the school-age child, the body develops a lower center of gravity than it had in preschool years.
- The loss of primary teeth begins at about age 6, and approximately four permanent teeth erupt each year.
- Regular dental checkups are an important part of routine health care.
- Visual maturity is complete between preschool age and 6 years, and therefore large-print books are no longer necessary at this time.
- Excessive time spent with computer and video games can contribute to a sedentary lifestyle, which may result in obesity, poor health, and poor social development.
- By ages 9 and 10, an understanding of rules and teamwork enables the child to participate in competitive team games.
- School-age children, according to Piaget, are concrete thinkers, and hands-on learning is retained best.
- School-age children often tell jokes to entertain peers and to tease elders.
- School-age children are less egocentric than they were at earlier ages, and they can understand how their actions affect others.
- Moral behavior is based on logical understanding and feeling pride or guilt as a result of the behavior. Knowing a rule is right does not guarantee behavior according to that rule.
- In later childhood, the 10-year-old may enjoy creating new rules or changing the rules of a game.
- Kohlberg believed that moral reasoning develops as cognitive skills mature.
- A school-age child may have a maximum attention span of 45 minutes.
- School-age children use language as an effective communication tool in relationships with others.
- Intelligence tests were designed for use in predicting scholastic ability and future performance.
- The primary developmental task of the school-age child is to attain a sense of industry by mastering skills and achieving goals.
- Belonging to a peer group is very important to a school-age child.
- The home, school, and neighborhood each affect the growth and development of school-age children.
- Creativity should be encouraged, because it helps develop problem-solving skills.
- Information concerning sexuality should be age appropriate, culturally relevant, and treated as a healthy aspect of life.
- Discipline should be used for teaching and reinforcing good behavior, which plays an important role in social and emotional development.
- Strength, endurance, and coordination can be nurtured by daily physical activity. Physical activity can also decrease risk factors for illness in later life.
- The major health-teaching needs of the school-age child include prevention of injury; maintenance of adequate nutrition; providing regular dental care; screening for scoliosis, vision, and hearing problems; and developing an active lifestyle.

Critical Thinking

A child is enrolled in public school for the first time. Discuss some advice a school nurse or health-care worker can offer the child's parent to help this child to be successful in school.

REVIEW QUESTIONS

1. Middle childhood includes children between the ages of:
   a. 3 and 5 years.
   b. 6 and 12 years.
   c. 13 and 15 years.
   d. 16 and 19 years.

2. A major developmental task of middle childhood includes:
   a. developing positive self-esteem and a positive self-image.
   b. eruption of permanent teeth.
   c. ability to play video games.
   d. prevention of injury.

3. The type of play activities typical in the middle-childhood age group include:
   a. parallel play.
   b. competitive games.
   c. solitary play.
   d. reading and fantasy.

4. The Wechsler intelligence test is used to determine:
   a. the overall intelligence of the child.
   b. verbal and nonverbal intelligence.
   c. presence of mental retardation.
   d. whether the child has college potential.

5. Middle childhood includes Erikson's stage of:
   a. trust.
   b. autonomy.
   c. industry.
   d. identity.

CHAPTER 10

Adolescence

http://evolve.elsevier.com/Leifer/growth

OBJECTIVES

1. Define adolescence.
2. State the three phases of adolescence.
3. State the physiological changes that occur during adolescence.
4. Define puberty.
5. Identify the major developmental tasks of adolescence.
6. Discuss the adolescent's stage of development according to Erikson and Piaget.
7. Discuss how to determine the fertile period of a female adolescent.
8. Summarize the nutritional requirements during adolescence.
9. Identify how a person's cultural background might contribute to behavior.
10. Discuss the impact of peers, cliques, and best friends on the growth and development of the adolescent.
11. Discuss the role of dating in the development of cognitive and social behavior.
12. Discuss the role of parents in fostering the positive growth and development of the adolescent.
13. Describe the physical-activity guidelines for adolescents.
14. State two specific health risks in the adolescent age group.

KEY TERMS

abstinence
adolescence
asynchronous
clique
cultural competence
ejaculation
empathy
menarche
menstrual cycle
nocturnal emissions
ovulation
puberty
secondary sex characteristics
spermatogenesis
vigorous exercise

DEFINITION

The origin of the word adolescence is from the Latin word *adolesere*, which means "to grow and mature." Adolescence is considered to be the bridge between childhood and adulthood. It is a unique stage of development characterized by many physiological, cognitive, psychosocial, and sexual changes. The health habits and coping skills formed during this period last a lifetime, and mastery of developmental tasks during this period helps prepare the adolescent for adulthood.

Health Promotion

The teen death rate has declined from 98 per 100,000 in 1980 to 62 per 100,000 in 2007. However, the latest rate did not meet the *Healthy People 2010* goal of 39.8 per 100,000, which remains a target for *Healthy People 2020* (Kelland, 2011).

DEVELOPMENTAL TASKS

Developmental tasks encountered during adolescence include establishing a stabilized sense of identity, separation from family, career planning, and establishing close peer relationships and intimacy.

Adolescence is often separated into three phases: *early adolescence* (10 to 13 years), *middle adolescence* (14 to 16 years), and *late adolescence* (17 to 20 years). The 13-year-old adolescent differs greatly from the 18-year-old adolescent. Each of these three distinct phases of adolescence has its own set of challenges (Table 10-1).

PHYSIOLOGICAL CHANGES

Early adolescence (also called preadolescence) is characterized by physical changes in the structure and function of various parts of the body. Weight gain is caused by an increase in musculoskeletal mass. However, growth is asynchronous, which means that different parts of the body mature at different times, possibly resulting in the temporary appearance of awkwardness. A growth spurt occurs during adolescence, and adult height is reached by approximately age 18. Because the sweat glands are more active, various skin problems such as acne can occur, which may have social consequences and may challenge teens' coping abilities. A facial pimple on the day of an important social event can cause chaos in the family.

The stomach and intestines increase in size and volume during adolescence, resulting in increased appetite and food consumption. The second and third molars, and often the wisdom teeth, erupt in early adolescence, and the jaw reaches adult size in mid- to late adolescence. Orthodontic braces are often prescribed for tooth alignment.

The weight and volume of the lungs increase, resulting in improvement of respiratory function. Improvements in eye–hand coordination and motor function enhance manual dexterity. Motor function also improves, and these factors contribute to the development of an interest and skill in sports activities and interactive computer games.

Physical Activity

The physical-activity guidelines for adolescents are the same as those for children (60 minutes or more of physical activity every day). At least three days per week, the activity should include vigorous exercise, which is defined as at least 20 minutes of exercise that causes sweating or breathing hard (CDC, 2006). Exercise activities should include warm-up and cool-down sessions. Because of decreased amounts of physical education opportunities in school, extracurricular physical activities become increasingly important during adolescence. Exercise activities can be performed individually or in groups and should be selected for personal enjoyment with consideration of individual capabilities and limitations.

TABLE 10-1 Three Phases in the Growth and Development of the Adolescent

	Early (10 to 13 years)	Middle (14 to 16 years)	Late (17 to 20 years)
Physical Growth	Appearance of secondary sex characteristics	Growth spurt in height	Growth slows
Body Image	Self-conscious; adjusts to pubertal changes	Experiments with different images and looks	Accepts body image; personality emerges
Self Concept	Low self-esteem; denial of reality	Impulsive, impatient; identity confusion	Has positive self-image; empathetic; independent thinker
Behavior	Behaves for rewards	Behaves to conform	Shows responsible behavior
Sexual Development	Sexual interest	Sexual experimentation	Sexual identity emerges; develops caring relationships
Peers	Unisex cliques of friends; has best friend; engages in hero worship; has adult crushes	Begins dating; has need to please significant peer; develops heterosexual peer group	Values individual relationships; begins partner selection
Family	Is ambivalent to family; strives for independence	Struggles for autonomy and acceptance; rebels/withdraws; demands privacy	Achieves independence; reestablishes family relationships
Cognitive Development	Concrete thinking; here and now is important	Early abstract thinking, daydreams, fantasies; starts inductive and deductive reasoning	Abstract thinking; idealistic
Goals	Socializing is priority; goals may be unrealistic	Identifies skills/interests; becomes a superachiever or dropout	Identifies career goals; enters work or college
Health Concerns	Concerned about normalcy	Concerned about experimenting with drugs or sex	Idealistic; decision making for lifestyle choice
Interventions	Convey limits; encourage verbalization	Help adolescents solve problems resulting from choices; use peer-group sessions; provide privacy	Discuss goals; allow participation in decisions; provide confidentiality

Modified from Leifer G: *Introduction to maternity & pediatric nursing*, ed 6, Philadelphia, 2011, W.B. Saunders.

Adolescents engaging in competitive sports can benefit from strength training (Faigenbaum, 2007). Under proper supervision, a comprehensive and systematic strength-training program can improve motor fitness and sports performance while decreasing incidences of injury. Strength training can increase muscle and bone mass and can also play an important role in weight management throughout adolescence and adulthood.

Puberty

Puberty refers to sexual maturity or having the functional ability to reproduce and involves physical and psychological changes.

Boys

For boys, puberty begins with hormonal changes between the ages of 10 and 13. Secondary sex characteristics are not involved in the reproductive process but appear at this time. Increases in androgens (testosterone and androsterone) are responsible for producing the male secondary sex characteristics. These include growth of pubic, facial, and body hair; enlargement and darkening in color of the scrotum; and an increase in penis size. The vocal cords also lengthen and thicken, resulting first in voice instability (voice cracking) and then in a deepening of the voice.

An area in the brain, called the hypothalamus, secretes gonadotropin-releasing hormone (GnRH), which stimulates the anterior pituitary gland to secrete gonadotropins, follicle-stimulating hormone (FSH), and luteinizing hormone (LH). These gonadotropins stimulate the testes, which are located in the scrotum, to produce testosterone, and under normal conditions a stable level of testosterone is maintained in the blood throughout most of the life span. FSH and testosterone stimulate spermatogenesis, which is the production of sperm. Sperm production starts during midpuberty and continues throughout the male life span. Sperm production requires a temperature of about 3° F below normal body temperature. This cooler temperature is possible because the testes are located outside the abdominal cavity in the scrotum, which hangs between the legs. Males of all ages should be counseled against wearing tight undergarments or sitting on enclosed plastic or leather seats for prolonged times, because fertility can be reduced if the temperature around the testes is too high.

Ejaculation is the release of sperm during an orgasm. This ability indicates the testes are mature. Most boys experience nocturnal emissions, also known as "wet dreams," when they ejaculate semen during sleep. This experience is part of normal sexual development and is not necessarily related to sexual activity.

Because of the enlargement of the scrotum and the penis during puberty, an athletic scrotal support (jock strap) should be worn by boys participating in sporting events to prevent injury to these vulnerable organs. Good personal hygiene is necessary to prevent friction rashes (known as jock itch), which is a fungal infection. Sharing of athletic supporters creates a risk for spreading these infections and is strongly discouraged.

Girls

For girls during puberty, hormone secretions begin to establish a pattern within a monthly cycle. This pattern can typically be 28 to 32 days apart. Menstrual cycles begin at puberty and last about 40 years, when the hormone cycles stop and menopause begins.

The hypothalamus gland produces a gonadotropin-releasing hormone (GnRH), which stimulates the pituitary gland to release luteinizing hormone (LH) and follicle-stimulating hormone (FSH). These hormones then stimulate the release of the female sex hormones (estrogen and progesterone) from the ovaries. Many thousands of eggs are present in the ovaries at birth. During ovulation, which typically happens once each menstrual cycle, one of the eggs finally matures and is released from the ovary (ovulation) into the fallopian tube, which leads to the uterus. As the egg travels in the fallopian tube toward the uterus, it can be fertilized if a sperm is present. If a sperm does not fertilize the egg, the egg enters the uterus and is expelled from the body with the blood and mucus that had thickened the walls of the uterus to prepare it for pregnancy. This blood, mucus, and unfertilized egg expelled from the body are called a menstrual flow (menstruation, or "period").

The very first menstrual period is called the menarche. The menarche usually occurs between ages 12 and 13 but can occur between 10 and 15. The menstrual cycle consists of (1) maturing the egg in the ovary, (2) formation of blood and mucus in the lining of the uterus, (3) ovulation, and (4) expelling the unfertilized egg with the blood and mucous lining from the uterus. This cycle lasts approximately 28 days and repeats until menopause. The menstrual flow typically lasts from 2 to 5 days, with a blood loss of about 1 ounce along with 1 to 2 ounces of serous fluid.

Ovulation occurs about 14 days *before menstruation starts*, and the egg lives for 1 day. Therefore this time is considered the most fertile period of a woman's cycle, when pregnancy can occur if sperm are present. Unwanted pregnancy can be prevented using one of several methods (Table 10-2). The best way to prevent an unwanted pregnancy is to avoid sexual intercourse, referred to as abstinence. Birth control pills prevent ovulation but can have systemic side effects. Intrauterine devices (IUDs) prevent a fertilized egg from adhering to the wall of the uterus; and condoms, if used correctly, can prevent the sperm from entering the vagina. Condoms also have the benefit of helping to prevent the spread of sexually transmitted diseases (STDs), such as chlamydia, gonorrhea, syphilis, and human immunodeficiency virus (HIV). In some research studies the term sexually transmitted infections (STIs) is replacing the term STDs. However, the Centers for Disease Control and Prevention (CDC) still use the term STD. Condoms are best used in combination with other methods, such as spermicides, to increase protection against pregnancy. Various hormone shots, such as Depo-Provera, prevent ovulation from occurring but require repeated injections.

In girls, secondary sex characteristics often become apparent before menarche. Hair develops in the pubic area and the axilla or underarms. Breasts begin to develop, fat begins to deposit more in the hips and thighs rather than being evenly distributed, and body contours change. At this time, adolescent girls are ready for their first bra to support their developing breasts. The bra straps should not fall from the shoulders but should not be too tight and the bra cup should support the fullness of the breasts near the underarms. Sports bras may be more desirable for girls who participate in athletics. A balance of diet and exercise is important for menstrual regularity and overall health.

Patient Teaching

Adolescence is the best time to teach preventative health measures such as testicular self-examination (TSE) for boys and breast self-examination (BSE) for girls. Sex education classes should include information about safe sex, family planning, and prevention of STDs. The school nurse can be a valuable resource person to help locate family planning services, such as Planned Parenthood, that may be available in the local community.

TABLE 10-2 Birth Control Options*

Method	How Used	Protects Against STDs?
MOST EFFECTIVE		
Abstinence	Avoid sexual intercourse.	Yes
HORMONAL		
Oral contraceptive ("the Pill")	Usually taken once daily. Extended dose regimens can delay menstruation up to a year.	No
Contraceptive injections (Depo-Provera)	Can take injection at specific intervals (e.g., every 3 mo).	
Implanon	Matchstick-sized capsules placed underneath skin of the arm provides contraception for up to 3 yr. Can be removed by a health-care provider at any time.	No
Vaginal ring	Inserted monthly; stays in for a 3-wk period and removed for 1 wk (to allow for menstruation).	No
Intrauterine devices	Inserted into the uterus (to allow for menstruation) can be effective for 5 yr.	No
Skin patch	A new patch is applied to skin once weekly for 3 wk, not worn for 1 wk (to allow for menstruation).	No
NONHORMONAL		
Male condom	New condom must be applied before each act of coitus or sexual encounter.	Yes
Female condom	New condom must be inserted before each sexual encounter.	Yes
Spermicidal foams	Must be applied or inserted before each sexual encounter.	No
Cervical cap	Used with spermicide at every sexual encounter.	No
Copper IUD	Must be inserted by health-care provider; lasts up to 10 yr.	No
PERMANENT		
Vasectomy	One surgical procedure provides permanent prevention of pregnancy (can be reversed in some cases).	No
Tubal ligation	One surgical procedure provides permanent prevention of pregnancy (can be reversed in some cases).	No

*It is important to understand that a woman's fertile period (when pregnancy can occur if sperm is present) is 14 days ***before the beginning*** of the next menstrual period. This is not necessarily the same as 14 days after the last menstrual period if the cycle is fewer than or more than 28 days apart.

Adolescents often have emotional reactions and concerns about their changing bodies. Boys may have socially embarrassing erections, and comparison of penis size can be a normal part of social interaction and exploration. Girls are often concerned with their breast size and menstrual discomforts. Teen magazines often exploit the ideal female figure and the muscular male body with standards that are very difficult for the average teen to meet. The changing body plays an important role in the development of an adolescent's self-image. Research suggests that males who develop early may enjoy more social success and positive self-esteem, whereas girls who develop early may be at more risk for lower self-esteem and a drop in school performance (Kleigman, 2011).

Teen Pregnancy

The teen pregnancy rate was 34.3 pregnancies per 1000 women in the year 2010, and many of these adolescents had multiple partners (CDC, NCHS, 2011). About 400,000 teenagers give birth each year according to the CDC, but this is a decline of 37% over the last two decades, which translates to 4% of all teen girls and 10% of total births. The decline may be attributed to sex education classes in schools, access to modern birth-control techniques, and the emergence of TV programs that focus on the plight of pregnant teens and bring the issue to the forefront of conversation and discussion.

In many cultures a ritual rite of passage occurs at the onset of puberty. In the United States, sex in movies, television, and other media may influence the behavior of adolescents, who are beginning to explore dating.

Patient Teaching

Health-care professionals, educators, parents, school nurses, and counselors are challenged to provide guidance and education that will promote healthy behaviors.

Sexual topics are a high priority for the adolescent. Boys may seek sexual experience because of social role expectations. Girls and boys seek sexual activity because of coercion, peer pressure, or curiosity. For these reasons, sex education is important before adolescence and must continue throughout adolescence. Accurate information from an authoritative source about the prevention of pregnancy and STDs can help teens make responsible and informed choices related to sexual matters. Too often, teens obtain misinformation from peers or other unreliable sources and become vulnerable to unsafe practices or abuse. For example, many young girls believe they cannot become pregnant the first time they have sexual intercourse, which is false.

Patient Teaching

Teens who become pregnant must cope with their own developmental tasks, as well as the tasks of parenthood. Counseling concerning their options and close health supervision are essential for a positive outcome in a teen pregnancy. Teens are at high risk for date rape and other sexual abuses, and therefore education concerning safe practices and preventative strategies is essential. Community resources that provide special programs for sexually active or pregnant teens are available, and school-based resources, such as education programs, provide opportunities for individual counseling.

COGNITIVE DEVELOPMENT

According to Piaget, young adolescents are in the *concrete phase* of thinking, which means they interpret words and concepts literally. By middle adolescence they begin to think more abstractly. This second stage of cognitive development is called the *formal operation stage*. Adolescents in this stage can process information quickly and efficiently, and their thinking becomes more complex. Adolescents can be self absorbed and self-conscious. They may feel that everyone is looking at them and worry that others may notice even slight blemishes on their skin. They can spend hours examining and experimenting with hairstyles and dress, feeling they are on a stage with all the world as their audience (Figure 10–1).

At times adolescents can also see themselves as unique and powerful. They may try to manipulate rules, engage in risky behaviors, or deny their own mortality. Some adolescents admire "idols" and can be disappointed or confused when they discover that their idols are not perfect. It is healthy for adolescents to discover their own uniqueness and to separate from their families. However, teens can sometimes become isolated, which may raise the risk of depression or self-harming behavior when problems arise.

Debate is a healthy mental exercise that can sharpen cognitive and social skills and defuse intense emotions for most adolescents. School debate teams help teens express varying views in socially acceptable ways. Debate is often interpreted as argumentative by parents and teachers, who may find teenagers difficult and challenging to get along with.

Teenagers often daydream, which may be the imaginary acting out of what would be said or done in various situations. Daydreams help the adolescent think through how he or she might respond in situations and can be a safety valve for strong emotions. Daydreams in the adolescent are harmless unless they interfere with functioning in school or relationships. Young adolescents fantasize about unrealistic career ideas, but by middle adolescence they may realize their true strengths and limitations and thus may set more realistic goals.

Kohlberg described the adolescent as moving toward the postconventional stage of moral judgment (see Chapter 5). The early adolescent is motivated by the need to conform and to please others. As later adolescence approaches, moral principles are based on one's own individual thinking and beliefs.

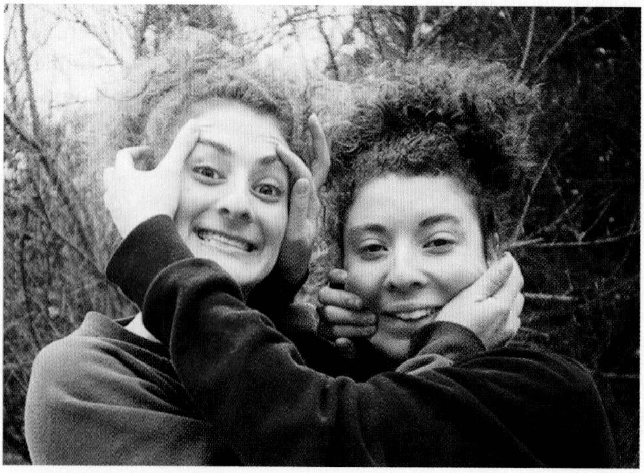

Figure 10–1 Best friends experiment with hairstyles, expressions, and make-up. Best-friend interaction supports growth and development.

Psychosocial Development

According to Erikson, one of the major tasks of adolescence is achieving a stable self-identity (see Chapter 5). Adolescents may try out various temporary styles and social roles in the process of finding their own individual identities. This process of identity exploration can lead to role confusion. In role confusion the adolescent can overcommit to many causes and can appear to go through personality changes. To achieve a sense of their own identity, adolescents must believe their identities are separate from their role as children in their families. The family can help secure a positive outcome in achieving this task by offering support and guidance and by giving adolescents freedom to discover their own interests. Close relationships with peers are helpful for adolescents exploring different roles and ideas. Close friendships develop mainly with same-sex friends in the early adolescent phase. They validate each other's thoughts and actions and may imitate each other's traits and habits. Middle adolescents (14 to 17 years) are concerned with how they look and who they date. Experimentation with sex and other social behaviors often occurs at this age, and a sense of omnipotence combined with curiosity may lead to risk-taking behaviors. As teens approach late adolescence, school performance, interaction with teachers and counselors, and participation in extracurricular activities can positively influence the successful achievement of adolescents' career goals.

Problem-solving approaches are used in the task of establishing a first date. Social skills and cognitive reasoning are aided by good coping skills to meet the challenges of achieving many developmental tasks of adolescence. There may be some subtle gender differences in initiating a date. Boys typically take a more active role, but girls may use techniques to attract attention and to encourage a boy to ask for a date. Not having a boyfriend or girlfriend may be considered just as stressful as the stress of initiating a relationship. In later adolescence, relationships may become less experimental, more affectionate, and longer lasting (Figure 10–2). A feeling of abandonment may occur in early adolescence if one of two best friends leaves the other for a dating relationship. Feeling left out or guilty is common in early adolescence despite the understanding that a relationship with a significant other need not be exclusive of other friends.

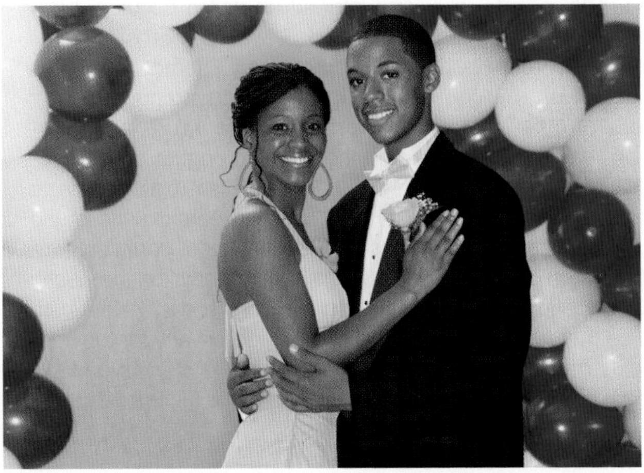

Figure 10–2 Dating is popular. Relationships may become less experimental, more affectionate, and longer lasting. (Courtesy of Photos.com)

Teen Violence

The United States rates highest in the industrialized world in violent death rates, and violent crimes involving teenagers are an increasing problem in our society. In 2009, 19% of youths in grades 9 through 12 reported being bullied, and juveniles accounted for 16% of all crime arrests and 26% of all property crime arrests (CDC, 2010). Children and adolescents often use violence to handle conflicts, because they may not have been effectively taught nonviolent techniques of managing conflicts during the formative years of developing socialization skills. Many children also witness their parents using physical violence at home to settle disputes.

Both parents working and thus being absent from the home after school hours, and the increasing availability of guns and drugs on school campuses, each contribute to the occurrence of violence in schools. Episodes of fighting often precede homicides. The impulsive nature of teenagers, their feelings of invincibility and immortality, their immaturity, and their exposure to violence on television and in interactive computer and video games and other media all combine to form a deadly vulnerability that includes violence in their lifestyles.

Adolescents who are homeless, abused, or disadvantaged may not be able to cope with the other developmental tasks of adolescence, such as dating, social development, or personal identity development, and they may act out in socially unacceptable ways. They may abuse drugs, exhibit violent behavior, engage in risky sexual practices, or even attempt suicide.

DEVELOPMENT OF RESPONSIBILITY

Adolescents look forward to challenges and often feel humiliated when placed in the dependent role. Independence in transportation can be achieved by riding a bicycle or driving a car. Babysitting or routine jobs to earn and learn to manage money is important to the

Cultural Considerations

Culture and the Adolescent

Culture plays a role in how adolescents think and interact. In some cultures, body piercing and tattoos are an accepted or expected practice, whereas other cultures view them as inappropriate or deviant. Health-care workers who interact with teens must be culturally competent. **Cultural competence** involves recognizing how your own values differ from those of other cultures and respecting the values and practices of others. Focusing on the cultural values and individual strengths of the adolescent, rather than the differences or variations, can help establish relationships to achieve positive health-teaching outcomes. Culture affects health-care practices and modes of communication. In most cases, the adolescent requires strict confidentiality. Maintaining this confidentiality can be a challenge when parents pay for the health insurance and control transportation access. It is important for nurses, health-care workers, and educators to be truthful, keep promises, and provide privacy for the adolescent. Cultural and religious traditions can help stabilize identity and involve rituals that celebrate the transition from childhood to the adult phase of life (Figure 10-3 and Chapter 3).

teenager. Using their own savings account, checking account, or debit or credit card to purchase some of their own clothes and supplies are important personal management skills for adolescents to learn.

It is important for the adolescent to be responsible for making decisions, especially those relative to career, politics, and religion. The role of parents should be to listen to and guide the adolescent rather than to mandate behavior. According to the behaviorist B.F. Skinner, teens will repeat behavior that is positively reinforced (see Chapter 5). Bandura, a social cognitive theorist, suggests that setting an example for the teen will motivate positive behavior (see Chapter 5).

PEER RELATIONSHIPS

Peer group affiliation has a major impact on adolescent growth and development. School plays an important role in psychosocial development, because it provides the opportunity for social interaction, peer group association, and clique formation. A clique is a social group with a fixed exclusive membership, whose members share similar interests, values, and tastes. Belonging to a group is of utmost importance to adolescents. From this social group, the adolescent chooses a best friend who enables the teen to experience mutual sharing of private thoughts and feelings. This may be helpful in normalizing and validating experiences and in forming successful relationships later in life.

During this period in adolescence, it is normal for openness and time spent with peers to increase and contacts with family to decrease. The teen may feel compelled to conform to peer pressures, which can cause problems and conflicts with the family if the values of the peer group conflict with family values or traditions. If the adolescent and the family relocate to a new neighborhood or a new state during this phase of the life cycle, the adolescent may experience more difficulty in joining an exclusive clique or group of friends in the new school. Failure to connect in a clique or a peer group can cause feelings of loneliness,

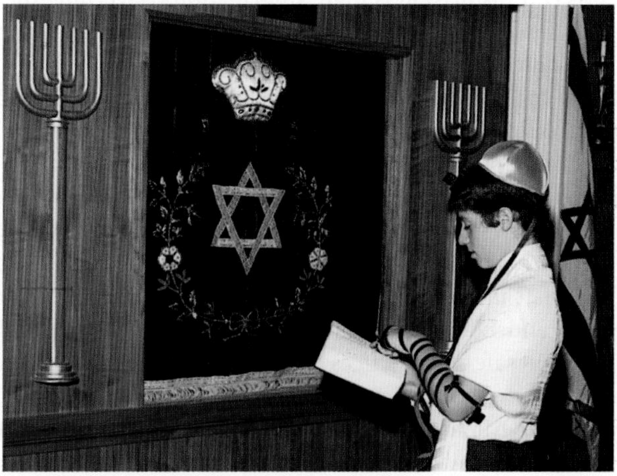

Figure 10-3 Cultural practice. Many childhood and religious traditions involve rituals that celebrate movement from childhood to the adult phase of life. Here a boy participates in the Bar Mitzvah ceremony marking his thirteenth birthday, when he is considered as entering adulthood.

loss, and interpersonal failure. This may contribute to lower self-esteem or to feelings of inadequacy. School performance may decrease as a result of social difficulty, independent of academic ability, and the adolescent may become vulnerable to risky behaviors such as self soothing with illegal substances or cutting classes. The dynamics of peer interaction are essential for the adolescent. Parents who accept and welcome peers into their homes can help encourage the formation of healthy peer relationships and may have fewer conflicts in their relationships with their adolescents. Peer counselors can be helpful in redirecting a troubled teen.

Erikson's sixth stage of psychosocial development, intimacy versus isolation, starts in late adolescence. After the middle adolescent establishes a fairly stable identity, the next developmental challenge is to share with another and develop a sense of intimacy. Empathy (understanding how others feel) is a quality essential to establishing a meaningful relationship with another person. This intimate relationship can be sexual, intellectual, or social. In late adolescence, a childlike dependence on the family is sometimes seen in times of illness or stress, but relating to the adolescent as a young adult is the best means of supporting adolescent development.

SEXUALITY

Developing a sexual identity is an important part of the adolescent's sense of self. Masturbation is one way for an individual to explore and learn about his or her body. Petting, or mutual masturbation, is a form of physical, erotic, and genital stimulation that teens may engage in with each other, and often petting does not include sexual intercourse (coitus). Petting or groping can lead to orgasm and is a common sexual outlet for young teens. This type of experimental behavior helps the adolescent learn about sexual responses that are pleasurable and about behavior patterns that may contribute to later relationships.

Sexually active and exclusive relationships often develop during later adolescence. Health-care workers must be aware that many teenagers may not consider oral sex a sexual act, but the risk of STD transmission is high. Information concerning the risks of oral sex should be included in sex-education programs, which should begin early, because learning about sex 2 years too soon is better than 1 day too late.

The adolescent's sexual exploration creates risk for unplanned or unprotected sexual activity, which increases adolescents' vulnerability for developing sexually transmitted diseases. In cases of extreme poverty, poor problem-solving skills, or drug dependence, an exchange of sex for food or drugs may occur, increasing the risk for HIV or acquired immunodeficiency syndrome (AIDS) infection. Adults must remember that sexually abused adolescents or those who are victims of rape do not consider themselves sexually active and thus may need appropriate interventions after such events to educate and protect them. The Sexuality Information and Educational Council of the United States (SIECUS) provides facts and guidelines about safe-sex practices and many other health topics for children from kindergarten through high-school age (www.siecus.org).

Sexual fantasy and experimentation is normal for both heterosexual and homosexual individuals. Homosexual behavior in adolescence is common. Sometimes experimentation with homosexual behavior has a relationship to future sexual identification and behavior, but it also may simply be part of an exploration of identity and lifestyle options. Homosexual behavior is reported in about 5% of adolescent boys and girls (Kleigman,

2011). Homosexuality is no longer considered a sexual deviance or mental disorder by the American Psychiatric Association (APA 2000). The role of the health-care worker is to help the adolescent understand how to cope with confused or prejudiced reactions of others rather than to make attempts at changing behaviors.

TEACHING TECHNIQUES

Teaching adolescents can be a challenge. There is enormous variability in the rates of physical, cognitive, and psychosocial maturity between early, middle, and late adolescence. Some adolescents pass slowly through the changes of puberty and cognitive development, yet may be advanced in physical development. The adolescent who appears physically mature but is not yet an abstract thinker does not learn or interact in the same way as an adolescent who is cognitively or emotionally mature and may be at high risk for destructive peer influences. Often adolescents who are physically mature before they are cognitively mature may be lured into an older peer group that engages in risky behaviors, and the teens may not be able to make responsible decisions concerning these actions.

Patient Teaching

The health-care worker who understands the characteristics of each adolescent phase of development can be a very effective teacher or source of information for teens and their parents. Identifying health risks of the adolescent is essential in planning teaching that is relevant to preventative health care. Rapid body changes can result in poor coordination that can result in sports injuries. Adolescents are capable of logical thought and abstract reasoning. They can understand cause and effect, health and illness, and disease prevention. However, healthy teens may have difficulty picturing themselves as sick or injured and may engage in high-risk behavior. They may have an "it will never happen to me" attitude toward illness or injury. Many adolescents have at least one serious health problem, such as asthma, allergies, or diabetes. Health conditions that benefit from preventative measures and early intervention include pregnancy, STDs, substances abuse, and depression. Motor vehicle accidents (MVAs) continue to be the leading cause of teenage morbidity and mortality and are preventable with appropriate education and training.

The first step in effectively teaching adolescents involves establishing a trusting relationship. Communication must be supportive and not threatening to adolescents' sense of independence or autonomy. If they are informed in a respectful way and understand the value of healthy behavior, they are more likely to use the information wisely. This approach is better than just telling them what they need to do. Providing privacy and one-to-one consultation can open up communication and reduce defenses. However, peer group teaching sessions may be more helpful and practical for discussing common problems such as smoking, sexual activity, substance abuse, and other health-related challenges. Discussion of options and decision making must be shared, and options that support the adolescent in thinking and acting as an adult and staying open to learning should be offered. Confrontation should be avoided. Often the health-care worker, counselor, or nurse can help guide the family concerning parenting strategies relating to their teens. Setting realistic limits without damaging the sense of independence is a delicate balance and a learned skill for most parents.

Health Promotion

The Society for Adolescent Medicine identified seven characteristics critical to providing effective health education and care for adolescents: *availability, visibility, quality, confidentiality, affordability, flexibility, and coordination* (Kleigman, 2011). One of the goals of *Healthy People 2020* is to provide community resources with these characteristics to increase access to health care and education for all adolescents.

KEY POINTS

- Adolescence is the bridge between childhood and adulthood.
- Adolescence is divided into three phases: early adolescence (10 to 13 years of age), middle adolescence (14 to 16 years of age), and late adolescence (17 to 20 years of age).
- The major tasks of adolescence include establishing a sense of identity, separation from family, establishing intimacy and peer relationships, and career planning.
- The physical, psychological, cognitive, and emotional aspects of development may mature at different rates.
- Puberty refers to sexual maturity.
- The reproductive system is controlled by hormones regulated by the hypothalamus and secreted by the anterior pituitary glands and the ovaries or testes.
- Ovulation occurs 14 days before the menstrual period begins.
- The changing body plays a role in the adolescent's development of self-image, self-esteem, and social interactions.
- Adolescents should engage in at least 60 minutes of physical activity every day and activity of vigorous intensity at least 3 days per week.
- Adolescents engaging in competitive sports can benefit from strength training.
- Young adolescents are in the concrete phase of thinking.
- Daydreaming can be developmentally appropriate and a useful safety valve for strong emotions.
- By middle adolescence, career goals may become more practical and realistic.
- In late adolescence, moral principles are based on the adolescent's own beliefs.
- Culture plays a role in how adolescents think and interact, and traditions can help stabilize identity.
- It is important to allow adolescents to begin to behave independently and to make their own decisions.
- Peer groups have a major impact on the social and emotional growth and development of adolescents.
- In late adolescence, intimacy with a peer can be sexual, intellectual, or social.
- Effective health education and care include *availability, visibility, high quality, confidentiality, affordability, and flexibility*.

Critical Thinking

Sexual topics are an important part of adolescent teaching. Outline a plan that will discuss menstrual health, help the adolescent girl understand her "fertile period," and create an awareness of birth control options.

REVIEW QUESTIONS

1. **A developmental task of adolescence includes:**
   a. concrete thinking.
   b. stabilizing identity.
   c. accepting competition.
   d. social interaction.

2. **The definition of puberty is:**
   a. exhibiting secondary sex characteristics.
   b. having the ability to reproduce.
   c. the decrease of gonadotropic hormones.
   d. becoming fertile.

3. **Which method of contraception, if used properly, can prevent the transmission of sexually transmitted diseases?**
   a. Condoms
   b. Birth control pills
   c. Intrauterine devices
   d. Spermicides

4. **A women's fertile period occurs:**
   a. 14 days after the last menstruation.
   b. 14 days before the beginning of the next menstruation.
   c. midway between menstrual periods.
   d. right after menstruation ceases.

5. **Which social group form is typical during the teenage years?**
   a. Cliques
   b. Same-sex peers
   c. Heterosexual peers
   d. Parallel groups

CHAPTER

11 Young Adulthood

http://evolve.elsevier.com/Leifer/growth

OBJECTIVES

1. Define young adulthood.
2. State the developmental tasks of young adulthood.
3. Name the physiological changes that occur in young adulthood.
4. State at least four priority health issues related to the young-adult stage of the life cycle.
5. List the reproductive health issues of young adulthood.
6. Use a knowledge of men's health needs in applying gender-appropriate care and guidance.
7. List two health-screening preventative programs that are important during young adulthood.
8. Discuss the role of schools in helping individuals adjust and cope with tasks and challenges of young adulthood.
9. Describe the psychosocial tasks of young adulthood as described by Erikson.
10. Explain Piaget's theory of cognitive thinking in young adulthood.
11. Describe Kohlberg's theory of moral development in the young adult.
12. Discuss Piaget's formal operational thinking as it applies to the young adult.
13. Trace the growth and development of a parent.
14. Design teaching techniques that will contribute to successful learning in the young adult.

KEY TERMS

ectopic pregnancy
exercise
hysterectomy
intimacy
intimate partner violence (IPV)
pelvic inflammatory disease (PID)
physical activity
postformal operational thought
sexually transmitted diseases (STDs)
structure
testicular self-examination (TSE)
transitional phase
vaginal birth after cesarean (VBAC)
young adulthood

DEFINITION

Young adulthood is most often defined as the age between 20 and 40 years. The stage may also be referred to as *early adulthood.* The legal age of adulthood in the United States is 18 years, when the individual can vote, be drafted into the military, and enter into marital relationships without parental consent. Until an individual reaches age 21, however, there may still be legal limitations on some activities, such as the use of alcohol.

DEVELOPMENTAL TASKS

According to Erikson, the major developmental task or crisis of young adulthood is *intimacy versus isolation*. The young adult makes the transition from the safety of the parents' home and the structure of the high school to achieve the tasks of self-support, independence, developing intimate relationships, and establishing a stable family and lifestyle. By age 21, some adults live separately from parents, establish a commitment to a work identity, and develop an adult social role of their own design. Others do not take on these adult roles and responsibilities until after they pursue a college education to achieve a career goal. In some cases, social and political events such as war or an economic crash can interrupt the progress toward career goals or financial or social independence. The developmental process from adolescence to adulthood is most often a gradual one, but in many cultures there are traditional expectations during this transition.

PHYSIOLOGICAL CHANGES

Physical growth in height and weight and organ and sexual maturation are generally complete by young adulthood. Physical health, motor coordination, and physiological performance typically peak between the ages of 20 and 30 (Figure 11-1). The epiphyses of the long bones fuse by the early twenties, and muscular strength is at its peak.

Health Promotion

By age 30, muscle mass and body water may naturally decrease, and fatty tissue increases, resulting in increased vulnerability to injuries. Efforts toward maintaining good physical fitness can prolong peak functioning or reestablish good health and fitness at an older age (Gerber, 2011). Poor health habits can compromise health at any age.

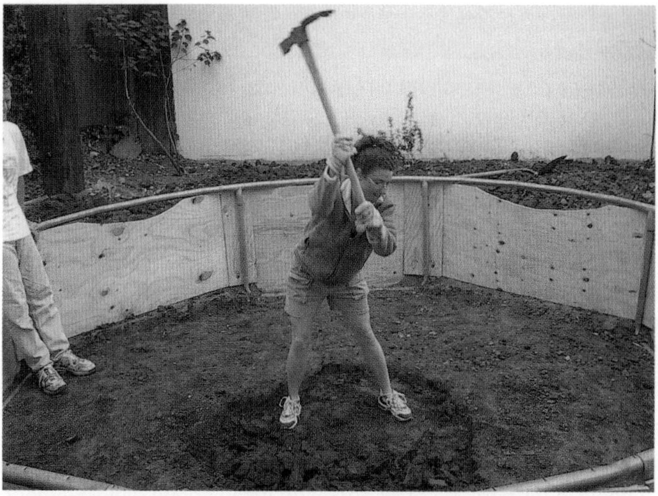

Figure 11-1 Physical health, motor coordination, and physiological performance are at their peak in young adulthood. Hard physical work and exercises are often enjoyed and are productive.

The heart and lungs are also at their peak capacity during young adulthood. Lifestyle choices made during the young-adult years will dramatically affect heart and lung health in middle age and beyond.

PHYSICAL ACTIVITY

The benefits of physical activity throughout adulthood are numerous and undisputed (Gerber, 2011). Among the benefits of regular exercise are decreased risk of heart disease, stroke, and diabetes; decreased cholesterol levels and blood pressure; increased insulin sensitivity; and increased muscle and bone mass. Active adults also display higher energy levels and less anxiety and depression. Physical activity is also a key component of weight control. These benefits can be achieved through moderate levels of exercise, and there is a dose–response relationship so that more exercise leads to even stronger benefits.

A sedentary adult should begin to increase activity levels slowly, with light to moderate intensity for a short duration (e.g., 10 minutes of walking). This can be gradually increased in *duration*, *intensity*, and *frequency* until minimum guidelines can be met.

According to the *Physical Activity Guidelines for Americans* (USDHHS, 2011), adults should perform at least 2.5 hours of moderately intense aerobic exercise every week, which should be spread throughout the week (30 minutes/day for 5 days/week or broken into shorter sessions of as little as 10 minutes at a time). Adults already achieving 2.5 hours per week should increase to 5 hours (60 minutes/day for 5 days/week) to gain more extensive health benefits. Vigorous-intensity exercise also increases the level of benefits achieved.

Muscle-strengthening activities such as weight training, body-weight calisthenics, and manual labor provide additional health benefits. These types of exercises should be moderate to high intensity, involve all major muscle groups, and be performed two or more days per week.

Exercises involving balance and coordination such as backward walking, standing on one foot, and stretches for flexibility in all major muscle groups should be performed two or more days per week.

Health Promotion

Wise food choices provide optimum nutrition, and regular exercise can help maintain health and prevent obesity or cardiovascular disease (Figure 11-2). **Physical activity** is the daily actions that use energy such as dog walking or gardening, whereas **exercise** consists of specifically planned and structured repetitive activities designed for a level of calorie burning that aids *endurance* (dancing, jogging, or swimming) (Table 11-1), *balance* (Tai Chi, heel-toe walk), *strength* (weight lifting), or *flexibility* (yoga or pilates). *Moderate physical activities* include walking at 3 mph (Rowe, 2011), golf, water aerobics, or dancing. *Vigorous activities* include aerobics, walking at 4 mph, competitive basketball, or bicycling at 10 mph (U.S. Department of Agriculture [USDHHS], 2011).

MyPyramid was developed in 2005 by the USDA as a guide for healthy daily food choices and was replaced in 2011 with MyPlate (Figure 11-3, *A*). MyPlate reflects healthy food choices and does not include foods that supply empty calories such as cookies, cakes, sugary drinks, and most fast foods. Research regarding optimum food choices for persons of all ages and with various diet limitations is ongoing (Figure 11-3, *B*).

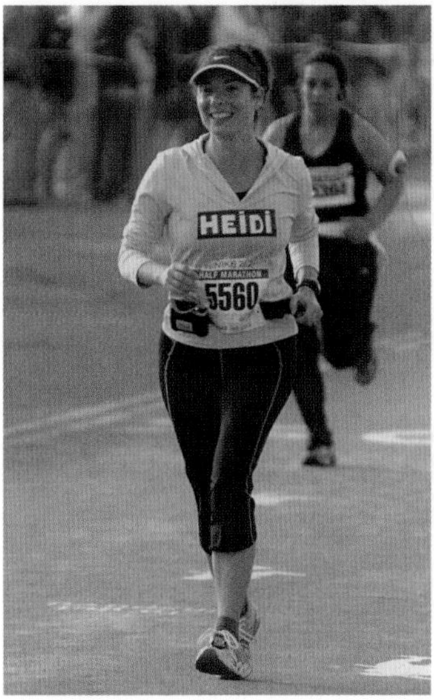

Figure 11-2 Young adults benefit from regular physical exercise such as running.

TABLE 11-1 Approximate Energy Expenditure for Levels of Activity Expressed as Multiples of Resting Energy Expenditure (REE)

Activity Category	Energy as Multiple of REE	kcal/min
Resting (sleeping, reclining)	REE × 1.0	1–1.2
Very light (seated and standing activities, painting trades, driving, laboratory work, typing, sewing, ironing, cooking, playing cards, playing a musical instrument)	REE × 1.5	Up to 2.5
Light (walking on a level surface at 2.5 to 3 mph, garage work, electrical trades, carpentry, restaurant trades, house cleaning, child care, golf, sailing, table tennis)	REE × 2.5	2.5–4.9
Moderate (walking 3.5 to 4 mph, weeding and hoeing, carrying a load, cycling, skiing, tennis, dancing)	REE × 5.0	5.0–7.4
Heavy (walking with load uphill, tree felling, heavy manual digging, basketball, climbing, football, soccer)	REE × 7.0	7.5–12.0

Data from Rowe D, Welsh G, Hell D. (2011) Stride Rate Recommendations for Moderate Intensity Walking, *J Med Sci Sports Exercise* 43(2):312-18; and Troino R, et al. (2008) Physical Activity in the US Measured by Accelerometer, *Med Sci Sports Exercise* 40(1):181-188; and Dong L, Block G, Mandel S. (2004) Activities Contribution to Total Energy Expenditure in US: Results of NHAPS Study, *Int J Behavioral Nutrition and Physical Activity* 1(4):1-4; and Ainsworth B, et al. (2000) Compendium of Physical Activity: Classification and update of energy costs, *J Med and Sci in Sports and Exercise* 32(9):498s-504.

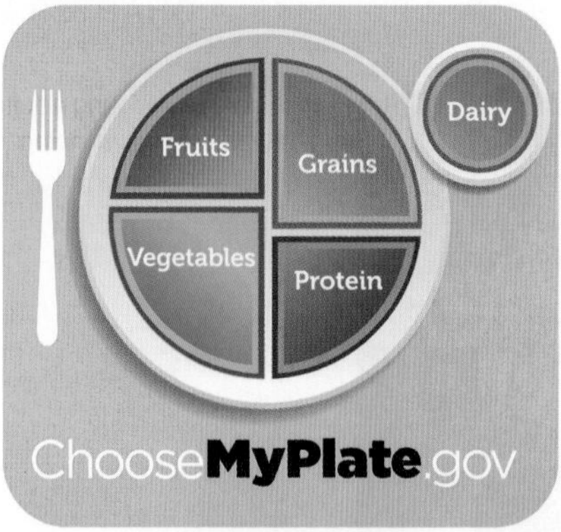

A

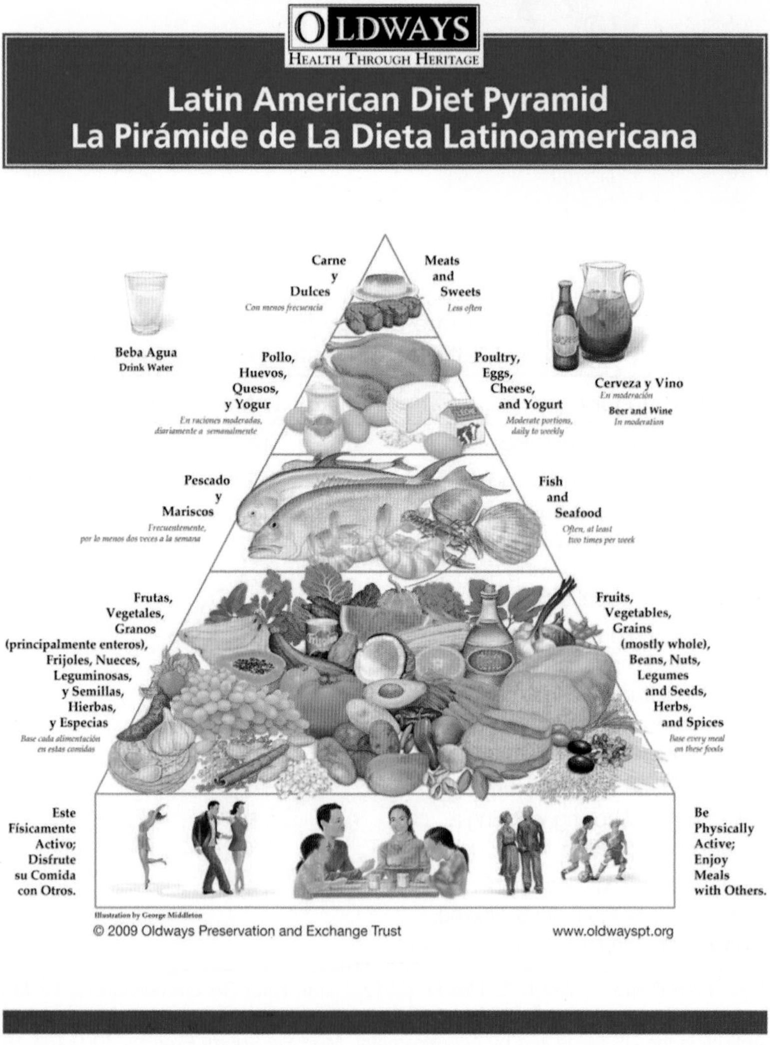

B

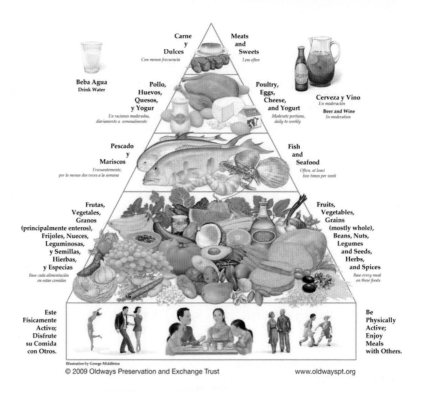

Figure 11-3 MyPlate. **A,** MyPlate.gov offers guidelines for good nutrition. (From U.S. Department of Health and Human Services/U.S. Department of Agriculture, 2011.) **B,** The traditional healthy Latin-American food pyramid has daily physical activity as its base and includes foods common to the Latin-American diet. The Latin-American Diet Pyramid can be accessed at www.oldwayspt.org/resources/heritage-pyramids/latino-diet-pyramid. *(Courtesy of Oldways Preservation and Exchange Trust.)*

Health Promotion

Smoking or substance abuse can contribute to a more rapid decline in health, beginning when the habit originates and extending throughout the lifespan. The eruption of the wisdom teeth and the development of gum disease are potential dental problems that commonly arise in this age group, and they must be addressed during the young-adult years. Conscientious brushing, flossing, and regular preventive dental care can help ensure good dental health. As the individual approaches age 30, gastric secretions may decrease, resulting in increased gastric discomforts. Junk foods, highly spiced foods, foods high in fat, and irregular eating habits established in adolescence may be more difficult to tolerate as a young adult progresses toward middle age. Visual acuity may begin to decline as the individual approaches middle age, and corrective lenses may be needed for reading or driving. Visual habits, such as taking breaks from reading to focus eyes on a distant point, can minimize visual decline associated with reading and frequent computer work.

Healthy People 2020 (see Chapter 1) has identified priority areas for health promotion during the young adulthood years. The priority areas include maintaining physical activity, fitness, and nutrition; decreasing the use of tobacco and alcohol; encouraging positive mental health practices; and providing adequate information concerning family planning options. It is easier to develop positive health habits at a young age than to change or compensate for bad habits later in life. Most lifestyle choices and health habits are made during the young adult years.

Often, entrance into college provides the final opportunity for parents to initiate a health checkup and to provide education concerning lifestyle choices. After the precollege physical examination, the young adult often does not seek health assessment unless a problem arises. The major causes of death in young adulthood are most often related to accidents or violence, both of which often are preventable.

WOMEN'S HEALTH

Women have a great influence on childrearing and early learning. Maintaining women's health, therefore, may enable women to influence a generation of children to practice good health habits and to choose healthy lifestyles. Education concerning women's health issues and access to care have increased dramatically in the past few years. Women's health clinics and women's health specialists are available at most health-care facilities.

Cultural Considerations

Wide variations exist in cultural practices (Figure 11-4). Health-care workers must be alert to individual differences within a cultural group and must avoid stereotyping patients from specific cultural backgrounds. A strong belief in fate may prevent some women from seeking health care early. Diet, religious objects, and the use of folk medicine also play roles in preventing illness in some cultural groups. Modesty can influence the desire to avoid genital examinations, and so maintaining privacy is very important during examinations. Communication between the health-care worker and the patient is important, because eye contact, touch, and use of personal space influence the rapport between patient and caregiver. Some women prefer to receive health care from female providers. Cultural response to a change in gender function may influence a women's acceptance of contraception or sterilization practices. In some cultures, women

(Continued)

Cultural Considerations—cont'd

who are menstruating are considered unclean and are isolated and forbidden to have contact with males. In other cultures, women consider menopause as a nonevent and do not suffer from anxieties related to aging (see Chapter 3).

Cultural beliefs concerning women's health care influence preferred labor management, position for birth, location of delivery, and the role of family members during labor and delivery. Ethical issues also influence women's health care. Ethical issues include abortion, surrogate parenting, infertility treatment techniques, adoption, stem cell research, gene therapy, cord blood banking, and organ transplantation. Social issues such as homelessness, access to health care, and poverty also need to be considered as issues related to women's health care.

Pregnancy

Because a unique risk to health occurs during pregnancy, providing family-planning services and birth control options for the young adult is essential (see Table 10-2). Maternal mortality rates have continued to decline during the past decade thanks to the availability of health care. The major risk factors contributing to the mortality rate include lack of prenatal care, inadequate knowledge of health needs, and poor nutrition. The death rate for young mothers obtaining legal abortions in the United States is low, but those performed outside an accredited facility often have negative outcomes. Therefore the health-care worker can play an important role in referring the young adult to available community resources. Recommended exercise during pregnancy is discussed in Chapter 6.

Health Promotion

The practice trial of vaginal birth after cesarean (VBAC) remains controversial, but *Healthy People 2020* goals include reducing the rate of cesarean births by the year 2020.

Ectopic pregnancy (pregnancy in the fallopian tube instead of the uterus) can be the result of malformation of the fallopian tube or from damage caused by pelvic inflammatory disease (PID). Sexually transmitted diseases (STDs) are the major causes of PID. Therefore, promoting healthy behaviors related to safe-sex practices during adolescence and young adulthood can reduce maternal morbidity and mortality.

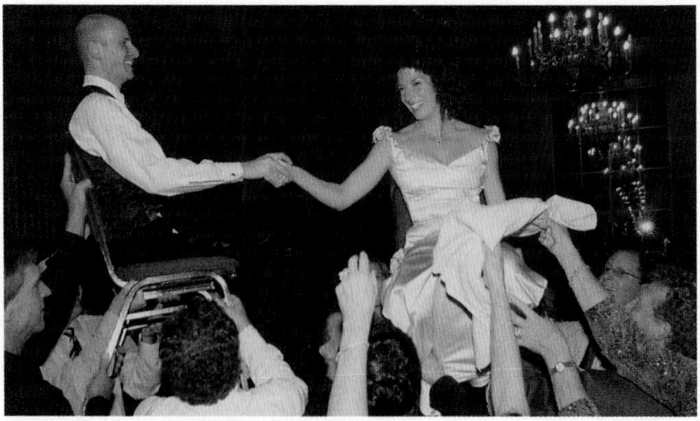

Figure 11-4 A typical cultural practice in a Jewish religious wedding ceremony. Cultural beliefs and practices are learned in childhood and can be carried throughout generations.

Hysterectomy (removal of the uterus) is the most common surgery performed on women during the reproductive years. The increasing use of laser techniques to treat uterine fibroids may decrease the need for this surgery.

Annual Papanicolaou (Pap) smears are encouraged for sexually active young women, because human papillomavirus (HPV) is also known to be a cause of cervical cancer, and both Pap and HPV tests are done at the same time. Encouraging breast self-examinations and mammograms at appropriate intervals can lead to early detection and early intervention for breast cancer (Box 11-1).

BOX 11-1 Breast Self-Examination

Perform breast self-examination monthly. If you are menstruating, do the examination 1 week after the beginning of your period, because your breasts are less tender at this time. If you are not menstruating, choose any day that you can easily remember, such as the first day of each month. Examine your breasts in three ways: in front of a mirror, lying down, and in the shower.

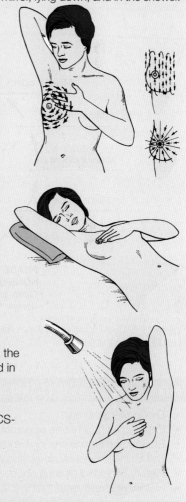

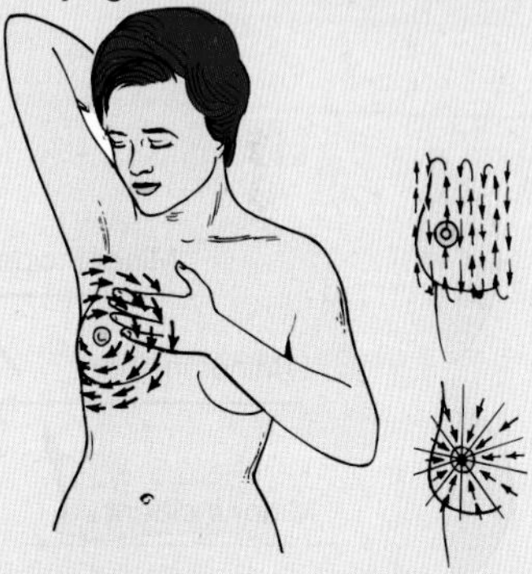

IN FRONT OF A MIRROR

Inspect your breasts in four steps:

1. With arms at your sides.
2. With arms over your head.
3. With your hands on your hips, pressing them firmly to flex your chest muscles.
4. While bending forward. Note any change in shape or appearance of your breasts, and note skin or nipple changes such as dimpling of the skin. Squeeze each nipple gently to identify any discharge.

LYING DOWN

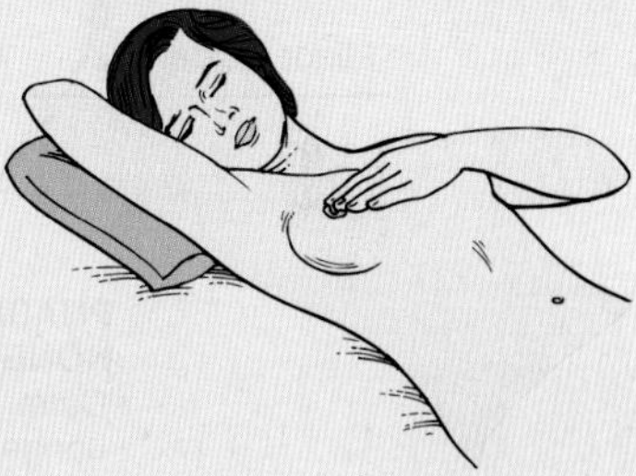

Place a small pillow under your right shoulder and put your right hand under your head while you examine your right breast with your left hand. Use the sensitve pads of your fingers to press gently into the breast tissue. Use a systematic pattern to check the entire breast. One pattern is to feel the tissue in a circular pattern, spiraling inward toward the nipple. Another method is to use an up-and-down pattern. Use the same systematic pattern to examine the underarm area, because breast tissue is also present here. Repeat for the other breast.

IN THE SHOWER

Raise your right arm. Use your soapy fingers to feel the breast tissue in the same systematic pattern described in the "Lying Down" section.

FOR ADDITIONAL INFORMATION

Contact the American Cancer Society at 1-800-ACS-2345, or visit www.cancer.org.

Illustrations from Lowdermilk DL, Perry SE, Bobak IM: *Maternity and women's health care*, ed 7, St Louis, 2000, Mosby.

Stress, Coping, and Domestic Violence

The multiple roles of women in the young-adult phase of life can contribute to stress and the potential development of depression or anxiety. A single working mother may have the combined responsibilities of running a household, earning enough money to cover basic expenses, finding adequate and affordable day care for young children, and caring for an elderly parent. These responsibilities may cause the young woman to delay seeking health care for herself, which can lead to devastating results.

Violent behavior against women is an epidemic that contributes to the morbidity and mortality statistics of young adult women (Figure 11-5). Domestic violence can include psychological, physical, sexual, financial, and social abuses between intimate partners. The result is often social isolation and physical trauma. The CDC now refers to domestic violence as intimate partner violence (IPV). IPV involves all ethnic, racial, socioeconomic, and educational levels of the population (Box 11-2).

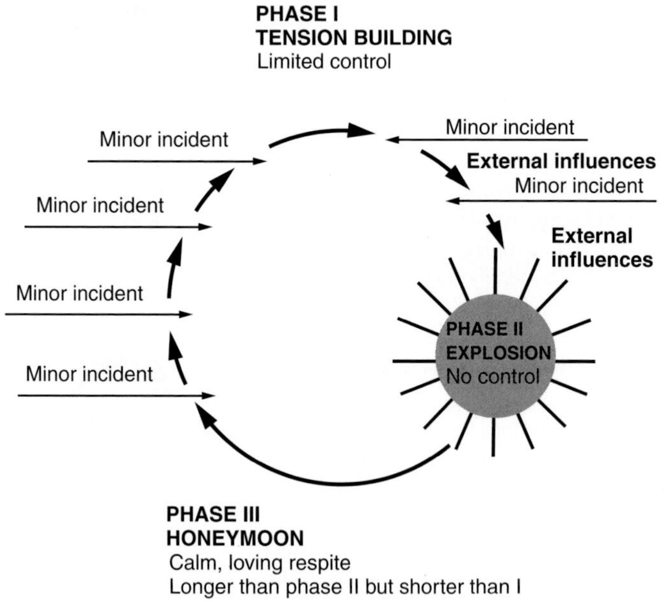

Figure 11-5 Cycle of violence. (From Rawlins P, Williams S, Beck C: *Mental health psychiatric nursing*, St Louis, 1993, Mosby.)

BOX 11-2 Signs of Intimate Partner Violence

- Erratic prenatal care
- Erratic child health-care appointments
- Bruises and lacerations in various stages of healing
- Self blame for marital or relationship problems
- History of alcohol or drug abuse in partner
- History of abuse as a child (cycle of violence)
- History of minor battering incidents

Health Promotion

Many communities have programs to address domestic violence and other crimes targeting women. *Healthy People 2020* lists specific objectives related to prevention and treatment programs (see Chapter 1).

MEN'S HEALTH

Men currently do not have gender-specific health-care providers as women do. Men's health as a specialty may be a future trend but is not yet established in most health-care facilities. Young male adults appear to seek health care or guidance less frequently than women within this age group. Although they may accompany their pregnant partners to the obstetrician, unless they have fertility issues, men rarely seek medical assistance until a specific problem presents itself.

The high testosterone levels in males may contribute to a lower cholesterol level than in women. Statistically, men may be at a higher risk for injury because of their work environment. Men may also smoke and drink alcohol more often than women, contributing to the development of many health problems.

Some men may resist seeking health care even when a health problem is present, or they do not seek preventative screening programs. However, recent public education has increased the awareness of the need for testicular self-examination (TSE) by all young adult males as part of a preventative program. The highest rate of testicular cancer is within the 17- to 35-year-old age group; thus TSE is an important aspect of preventive health care.

Free clinics are available within many communities for STD testing and treatment and human immunodeficiency virus/acquired immunodeficiency syndrome (HIV/AIDS) counseling. Physical examinations have become routine requirements at colleges before a student can enter sports programs and can be the initial access route to health care. Education concerning the harmful effects of smoking, alcohol, substance abuse, and obesity, and ways to reduce these problems, has increased awareness of health in men. Health and fitness clubs have become popular and lucrative businesses and have led to improvements in the health status for men and women. However, health-care workers must caution men concerning the adverse effects of overtraining, which are manifested by body and muscle fatigue, joint or muscle injury, dehydration, or loss of strength.

Increasing access, within the community and workplace, to health education and screening can be very advantageous. Studies have shown that community education and federal intervention concerning issues such as the need for seat-belt use, the dangers of smoking and drinking, and the use of condoms may have contributed significantly to healthier behavior choices. Many colleges and community groups host health fairs where blood pressure checks and education concerning various lifestyle choices are offered.

PSYCHOSOCIAL DEVELOPMENT

Schools play significant roles in helping the adolescent prepare for the developmental tasks and challenges of young adulthood. Parenting and family-life classes and money-management workshops are examples of courses that can help prepare for the transition into adult life. Students who plan to attend college often do not participate in these preparatory courses, because their focus is on college prerequisite courses. Some colleges have designed survival programs that help freshman students adjust to their new environments and adult responsibilities. Most colleges also offer career counseling and support services for young adults to help them achieve their educational goals. Work-study courses introduce young adults to the work environment and help them adapt to the work milieu.

There are many developmental tasks and challenges that occur during the young-adult years. These tasks include developing a mature sense of right and wrong, successful separation from family control, initiating a preferred lifestyle, establishing friends and intimate relationships, deciding on marriage, pursuing career goals, and developing parenting skills. The sense of identity should be formed and stable by young adulthood and will start the individual on a path toward specific goals. These specific goals can change in later stages of the lifespan, when unexpected events, further self learning, or periods of transition allow time for reflection and reevaluation of accomplishments, and new goals can be formulated.

Intimacy

Erikson described establishing intimacy as one of the major tasks of young adulthood (see Chapter 5). Intimacy involves more than sexual behavior. It includes the ability to develop a warm, trusting, honest relationship with another person with whom it is safe to be open and to express and share private thoughts. If a clear sense of identity has not been achieved during adolescence, then the young adult may feel guarded and only form casual relationships. Eventually this may contribute to isolation or difficulty in forming deep, long-term commitments.

Cognitive Ability

Intellectual and creative skills and abilities peak during young adulthood and improve with expanded education and experience. Piaget was a theorist (see Chapter 5) who believed that the development of the formal operation as a method of thinking begins in adolescence and extends into young adulthood. The level of abstract thinking and logical reasoning is enhanced by the technology that is available in everyday life. The formal-operation type of thinking is necessary in the techniques of effective problem solving.

The young adult's cognitive process involves realizing that knowledge is the integration of multiple points of view. This process of integrating various points of view to develop knowledge and understanding is sometimes referred to as postformal operational thought (Commons et al., 1982). Individuals who have a well-developed postformal thought process are best able to problem solve in general, including choosing between multiple-choice answers on a test. Therefore school performance may be best in the young-adult age group.

Levinson was a psychologist who described four seasons of life (see Chapter 5). He believed that each season had a structure that is separated by transitional periods. During the structure period of young adulthood, significant choices such as a marriage partner and commitment to a career are made. During the following transitional phase, those choices are reviewed and reevaluated, and changes may be made. During one of the later transitional phases, individuals may reflect on past activities and may become unhappy because of missed opportunities or what they perceive as wrong choices. This may contribute to a midlife crisis experience.

Moral Reasoning

Kohlberg was a theorist who believed that the individual must be capable of the formal operational level of thought before achieving mature moral reasoning. Life experiences in an adult role or a college milieu can enhance the development of moral reasoning. Taking responsibility for the care of others, handling the differing points of view of others, and understanding how their own actions affect others all contribute to the development of mature moral reasoning.

Sexuality

Young adults who are significant in a child's life can model positive displays of affection. Having young children see loving and joyous contact, such as hugging and kissing between parental role models and close family members, can help a child understand caring behaviors. Although allowing nudity in the home is a personal choice for parents, the concept of demonstrating comfort with their own bodies helps children to develop a positive body image. Treating one part of the body as dirty or naughty may result in having to readjust these beliefs when the child reaches maturity in order to achieve a sense of comfort in intimacy, and therefore the mature child's mastery of this task of attaining intimacy may be delayed.

Sexual intimacy in young adulthood differs from that in adolescence. By young adulthood, identity and cognitive function have reached the level that allows intimate sharing, controlled but honest emotional expression, caring about the partner, and the ability to make compromises and commitments. Sexual behavior and expectations are influenced by culture, customs, and environment. However, the ability to develop a sense of intimacy and the attachment required for a long-term commitment is closely related to the individual's experience when he or she was an infant seeking attachment with a parent. Healthy parent–child bonding produces a sense of security and trust. If relationships with parents in the early years did not produce a healthy, secure attachment, then achievement of a secure and stable intimacy with others in the young-adulthood phase of life may be more difficult or delayed.

Marriage

Many young adults who pursue higher education in college either postpone marriage or choose careful family-planning or child-care arrangements that allow them to continue to pursue their goals. See Table 10-2 for contraceptive options available for effective family planning. Marriage most often occurs during the young-adult phase of the life cycle. However, many individuals delay marriage until they are established in their careers. Today childbearing can be achieved at a later age due in large part to the advances in research and technology. People often select partners who are similar to themselves in interests, values, religious beliefs, and education. Family pressures or cultural traditions may also play a role in choosing a marriage partner.

Partner choice is thought to be based on a three-stage process (Murstein, 1982). The first stage is the *stimulus stage,* which involves initial impressions and awareness of characteristics that attract each partner in the couple to each other. The *value-comparison stage* follows and involves getting to know one another better. The *role stage* involves evaluating long-term compatibility and deciding on a long-term commitment.

Gender roles and career issues play an important part in early adjustment to marriage. Balancing work, marriage, family, and parental roles is a challenge for young adults.

TABLE 11-2 Growth and Development of Parents

Child's Task (Erikson's Stages)	Parents' Task	Intervention
FIRST PRENATAL TRIMESTER		
Growth	Develop attitude toward newborn. "Happy" about child? Parent of one disabled child? Unwed mother? These factors and others will affect the developing attitude of the mother.	Develop positive attitude in both parents concerning expected birth of child. Use referrals and agencies as needed.
SECOND PRENATAL TRIMESTER		
Growth	Mother focuses on infant because of fetal movements felt. Parents picture what infant will look like, what future he/she will have, and other ideas.	Parents' focus is on child care and needs and providing physical environment for expected infant. Therefore information concerning care of the newborn should be provided at this time.
THIRD PRENATAL TRIMESTER		
Growth	Mother feels large. Attention focuses on how fetus is going to get out.	Detailed information should be presented at this time concerning the birth process, preparation for birth, breastfeeding, and care of sibling at home.
BIRTH		
Adjustment to external environment	Elicit positive responses from child and respond by meeting child's need for food and closeness; if parents receive only negative responses (e.g., sleepy infant, crying infant, difficult feeder, congenital anomaly), positive development of the parent may be inhibited.	Encourage early touch, feeding, and other practices. Explain behavior and appearance of newborn to allay fears. Help parents to identify positive responses. (Use infant's reflexes, such as grasp reflex, to identify a response by placing mother's finger into infant's hand.)
INFANT		
Trust	Learn "cues" presented by infant to determine individual needs of infant.	Help parents assess and interpret needs of infant (avoid feelings of helplessness or incompetence). Do not let in-laws take over parental tasks. Help parents cope with problems such as colic.

TABLE 11-2 Growth and Development of Parents—cont'd

Child's Task (Erikson's Stages)	Parents' Task	Intervention
TODDLER		
Autonomy	Try to accept the pattern of growth and development. Accept some loss of control, but maintain some limits for safety.	Help parents cope with transient independence of child (e.g., allow child to go on tricycle, but don't yell "Don't fall," or anxiety may be radiated.)
PRESCHOOL		
Initiative	Learn to separate from child.	Help parents show standards but let go so child can develop some independence. A preschool experience may be helpful.
SCHOOL AGE		
Industry	Accept importance of child's peers. Parents must learn to accept some rejection from child at times. Patience is needed to allow children to do things for themselves, even if it takes longer. Do not do the school project for the child. Provide chores for child appropriate to his/her age level.	Help parents to understand that child is developing his/her own limits and self-discipline. Be there to guide child but do not constantly intrude. Help child achieve results from his/her own efforts to perform.
ADOLESCENT		
Establishment of identity Acceptance of pubertal changes Development of abstract reasoning Examination of career choices Investigation of lifestyles Controlling of feelings	Parents must learn to let child live his/her own life and not to expect total control over the child. Expect at times to be discredited by teenager. Expect differences in opinion and respect them. Guide but do not push.	Help parents adjust to changing role and relationship with adolescent (e.g., as child develops his/her own identity, child may become a Democrat if parents are Republican). Expose child to varied career fields and life experiences. Help child to understand emerging emotions and feelings brought about by puberty.

Modified from Leifer G: *Introduction to maternity & pediatric nursing*, ed 6, Philadelphia, 2011, Saunders.

This period is known as the beginning task of *generativity,* as described by Erikson (see Chapter 5). It should be noted that generativity can be achieved by means other than parenting, such as involvement in a career, close interactions with family, or participation in community activities.

Parenting

Not all adults achieve or desire marriage and family. Some pursue careers that are fulfilling, thereby leaving little time for the responsibilities that marriage and parenthood require. Others choose to be in long-term, committed relationships without children, and some choose to delay marriage and childrearing until later life stages. However, this chapter will include the development of parenting skills as one of the tasks of young adulthood (Table 11-2).

The most proactive development of parental skills begins at the time conception is confirmed. When parents learn they are to have a baby, both positive and negative feelings are normally evoked. Parents may want the baby and want to be perfect parents. However, they may worry about being inadequately prepared for the parental role, the time commitment, and the impact on their careers and lifestyle. In the second trimester of pregnancy, when parents begin to feel the fetus move, their focus turns to the baby and what it might be. By the beginning of the third trimester of pregnancy, parents ascribe personality traits to the fetus and are receptive to teachings about parenting and child care.

If the newborn arrives as a welcomed guest in the home, and the parents are supportive of one another, healthy parenting styles can be easily learned. At least 6 months of maternity leave, from work or from other routine activities, may be ideal in fostering attachment between parent and child, but often financial or career pressures require a shorter adjustment time. Close parent–child interactions during the early months of life can help in the formation of healthy attachments and positive parenting styles. Stepparents or parents who adopt older children may need extra time and effort to develop parent–child attachment and relationships.

The infant soon learns to associate the presence of the mother with feeding and relief of hunger and discomfort, and the baby soon calms whenever the mother is present. This behavior in turn strengthens the mother's sense of adequacy and effectiveness as a parent. Parent–infant attachment is best observed during feeding, when both mother and infant should be focused on each other. If either is preoccupied or inattentive, parent–infant bonding may not be successful. If the parent is an adolescent, some developmental tasks of adolescence may interfere with the developmental tasks of parenthood. Special interventions by the health-care worker can be helpful in prioritizing behaviors and in meeting the major needs of the infant and adolescent parent. Refer to Chapter 10 for more information on the adolescent stage of development.

TEACHING TECHNIQUES

Successful learning for adults always involves relating the information they are learning to the appropriate developmental tasks they are experiencing. For example, a new parent will likely be very receptive to information concerning parenting skills. An adult in a managerial position at work may be most receptive to learning about managing styles and techniques. The knowledge and skills learned should be applicable to the learner, should be realistic, and should help solve the problems currently encountered by the learner. Concepts presented to young adults should build on their previous knowledge and skills, rather than beginning below their level of understanding, or they will be "turned off". Teaching goals should be clear and should outline how the new knowledge can be applied and how it will benefit the learners' current life roles. Learning is a lifelong process. Teaching techniques for young adults should be interactive, problem oriented, and related to daily psychosocial tasks at work, home, or school.

KEY POINTS

- Young adulthood is most often defined as being from 20 to 40 years of age.
- Physiological performance has a natural peak between 20 and 30 years of age.
- Proper nutrition and exercise can prevent obesity and can contribute to health during the young-adult years and beyond.
- Most lifestyle patterns are established during the young-adult years.
- It is easier to develop positive health habits as a young adult to achieve a positive health status than it is to change habits later in life.
- The major causes of death in the young-adult age group are related to accidents and violence, and both are preventable.
- Promoting healthy behaviors relating to safe-sex practices during adolescence and young adulthood can reduce the incidence of sexually transmitted diseases.
- Recent public education efforts have increased awareness of the need for testicular self-examination (TSE) and breast self-examination (BSE) as part of gender-specific preventive health programs.
- Health and fitness spas have become lucrative businesses that help improve the health status of men and women. However, overtraining may adversely affect health and should be avoided.
- Developmental tasks of young adulthood include developing a stable sense of identity and a mature sense of right and wrong; successful separation from family control; establishing adult friendships and intimate relationships; choosing marriage partners and career goals; developing parenting skills; and initiating a preferred lifestyle.
- Piaget's formal operational thinking begins in adolescence and extends into young adulthood.
- Formal operational thinking is necessary for the establishment of effective problem-solving skills.
- Postformal operational thought involves integrating various points of view.
- In most cultures there are established expectations of adulthood.
- The task of generativity can be achieved by a means other than parenting.
- Development of a parent accelerates when conception is confirmed.
- When teaching young adults, the goals and how the new knowledge can be applied in the lives of the learners should be made clear.

Critical Thinking

Using Erikson's stages of growth and development, discuss how parents can apply positive parenting styles to help their children successfully achieve developmental tasks.

REVIEW QUESTIONS

1. Young adulthood includes the ages between:
   a. 12 and 16 years.
   b. 17 and 19 years.
   c. 20 and 40 years.
   d. 41 and 60 years.

2. The young adult is in Erikson's stage of:
   a. industry.
   b. autonomy.
   c. intimacy.
   d. identity.

3. An ectopic pregnancy is a(n):
   a. unplanned pregnancy.
   b. pregnancy occurring outside the uterus.
   c. pregnancy occurring in early adulthood.
   d. pregnancy consisting of twins.

4. Effective teaching techniques for the young adult should include information that:
   a. is realistic and helps solve problems.
   b. is exciting and dramatic.
   c. relates to world problems.
   d. is already understood.

5. The major cause of death in the young-adult age group is:
   a. congenital malformation.
   b. preventable accidents.
   c. heart disease.
   d. sedentary lifestyles.

CHAPTER 12

Middle Adulthood

http://evolve.elsevier.com/Leifer/growth

OBJECTIVES

1. Define middle adulthood.
2. List the physiological changes that occur during middle adulthood.
3. Define the major developmental tasks and challenges of middle adulthood.
4. State the complexities of the menopausal experience in women.
5. Discuss the male climacteric.
6. Define midlife crisis.
7. Discuss sexuality in the middle-adulthood phase of the life cycle.
8. List preventative health-care measures appropriate for middle adulthood.
9. Define the "sandwich generation."
10. Describe the benefits of regular exercise during middle adulthood.
11. List teaching strategies that may be effective for the patient in the middle-adult phase of the life cycle.

KEY TERMS

climacteric
"empty nest" syndrome
generativity
hot flashes
identity accommodation
menopause
middle adulthood
midlife crisis
reproductive health
sandwich generation
sexuality
stagnation

DEFINITION

Middle adulthood is defined as the period of development after the early adult years but before retirement (Levinson, 1978). Middle adulthood is often referred to as the period between 40 and 60 years of age. An individual's behavior during this period is influenced by genetics and the environment, and an interaction of biological, psychological, and social changes occur. By middle age, the adult has established roots in a community with ties to culture, religious groups, schools, neighborhood centers, and friends. Some culture-specific influences affect development, but the greatest current environmental influence is the worldwide political dynamic that reaches across oceans to influence life and lifestyles in the United States. Some theorists suggest that developmental changes are gradual and progressive, but others express the concept of passing through distinct stages (see Chapter 5).

Lifespan Considerations

Metabolic needs decrease during middle adulthood, and if diet and exercise are not part of a healthy lifestyle, excess weight begins to accumulate. A decrease in energy and perceived physical attractiveness may occur. A loss of muscle tone and skin elasticity may result in a less firm appearance of body contours. Body fat may redistribute to the hip area. Impacted wisdom teeth may require extraction, and periodontal disease is a risk if oral care is not meticulous. Hair may begin to gray and thin. Eye changes common to middle age can be easily corrected with glasses, contact lenses, or laser surgery. Diet, smoking, and lack of exercise influence cardiovascular changes that occur during midlife, but hormonal changes also influence risk factors for cardiovascular disease.

DEVELOPMENTAL TASKS

The main task or crisis of middle adulthood is generativity versus stagnation (Erikson, 1994). *Generativity* has been defined as contributing in a positive way to family or community. This contribution improves self-image and promotes subjective well-being. Failure to achieve generativity results in *stagnation,* which is total concern for self and denial of the developmental process. Generativity can be achieved in many ways and is not necessarily limited to having children and a family of one's own. There are many opportunities to achieve generativity through career and personal activities and achievements. Other developmental tasks of middle adulthood include managing a career and finances, managing a household, and nurturing marriage and family relationships.

Maintaining a positive self-image is important to the middle-aged adult. When individuals deny they are aging and cannot view themselves as middle aged, they often experience difficulty in adjusting to necessary changes, and depression may develop. Maintaining a positive self-image is a challenge when society and the media place high importance on looking and acting young. Another important task of middle age is identity accommodation, which is changing the concept of one's own identity to fit reality, rather than what was dreamed.

The effect of the spouse or significant other on continued development and life stability is important. The feedback of a spouse or significant other influences self-image in the midlife stage. New social experiences challenge the middle-aged adult. Involvement with child care, athletic events, parents of school friends, and parent–child relationships can also influence psychological well-being (Figure 12-1).

CHALLENGES

Maintaining optimum cognitive functioning is necessary to prevent a decrease in problem-solving skills. Adjusting to changes in relationships with coworkers, friends, and family are also important to maintaining psychological well-being. Many middle-aged adults find time to continue their education, which may have been interrupted by marriage and childrearing. The middle-aged adult may need more time to learn and assimilate new material, but once learned, the content

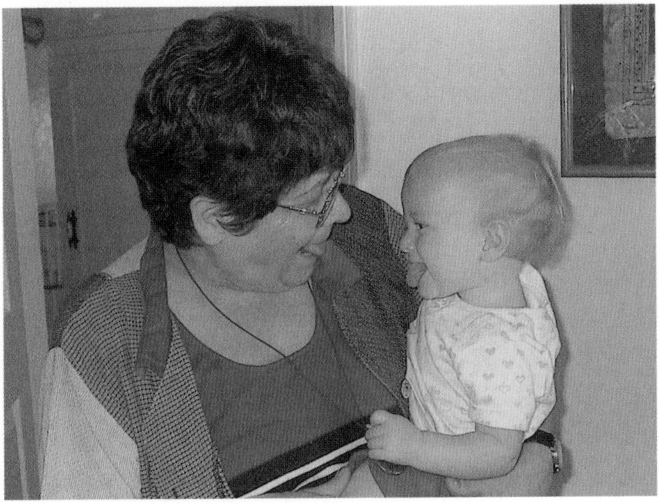

Figure 12–1 A grandparent enjoys remaining involved with the family and values interaction with grandchildren.

is remembered with more accuracy. Perseverance and patience may be needed to succeed in school. The stresses of middle adulthood often include marital separation, divorce, major illness or injury, loss of income, or unplanned pregnancy. The challenge of caring for aged parents while helping teen children into adulthood also offers challenges to this age group.

Women at midlife are at high risk for social isolation because of divorce, separation, or widowhood. The "empty nest" syndrome that can occur when grown children start to leave home for the first time may increase the feelings of isolation.

Midlife Crisis

Middle adulthood is a time of self-reflection, reevaluation, and prioritization. Looking back, the adult may grieve lost youth and missed opportunities. Looking ahead, adults may fear the inevitability of their own mortality, which may lead to despair. Sometimes during this stage of the midlife crisis, adults try to make up for lost opportunities of the past or challenge the inevitability of the future. They may start to engage in behaviors that are atypical for their character (Figure 12-2). Sometimes reflection and reinterpretation of past experiences bring new insights and may serve as turning points in self-perception.

The Sandwich Generation

Middle adults are said to be in the sandwich generation, which means they must handle increased financial and emotional responsibilities related to their children and their older and possibly dependent parents. These stressors contribute to the challenges of middle adulthood.

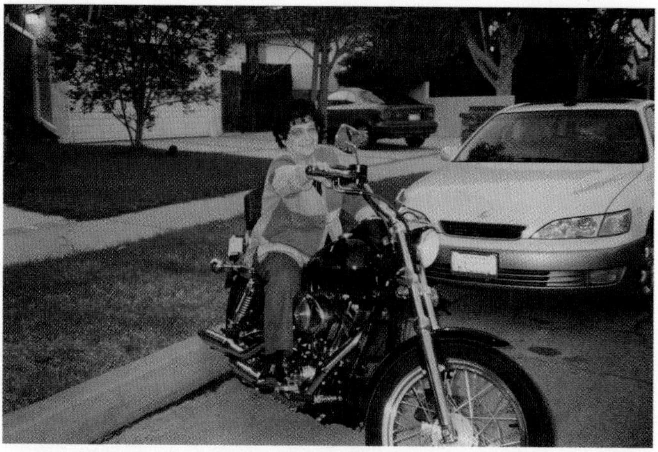

Figure 12–2 It is never too late to learn and to enjoy the skills of a new activity.

The family influences the adjustment to middle adulthood. A fulfilling marriage will help validate positive self-esteem, whereas divorce, separation, conflicts with adult children, or aging parents may impact the psychological functioning of middle-aged adults in a negative way.

SEXUALITY

Sexuality is a part of every phase of the life cycle and is not limited to the sex act. Sexuality involves beliefs and behaviors that surround physiological responses, emotions, and sociocultural values. Communication, a sense of closeness, and mutual comfort are key aspects of sexuality. Middle adulthood is a time when the adult is often focused on career goals and financial stability, and little time or energy may be set aside to fulfill sexual needs. Yet the middle-aged woman is at the peak of sexual desire and sexual pleasure, because the pressures of pregnancy prevention are often relieved by the approach of menopause.

A significant percentage of the population in the United States is living as single adults. The reasons can include postponing marriage for a career, divorces, or never entering into a long-term relationship. Options for sexual lifestyles for the single person can include celibacy, a sexually exclusive companion, or a long-term relationship with one or more partners. People may also live together without marriage for a variety of reasons, including the fact that a widow, widower, or divorced person may have to give up monetary benefits if he or she were to remarry. Less common situations that people engage in to satisfy sexual needs include open marriages, extramarital affairs, group marriages, and swinging (i.e., mate swapping) (Masters et al., 1986; Bergstrand, 2000).

Gradual hormonal changes in the woman occur before menopause and may start as early as age 35, although the age for actual menopause is closer to 50. Each woman responds to subtle menopausal changes in a unique way, and sexuality can be affected by these changes. Estrogen-sensitive skin can lead to dry skin. Breasts flatten and hair thins as estrogen-to-androgen ratios change.

The absence of children in the home, who may have left for college or marriage, may provide time to renew relationships between partners. A self-assured attitude, developed as a result of experience and age, may limit inhibitions and can create many enjoyable close moments with partners at this stage of life.

REPRODUCTIVE HEALTH

Reproductive health is a term used to describe the health of the reproductive organs in all persons. The climacteric refers to the time in life in which hormonal changes result in cessation of the reproductive ability in the female and a corresponding decrease in sexual activity in the male. Complex interactions exist among sex hormones, physiology, and physical and emotional well-being.

Structural differences in the male and female central nervous systems begin in the embryonic stage of development and are influenced by hormones. The reproductive years in the female involve a unique group of health issues. Sex hormones such as estrogen protect women from some illnesses that often affect men. As they age and as sex hormones decrease during menopause, women develop risks for disease that are similar to men's. Most clinical research concerning health has been conducted with male subjects, and the same findings were applied to women, which has not always been accurate.

Today women make up 40% of students in medical schools and more than 50% of minority graduates from medical schools (Boulis, 2010). Women are increasingly influencing the direction of research and the delivery of health care.

Women's Health

Menopause is the cessation of the menstrual period caused by hormonal changes in the body. Menopause usually begins between 45 and 55 years of age and is genetically controlled. The menstrual cycle becomes shorter and more irregular. Hot flashes may result when capillaries dilate and blood rushes to the skin surface. The body feels warm, the woman may sweat, and then vasoconstriction occurs and the woman feels cold. This can occur several times a day and is very uncomfortable and distracting. Hormone replacement therapy (HRT) may be prescribed, but is not appropriate for all women because of risks for developing blood clots and other complications. Complementary and alternative medicine (CAM) therapy is popular with many women during menopause. Health-care workers must assess any interactions between CAM therapy used by the woman and prescribed medicines or treatments.

The onset and experience of menopause is unique for each woman, and health-care approaches must be tailored to each (Box 12-1; see also Chapter 13). A detailed and accurate personal-health interview can uncover problems that require interventions.

Recent medical advances have prolonged the physical reproductive capabilities of some women. The psychosocial issues involved in childbearing at a later age, and the advantages and disadvantages of the middle-aged or older adult becoming a new parent, present new challenges to the parents, the child, and the health-care worker.

BOX 12-1 Signs of Menopausal Changes in Women

- Hot flashes
- Heart palpitations
- Headache
- Decreased vaginal lubrication
- Fatigue
- Insomnia
- Emotional lability (happy one minute, crying the next)

Men's Health

Sexual concerns of men are typically related to role changes, work-related stress, decreased physical fitness, and sexual performance anxiety. Indicators of health, as outlined in *Healthy People 2020,* include rates of longevity, morbidity, and mortality. Although longevity rates have increased for both men and women, women still generally live longer than men. In each leading cause of death in adults, men have a higher rate of mortality. The morbidity rate is generally higher for women in both acute and chronic conditions. A contributory factor may be that men perceive themselves as healthy and therefore delay seeking medical care and preventative care. Research has shown that there are explanations for gender differences in health and illness (Graham, 2009). Testosterone levels may lower high-density lipoprotein (HDL, lipid) levels, and body-fat distribution in men may predispose them to heart disease.

The male climacteric involves a gradual decline in the blood concentration of testosterone and other hormones. This results in a decrease in muscle mass and strength, a decrease in sex drive, and a decrease in a sense of well-being. Testosterone-replacement therapy has recently been studied and has been found to have positive influences on improving strength, decreasing fat accumulation, and increasing libido and sense of well-being. Testosterone-replacement therapy does not increase erectile function, because blood circulation plays a major role in erectile function. Some nonprescription medications have recently become available for use for specific symptoms related to the male climacteric. Many drugs decrease testosterone levels in the male, such as chemotherapy, ingestion of lead and exposure to certain insecticides, ethanol, and many illicit drugs. Disease such as cystic fibrosis, sickle cell anemia, anorexia nervosa, liver disease, and renal failure also decrease testosterone levels in men. Androgen therapy is used with caution in older men with enlarged prostates and urinary symptoms.

Generally, men remain in the workforce longer than women and may partake in activities that pose a higher potential for injuries. Men engage in sports and leisure activities that also have a high risk for injury, and some may use illegal substances to prove their masculinity. Young boys are often socialized to ignore symptoms of illness and are told not to "be a sissy"; so, to avoid being labeled as sickly, men may postpone seeking medical advice until the problem is more advanced.

It is well known that strenuous exercise suppresses ovarian function in women, and many champion athletes have *amenorrhea* (absence of menstrual periods). Strenuous exercise can also affect men by decreasing testosterone levels and decreasing the sperm count; this effect can last for several months. Middle-aged men who fear the aging process may begin to experience alteration in sexual performance, but the ability to procreate, or father children, remains intact.

Health Promotion

Gender-appropriate health education is important to provide vital information without damaging sex-role–stereotyped self-images. Men typically contact the health-care system via a pediatrician when young, a school nurse when school age, and a military doctor or company physician when a young adult. Men often do not choose a personal doctor until middle age. Recently, preventative care for men, in the form of testicular self-examination for testicular cancer and screening for prostate cancer, has been marketed and is included in routine health examinations. Men should be counseled concerning healthy lifestyles, sexually transmitted disease prevention, anticipated role changes, and job retraining when necessary. Expanded health promotion and early detection activities help achieve the goals of *Healthy People 2020* for men and women (Box 12-2). The recommended immunization schedule for adults is listed in Appendix A.

BOX 12-2 Essential Health Screening for Middle-Aged Women and Men

Healthy, middle-aged women and men should have the following screening tests performed at regular intervals:

- Vision testing
- Dental checkups
- Blood-pressure monitoring
- Lipid screening (cholesterol, triglycerides)
- Cardiovascular screening
- Colorectal cancer screening

WOMEN

- Breast examination and mammogram
- Papanicolaou (Pap) testing

MEN

- Testicular examination
- Prostate cancer screening

PHYSICAL ACTIVITY

In middle adulthood, the purpose of regular physical activity shifts focus from increasing fitness (as in young adulthood) to maintaining fitness and avoiding disease. Cardiovascular endurance, muscle strength, and bone mass all decrease naturally beginning around age 35, but regular physical activity can slow these changes. As in younger adulthood, middle adults should continue to strive for 2.5 hours of moderate physical activity per week.

Exercise can also be a social outlet for an otherwise isolated person. During middle age, people often are busy with work and family and may find it difficult to find time for exercise or socializing. Exercise groups, gyms, and personal trainers can all provide access to physical activities among peers.

It is important for middle-aged adults to find enjoyable activities to ensure compliance. Hiking, outdoor bootcamps, group exercise classes, and recreational sports such as soccer or basketball are all examples of physical activities with a social component.

TEACHING TECHNIQUES

Successfully teaching middle-aged adults depends on having an understanding of their typical concerns and potential sources of stress. Stress can inhibit learning or be the motivational force for learning. Misconceptions concerning menopause are common, and many adults want information related to preventing chronic illnesses. Teaching plans should be related to the problems and concerns of the individual and the age group.

Middle-aged adults may be concerned about the lives of their grown children, may want help adjusting to the role of grandparent, or may need help with designing strategies to care for their own older, frail parents. Middle-aged adults receive great personal satisfaction from contributing to the community and may start to plan their alternative lifestyles for retirement (Figure 12-3).

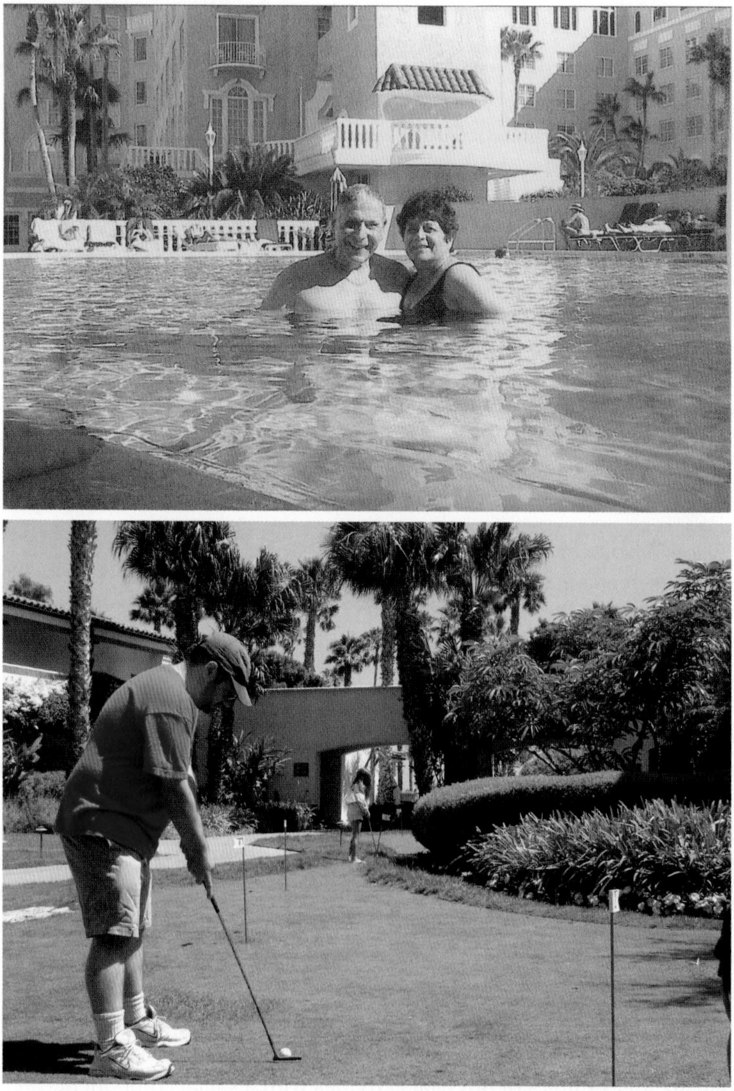

Figure 12–3 Retirement lifestyles can include many active and enjoyable leisure activities.

Middle-aged adults are often interested in learning about menopause and the teaching of coping styles that will help maintain a positive health status. Teaching strategies should incorporate the independence and competencies of the adult learner and should provide information that coincides with the concerns and stresses common to the age group. As with all age groups, a simple compliment (validation) concerning their learning competencies can also provide the reward needed to support motivation for further learning. An example of a creative group exercise related to helping the middle-aged adult accept the aging process in a positive way and to build self-esteem is reviewed in Table 12-1. Similar group exercises are helpful for the older adult who may be having difficulty coping with mental-health problems or the stresses of losing a spouse or partner.

TABLE 12-1 Creative Structured Group Exercises and Processing Suggestions

Structured Activity	Processing Focus
CRAFT PROJECTS	
Adapt project and level of supervision to person's skill level and safety needs. Use theme of craft as an object lesson. Link symbolically to mental health and healthy living.	
Foam or Felt Leaves	
1. Use foam or felt to craft individual leaves to serve as name tags, decorate with sequins or glitter.	Discuss how, like each leaf, each person is distinct. Link this concept to the special value of each person in the group . However, like a torn or crinkled leaf, no person is perfect. Parts, positive or negative, contribute to each unique self. Link this concept to the acceptance of self and disorder as the first step to taking charge and preventing relapse.
2. Make a plaque showing progression of seasons using varying shades of leaves.	Link seasons with turning points in life. Like seasons, people go through changes and losses. Change is a chance to start over. Link this concept to patients' situations (e.g., release from the hospital, change in living status). Process ways to cope with losses, holiday blues, or intense feeling experienced on the anniversary of a major change or crisis.
3. Piece together several leaves to: (a) Make a frame for each person's photograph. (b) Make a wall hanging using a branch of a tree to form a tree trunk, with each person attaching his or her individualized leaves.	Discuss that many leaves together are needed to frame the portrait or complete the tree. Likewise, each person may need to give or receive support by joining with others. Discuss deciding when to stand alone, "branch" out, or join together in a group.

(Continued)

TABLE 12-1 Creative Structured Group Exercises and Processing Suggestions—cont'd

Structured Activity	Processing Focus
4. Fashion leaves into a full wreath using the rim of a paper plate as a foundation. Decorate with items such as buttons, raffia, bows and pumpkin cutouts.	Like a wreath, life can be a circle, having continuity. Link this concept with decisions to continue to persevere despite having a mental illness (e.g., ability to choose each day to take medications, adhere to treatment, attend the group). Discuss crisis events and risks of staying in the circle (e.g., suicide attempts, stopping medications). Focus on using support systems, healthy self talk and healthy coping mechanisms.
Collage	
1. Using pictures and words from magazines or old greeting cards, paste together overlapping pictures and words representative of patients' qualities, favorite things, memories or values.	Relate pictures to person's strength and self-esteem. Discuss being different as associated with positive unique qualities vs. the perception of being different due to the stigma of mental illness. Link this concept to assertiveness skills and the need for advocacy.
2. Create a group mural representing the treatment group. Each member contributes pictures to form the whole.	Use the group collage to highlight commonalities and the group's shared history, present, and future. Link this concept to those of cohesion and support, as well as the need for separateness and skills to manage conflict. Discuss ways to manage on one's own during holidays or other times of separation.
3. Develop a collage depicting stressor and stress relievers.	Discuss what affects patient's perception of stressors. Discuss what can and cannot be changed, cognitive reframing, and healthy and unhealthy coping (e.g., addictions).
GAMES	
Use innovative and traditional games adapted to highlight mental-health concepts. Adapt complexity to client functioning and safety needs.	
Noncompetitive Games (Individual Participation)	
1. Fishing for feelings: Write "feeling" words (e.g., lonely, joyous, jealous, peaceful) on colored paper "fish." Attach a large paper clip to each fish. Place fish on the floor with some fish face up (with the feeling word visible) and some face down. With patients sitting around the "pond," have them use a fishing pole with a magnet attached to fish for a feeling.	Link fishing to recreation and discuss family times, both positive and negative. Ask patients to talk about a time when the feeling they "caught" was experienced. When a client "catches" a fish that is a less positive feeling, link that concept with facing the unknown and discussing the risk-taking and growth.

TABLE 12-1 Creative Structured Group Exercises and Processing Suggestions—cont'd

Structured Activity	Processing Focus
2. Stress Balloons: Inflate balloons. Have patients use felt-tip markers to write a number of stressors on his or her balloon. Ask patients to bounce their balloons in the air and try to keep all the balloons off the ground. Inevitably, the balloons will fall. Let all patients stomp stress away by stepping on the balloons.	Teach patient about physical and emotional signs of stress. Discuss how laughter releases stress. Link this concept to how it is easier for many hands to juggle the stressors than for one person to strive alone. When all the balloons finally fall, discuss patients' choices to let some things go (e.g., forgive, move on).
Competitive Games (Team Participation)	
1. Using a quiz-show format, create six categories with five questions in each category. The questions should be more difficult as the dollar value linked to each question increases. Use play money and a banker to add another arena for patient processing. Categories can focus on healthy living and self-care practices, signs, and coping strategies associated with mental illness, or psychotropic medications and managing side effects.	Discuss competition vs. cooperation, taking turns, and winning and losing. Discuss ways life is a game with rules. Discuss how one decides when to obey or when to step outside of the rules. Link the concept of changing rules with the need to reexamine some of the rules learned in childhood (e.g., giving oneself permission to succeed, choosing wellness).
2. Write a word or phrase on a sign. Cover each letter individually. Patient teams take turns guessing letters until the word or phrase is discovered. For example, phrases can center around holiday themes and traditions, medications, stress and coping mechanisms, type of mental illnesses, or signs of decompensation.	Discuss the specific content highlighted by the game (e.g., managing medication side effects, recognizing signs of decompensation, and met and unmet needs). Reinforce patients' personal power to choose how they view themselves or stressors, how to adapt, and how to ask for, receive, and provide support.
3. Using a bingo format, create 6-inch square boards on sheets of paper, with answers printed in each of 25 squares. The space in the middle of each sheet is a free space. Hand out bingo "cards" to teams. When an answer on the sheets is called, teams mark an X in that square. The first team to have five Xs in a row vertically, horizontally, or diagonally wins the game. Center the bingo games around themes, such as feelings, human needs, or communication tasks (e.g., shaking hands, saying one thing patients admire about the person to their right).	Like a printed bingo card, each person is given a genetic "bingo" card at birth, with some characteristics unchangeable (e.g., race, family of origin, gender, eye color, bone structure). Talk about patients' family roots, genetic "givens," body image or gender commonalities and differences, as well as the genetic component of some types of mental illnesses. Discuss feelings and what aspects of self care are within one's capacity to change. Share ways to empower oneself to gain control over how each patient chooses to play life's bingo card.

From Scheick D: Mastering group leadership. *Psychological Nursing and Mental Health Services* 40:35–36, 2002.

KEY POINTS

- Middle adulthood is the period after the early adult reproductive years and before retirement. It includes the period between 40 and 60 years of age.
- Erikson's developmental task of middle adulthood is generativity versus stagnation.
- Other developmental tasks of middle adulthood include managing finances and a career; nurturing marriage and family relationships; managing a household; and maintaining a positive self-image.
- Middle adulthood is a time of self-reflection, reevaluation, and prioritization.
- Gradual hormonal changes occur before menopause; these changes may begin as early as age 35.
- The climacteric is when hormonal changes result in cessation of menstruation in women and decreased muscle mass and sex drive in men.
- Concerns of middle-aged men are typically related to role changes, work-related stress, decreased physical fitness, and performance anxiety.
- Preventive health care for men includes testicular self-examination, annual dental examinations, blood pressure and blood-lipid levels, and prostate and colorectal cancer screenings.
- Middle age is referred to as the *sandwich generation*, where responsibilities include the care of children and older parents.
- Physical activity is important for maintaining fitness and preventing illness. Exercise with a social component can provide a social outlet for the busy middle-aged adult.

Critical Thinking

Gender-appropriate health education is important in middle adulthood. Outline two health-education plans, one for men and one for women. Include information about preventing illness, recognizing midlife mental-health issues, and managing the approach of the climacteric.

REVIEW QUESTIONS

1. **Middle adulthood includes the period between the ages of:**
   a. 20 and 29 years.
   b. 30 and 39 years.
   c. 40 and 60 years.
   d. 60 and 80 years.

2. **The main task or crisis of middle adulthood is:**
   a. intimacy versus isolation.
   b. generativity versus stagnation.
   c. identity versus role confusion.
   d. dependence versus independence.

3. **Menopause includes:**
   a. cessation of sexual activity.
   b. loss of sexual ability.
   c. cessation of menstrual period.
   d. the beginning of a midlife crisis.

4. **Preventative health care for men in middle adulthood should include:**
   a. annual chest X-rays.
   b. testicular self-examination.
   c. annual Pap tests.
   d. daily recording of pulse rate.

5. **The *sandwich generation* refers to people who:**
   a. do not have time to cook.
   b. care for children and grandchildren.
   c. prefer sandwiches to hot meals.
   d. care for elderly parents in addition to young children.

CHAPTER 13

Late Adulthood

http://evolve.elsevier.com/Leifer/growth

OBJECTIVES

1. Discuss the major goals of *Healthy People 2020* as related to late adulthood.
2. Identify common health concerns of late adulthood.
3. Describe challenges and developmental tasks of late adulthood.
4. Discuss lifestyle changes that may be necessary for late adulthood.
5. Discuss the relationship of physical activity to the aging process and cognition.
6. Define elder abuse and describe one means by which it can be prevented.
7. Discuss the ways menopause may affect women in the late-adulthood phase of the life cycle.
8. List the learning needs of later adulthood.
9. Select appropriate teaching techniques to promote effective learning and coping for late adulthood.

KEY TERMS

assistive devices
autonomy
competence
disengagement
elder abuse
late adulthood
polypharmacy
relatedness

DEFINITION

The U.S. government has traditionally defined old age as over age 65 or 67, when full Social Security benefits become available, retirement usually occurs, and a leisurely lifestyle is adopted. Late adulthood is considered as encompassing the ages between 65 and 74 years. This default definition, which focuses on chronological age only, does not take into consideration the functional or social dimensions of old age. Increased technology and improved health-care practices have enabled people to live longer and to remain active and productive. Today many people in the late-adulthood phase of the life cycle postpone retirement and remain active in the workforce as senior employees or part-time consultants.

Some health concerns of the older adult include:

- Development of osteoporosis
- Risks for falls and fractures
- Poor awareness of healthy behavior options
- Increased risk of influenza and pneumonia
- Development of cataracts
- Increased loss of hearing

Health Promotion

Some of the major goals of *Healthy People 2020* for older adults are to increase the lifespan and the quality of life by focusing on wellness and healthy behaviors, prevention of illness, and treatment of disease. Reducing the number of illnesses and deaths related to vaccine-preventable illness, reducing the occurrence of hip fractures from unintentional injuries, and early diagnosis and management of dementia are priority goals for late adulthood.

Maximizing health as much as possible promotes mobility and independence. The older adult can develop meaning and enjoyment in life despite physical limitations. *Healthy People 2020* goals related to independence include increasing certified specialists to care for the elderly; promoting services such as housing and transportation to increase accessibility to care while keeping the elderly in their communities; and understanding and studying elder abuse.

STATISTICS

According to the Department of Health and Human Services (USDHHS), in the year 2009 over 39.6 million Americans were 65 years old or older, which was an increase of 12% since the year 2000. It is estimated that the number will increase to over 86 million by the year 2050. Table 13-1 shows the elderly population in the United States according to census reports of 2005 and projections of the elderly population for the years 2015 and 2025.

Income

The income sources for older persons in the United States include social security, pensions, personal assets, and earnings. Approximately 1.3% or 4.6 million Americans more than 65 years of age are still actively employed. Approximately 3.4 million persons above age 65 were below poverty level, and 3.7 million required caregiver assistance in 2010. In the year 2010, 93% of persons above 65 years of age were covered by Medicare with 58% having private health insurance. A total of 1.8% of persons over 65 had no health coverage. These statistics will undoubtedly change because of the enactment of the Health Care Affordability Act of 2010 and other alterations to U.S. health-care laws that are under debate for future implementation.

Education Level

As of 2009, approximately 77% of people over 65 years of age were high school graduates and 15% of those over 75 were college graduates. About 475,000 grandparents over the age of 65 were primary caregivers of their grandchildren (USDHHS, 2010). Understanding these statistics enables the health-care worker to plan for the needs and limitations of the elderly population they serve in the twenty-first century. The living arrangements, support systems, income, and educational levels all influence the plan of care for the older person. The health-care worker can refer to the U.S. Department of Health and Human Services Administration on Aging for elder-care resources and other information concerning the geriatric population. The World Health Organization (WHO) has urged governments around the world to consider the health needs of the older adult in the general health programs of their countries.

(Text continued on p. 200.)

TABLE 13-1 Ranking of States by Projected Percentage of Population Age 65 and Older: 2000, 2010, and 2030

State	2000 Percent	2000 Rank	State	2010 Percent	2010 Rank	State	2030 Percent	2030 Rank
United States	12.4	NA	United States	13.0	NA	United States	19.7	NA
Florida	17.6	1	Florida	17.8	1	Florida	27.1	1
Pennsylvania	15.6	2	West Virginia	16.0	2	Maine	26.5	2
West Virginia	15.3	3	Maine	15.6	3	Wyoming	26.5	3
Iowa	14.9	4	Pennsylvania	15.5	4	New Mexico	26.4	4
North Dakota	14.7	5	North Dakota	15.3	5	Montana	25.8	5
Rhode Island	14.5	6	Montana	15.0	6	North Dakota	25.1	6
Maine	14.4	7	Iowa	14.9	7	West Virginia	24.8	7
South Dakota	14.3	8	South Dakota	14.6	8	Vermont	24.4	8
Arkansas	14.0	9	Connecticut	14.4	9	Delaware	23.5	9
Connecticut	13.8	10	Arkansas	14.3	10	South Dakota	23.1	10
Nebraska	13.6	11	Vermont	14.3	11	Pennsylvania	22.6	11
Massachusetts	13.5	12	Hawaii	14.3	12	Iowa	22.4	12
Missouri	13.5	13	Delaware	14.1	13	Hawaii	22.3	13
Montana	13.4	14	Alabama	14.1	14	Arizona	22.1	14
Ohio	13.3	15	Rhode Island	14.1	15	South Carolina	22.0	15
Hawaii	13.3	16	New Mexico	14.1	16	Connecticut	21.5	16
Kansas	13.3	17	Wyoming	14.0	17	New Hampshire	21.4	17
New Jersey	13.2	18	Arizona	13.9	18	Rhode Island	21.4	18
Oklahoma	13.2	19	Missouri	13.9	19	Wisconsin	21.3	19
Wisconsin	13.1	20	Oklahoma	13.8	20	Alabama	21.3	20

(Continued)

TABLE 13-1 Ranking of States by Projected Percentage of Population Age 65 and Older: 2000, 2010, and 2030—cont'd

State	2000 Percent	2000 Rank	State	2010 Percent	2010 Rank	State	2030 Percent	2030 Rank
Alabama	13.0	21	Nebraska	13.8	21	Massachusetts	20.9	21
Arizona	13.0	22	Ohio	13.7	22	Nebraska	20.6	22
Delaware	13.0	23	Massachusetts	13.7	23	Mississippi	20.5	23
New York	12.9	24	New Jersey	13.7	24	Ohio	20.4	24
Oregon	12.8	25	New York	13.6	25	Arkansas	20.3	25
Vermont	12.7	26	South Carolina	13.6	26	Missouri	20.2	26
Kentucky	12.5	27	Wisconsin	13.5	27	Kansas	20.2	27
Indiana	12.4	28	Kansas	13.4	28	New York	20.1	28
Tennessee	12.4	29	Tennessee	13.3	29	New Jersey	20.0	29
Michigan	12.3	30	Kentucky	13.1	30	Kentucky	19.8	30
District of Columbia	12.2	31	Oregon	13.0	31	Louisiana	19.7	31
South Carolina	12.1	32	Michigan	12.8	32	Michigan	19.5	32
Minnesota	12.1	33	Mississippi	12.8	33	Oklahoma	19.4	33
Illinois	12.1	34	Indiana	12.7	34	Tennessee	19.2	34
Mississippi	12.1	35	Louisiana	12.6	35	Minnesota	18.9	35

North Carolina	12.0	36	New Hampshire	12.6	36	Virginia	18.8	36
New Hampshire	12.0	37	North Carolina	12.4	37	Nevada	18.6	37
Wyoming	11.7	38	Virginia	12.4	38	Idaho	18.3	38
New Mexico	11.7	39	Illinois	12.4	39	Oregon	18.2	39
Louisiana	11.6	40	Minnesota	12.4	40	Washington	18.1	40
Maryland	11.3	41	Nevada	12.3	41	Indiana	18.1	41
Idaho	11.3	42	Washington	12.2	42	Illinois	18.0	42
Washington	11.2	43	Maryland	12.2	43	California	17.8	43
Virginia	11.2	44	Idaho	12.0	44	North Carolina	17.8	44
Nevada	11.0	45	California	11.5	45	Maryland	17.6	45
California	10.6	46	District of Columbia	11.5	46	Colorado	16.5	46
Texas	9.9	47	Colorado	10.7	47	Georgia	15.9	47
Colorado	9.7	48	Texas	10.5	48	Texas	15.6	48
Georgia	9.6	49	Georgia	10.2	49	Alaska	14.7	49
Utah	8.5	50	Utah	9.0	50	District of Columbia	13.4	50
Alaska	5.7	51	Alaska	8.1	51	Utah	13.2	51

From U.S. Census Bureau, Population Division, *Interim State Population Projections, 2005.* Internet Release Date: April 21, 2005. Accessed March 7, 2012, from www.census.gov/population/www/projections/projectionsagesex.html.

CHALLENGES AND PROBLEMS

Several factors influence the health and well-being of older adults:

- *Access to health care*—Access to health care to maintain optimum physical and mental health may be blocked by lack of transportation or knowledge of community resources. When access to health care is blocked, preventive care is neglected, and health care is only obtained after an illness or disease develops.
- *Reduced income*—Reduced income is a problem for many older adults. Social security and pension incomes may not cover daily living and health-care expenses. Working past retirement age is a potential solution for some older adults. In 1986, age-based mandatory retirement was abolished, but age-discrimination remains a problem for those seeking new jobs.
- *Changes in living arrangements*—Adjusting to changes in living arrangements can also influence the physical and mental well-being of the older adult. Evidence suggests that living as extended family, or near family members, is optimal. As another option, assisted-living communities help the older adult maintain independence, social interaction, and a positive self concept. Some older adults may live in inadequate housing, whereas others may be institutionalized in nursing homes and may lose independence and control over their lives.
- *Caregiver assistance*—According to the Centers for Disease Control and Prevention (CDC), the most common activities of daily living that require assistance by home health-care aides include body hygiene, bed-to-chair transfer, toileting, shopping, meal preparation, and light housework. Ambulatory-care clinics and home-care organizations can be helpful to the older adult.
- *Altered nutritional needs*—Dental problems, inability to cook, dislike of eating alone, pain or malaise because of a medical condition, or lack of accommodation for special needs related to cultural or religious food traditions may be causes for altered eating habits. Attention to diet and nutrition improves and maintains good health in the older adult. Caloric needs may decrease with age, but a balanced nutritional intake remains essential. Assessment of the nutritional needs of the older adult is essential, and community resources such as "Meals on Wheels" can be used.
- *Assistive devices*—Assistive devices may be needed to help the older adult maintain independent living. Assistive devices include such items as walkers, canes, respiratory equipment, hearing aids, and electronic emergency-response devices.
- *Preventing falls*—Preventing falls becomes more important as the older adult develops vision or hearing problems and slower response times. The use of certain medications can cause dizziness or imbalance that can also increase the vulnerability of the older adult to falling. The health-care worker can assess the older adult's environment and can help with securing loose rugs, improving tracking on slippery floors, clearing general clutter, and improving lighting, especially near stairways. Installing handgrips in showers and tubs can also be instrumental in preventing accidents. Reaching for items on high shelves, changing light bulbs, going up and down stairs, and opening simple medicine bottles are some activities that may require assistance or improved safety strategies.
- *Polypharmacy*—The problem of polypharmacy arises with the use of medications by older adults. Polypharmacy is the ingestion of multiple medications in one day. Medications may be prescribed for various medical conditions or may be purchased over the counter. Drug–drug interactions, drug–food interactions, and drug–environment interactions (such as increased sensitivity to sun exposure) can occur. Optimal or average drug dosages are normally determined by research on young adults, and little research is

available concerning modifications of dosages required by older adults. In older adults, the decreased ability of the liver and kidneys to excrete drugs from the body can result in an accumulation of the drugs to toxic levels. The older adult may forget to take a dose of medication or may accidentally take an extra dose and therefore may be undermedicated or overmedicated and prone to undesirable side effects. Patient monitoring and education are essential. The use of memory aids such as notebooks, electronic reminders or labeled pill boxes may be helpful.

- *Elder or dependent abuse*—Elder abuse affects more than 2 million older adults each year. Elder abuse is defined as the infliction of harm or neglect through actions or acts of omission. Abuse can be physical, emotional, or financial and can include neglect or obstruction of personal rights. The family or health-care worker can observe interactions between older adults and the caregivers and alert other family members to potentially abusive situations. Referral of the caregiver to community agencies for respite care may decrease the stress that can often lead to abuse.

PSYCHOSOCIAL DEVELOPMENT

There are many developmental tasks and related challenges for the older adult (Box 13-1). Older adults with healthy attitudes and coping skills typically do not mourn their lost youth but are able to find fulfillment and meaning in their lives despite health limitations. However, weight gain, dental problems, diminished eyesight and hearing, decreased mobility, and changes in body image are some issues that create difficulty. Older adults may show a readiness for learning if they recognize old age is near and they realize that physical health and life circumstances may change. Developing a healthy lifestyle and healthy behaviors with access to preventative care is a primary goal in the education and care of the older adult.

PSYCHOSOCIAL ISSUES

The social network of friends usually narrows for the older adult because of the death of peers. This may result in fewer social experiences with peers unless older adults live in retirement communities or are connected with organized social activities specific for their age group. Remaining an integral part of an extended family provides valuable social activities and relationships, but family relationships may be different than peer relationships.

Basic needs for autonomy (self-direction), competence (effective interactions), and relatedness (a sense of belonging) motivate social activities that enhance general well-being. An environment that helps meet these basic needs enables the older adult to maintain positive social interactions (Figure 13-1).

BOX 13-1 Tasks and Challenges of the Older Adult

Older adults must adjust to the following:

- Menopause
- Retirement and redirection of goals and energy
- Decreased income
- Grandparenting
- Reentry into the job market

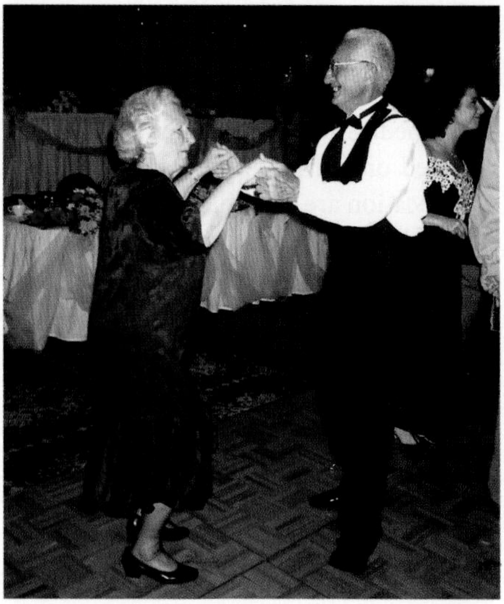

Figure 13-1 Social activities and positive social interactions enhance a feeling of well-being in the older adult.

Complete dependency often does not support *autonomy*, *social competence*, or *relatedness* in satisfying ways unless the situation is specifically designed to provide assistance in achieving these goals. Many assisted-living facilities for older adults are designed to offer assistance with living without taking away the fulfillment of these three basic needs.

Grandparenting

When healthy older adults assume the role of grandparents, they often do more for their children than their children do for their own parents. The grandparenting role can be satisfying for the older adult, because it enhances self-image, increases activity level, creates feelings of self-worth and usefulness, and contributes to the meaning and quality of life. Many older adults may enjoy their grandchildren more because they know the children's parents will take over when they tire. Some older adults serve as volunteer adoptive grandparents to children in need or seek useful volunteer activities in the community. The role of the grandparent in the home can be a positive experience for grandchildren when healthy relationships between all generations are maintained.

It is when grandparents become ill or disabled that the roles can reverse and the older adult needs more assistance. This role reversal can result in family stress and financial strain. Many families are not aware of community programs available for assistance with older adults and for caregiver support. Family education concerning the older adult's limitations and abilities can increase compassion and motivation to assist and improve verbal communication and the quality of the relationship. Health-care workers can educate and guide families concerning resources available to them before emotional stress, financial strain, caregiver burnout, and older adult alienation occur.

Postmenopause

There are more than 81 million women between the ages of 50 and 60 in the United States who may face transition to menopause with varying levels of support. Adjusting to the postmenopausal phase of life is an important developmental task of the older woman.

Menopause is defined as the absence of menstruation for a period of at least 1 year (due to decline or cessation of hormonal production and function).

Menopause is not a disease or illness; it is a natural occurrence in the life cycle. However, there are discomforts and risks associated with the postmenopausal phase that can be averted with healthy lifestyles and access to preventative medical care. Some discomforts associated with postmenopause include genital atrophy, vasomotor instability, heart disease, breast cancer, or osteoporosis. Hormone replacement therapy (HRT) was designed to relieve some of these discomforts, but controversy exists concerning the safety and advisability of routine HRT. Complementary and alternative medical therapies (CAM) are also available when HRT is not recommended. *Complementary therapy* refers to nontraditional therapies, such as relaxation or biofeedback, that are used with traditional therapy. *Alternative therapy* refers to nontraditional therapy, such as herbs and oils, that are used instead of traditional therapy. A healthy lifestyle is essential. See Chapter 3 for cultural aspects of aging. The *Physician's Desk Reference for Herbal Medicines* can be used as a guide in helping the older patient evaluate complementary therapies that they may choose to use.

Lifestyle Changes

Simple lifestyle changes for women experiencing menopausal and postmenopausal symptoms include dressing in layers to cope with hot flashes, using a portable fan, adjusting heat and air conditioning in the room, limiting alcohol and caffeine intake, and drinking more fluids. Vaginal dryness can be overcome by the use of water-based gels or lubricants. Mood swings can be recognized and managed by increasing self-awareness and reframing thoughts and interpretations of situations. Understanding partners can also be supportive. The use of CAM therapy such as herbal supplements to prevent the development of depression requires close evaluation for possible interaction with prescribed medicines or other treatments.

Decreases in estrogen often cause vaginal-wall thinning and urine leakage when sneezing or laughing. Panty liners, pads, and adult diapers can be of help in handling these embarrassing problems that can otherwise cause the woman to want to stay at home.

Driving Safety

Many adults over age 65 may have early undetected impairments that can affect their safety on the roads. Occupational and physical therapy can help maintain driving safety and delay loss of their driver's licenses, but when driving is no longer safe, the license must be taken away. Counseling concerning other methods of transportation available within their community is essential. Isolation, loneliness, stagnation, or depression may occur if alternative transportation options are not offered.

Health Screenings

Health screenings can identify developing health issues in early stages and can lead to early interventions and prevention of greater difficulties. Screenings should include dental and eye checkups and a physical evaluation that includes weight, blood pressure, thyroid, and blood glucose and lipid levels. It is useful to assess for substance abuse, overmedication, sexual dysfunction, urinary incontinence, and other indications that lifestyle changes are necessary. Papanicolaou (Pap) smears for cervical cancer are recommended at 1- to 3-year intervals in healthy older women. Mammography screening for breast lesions and screening for colorectal cancer and prostate cancer in men are also recommended. Routine cardiovascular screening should be performed for patients who present with two or more risk factors, such as increased lipid levels, hypertension, or smoking. Postmenopausal bone loss and osteoporosis should be assessed regularly, and preventive measures such as increased calcium intake, vitamin D, and daily weight-bearing exercise can be emphasized during routine office visits. A nutritional health assessment is essential. Referral for dental care or community services such as "Meals on Wheels" may be an option to assist in the maintenance of nutrition if transportation is an obstacle.

Health Promotion

In late adulthood, decreased organ size and function can cause increased toxic effects related to alcohol use. Assessing for alcohol abuse is therefore also an important aspect of health screening. A quick and simple assessment tool for alcohol abuse is the CAGE questionnaire, which includes four questions regarding the patient's feelings about his or her drinking or specific habits. Two affirmative answers to the specific questions related to alcohol intake may indicate a need for further evaluation or follow-up (Ewing, 1984; O'Brien, 2008).

Sexuality

As people age, specific changes in sexual responses occur. However, the notion that the older adult is sexually inactive is untrue. Some older adults may feel guilty or abnormal because they continue to have sexual feelings. The most common cause of sexual dissatisfaction is the lack of a partner. In this age group, divorces, widowhood, or ill or disabled spouses are common problems. Men may develop erectile dysfunction, which is now treatable with a high rate of success. Painful intercourse (dyspareunia) for women may be the result of atrophy of the vaginal tissues and a decrease in natural lubrications. Both problems can be easily overcome.

Health Promotion

HRT or CAM therapy can alleviate menopausal symptoms that interfere with sexual pleasure. A health-care provider must evaluate the suitability of HRT for individual patients before determining the appropriate approach to care. Sex therapy is available and can be helpful. The main obstacle in maintaining a healthy sexual lifestyle is the tendency to avoid talking about it because of embarrassment. Therefore it is the health-care worker's responsibility to assess sexual functioning in older men and women.

Memory Loss

The older adult experiences memory changes, particularly in remembering names and faces of people. Normal memory loss can be associated with aging, and temporary memory loss can be caused by depression or anxiety. Preclinical manifestations of Alzheimer's disease are a common worry when normal memory loss becomes increasingly noticeable (Boxes 13-2 and 13-3).

Health Promotion

Active lifestyles that routinely exercise memory skills are thought to help maintain memory function. Perhaps this is another "use it or lose it" phenomenon. However, studies have shown that older adults need more time to process thoughts and perform tasks than younger adults (Salthouse, 2006). Knowledge or information that is deeply processed rather than superficially memorized will be remembered longer. See Table 13-2 for a summary of memory decline resulting from normal aging, depression, or dementia.

BOX 13-2 Warning Signs of Problematic Memory Decline

- Memory loss affecting job functioning
- Difficulty remembering steps in familiar tasks
- Disorientation
- Lack of awareness of time, place, or date
- Decrease in abstract thinking (increased need for concreteness)
- Associated problems with mood, language, or personality changes

BOX 13-3 Preventable Causes of Memory Problems

- Drug toxicity
- Depression
- Metabolic problems (kidney or liver dysfunction, hypoglycemia)
- Sensory problems (difficulty hearing, seeing, or sensing information)
- Nutritional deficiencies (dehydration, B_{12} deficiency, iron deficiency)
- Illness (pneumonia and other infections)

Emotional Health

Emotions and emotional control develop during the growth and development process, as a person copes with the challenges in each phase of the life cycle. Earlier theorists believed disengagement was a task of the older adult. This implies that removing emotional attachments to people, places, and objects is part of the natural aging process. This may be true of the depressed older adult but is likely not a natural or healthy process. The aging healthy adult does not naturally disengage. Instead he or she continues emotional learning and emotional competencies. Past experiences from the long lives of older adults may influence their expression of emotional responses.

TABLE 13-2 Memory Decline Resulting from Normal Aging, Depression, or Dementia

Normal Age-Related Memory Decline	Depression-Related Memory Problems	Dementia-Related Memory Problems
Onset age specifically identifiable	Onset with depression	Difficult to establish onset
Slow progression of symptoms	Rapid or sudden progression of symptoms	Slow or stepwise progression
History of depression less common	History of depression less common	History of depression less common
Complains about memory loss	Complains about memory loss	Usually unaware of memory loss
May emphasize disability	May emphasize disability	Conceals disability
May decrease or increase efforts to perform	Decreases effort to perform	Struggles to perform
Uses notes and other memory aids	May not try to keep up	Needs instruction to use memory aids
No lasting mood change associated	Consistent depressive mood	Emotional lability and shallowness
Behavior may or may not change	Behavior change is greater than impairment	Behavior change may be appropriate for the impairment
Nocturnal drop in performance unusual	Nocturnal drop in performance unusual	Nocturnal drop in performance common
"Don't know" answers common	"Don't know" answers common	Guesses or "near miss" answers common
Recent and remote memory losses are equal	Recent and remote memory losses are equal; memory gaps for specific events common	Recent memory impaired, remote is intact; memory gaps for specific events unusual

Cultural Considerations

Culture and expectations play a role in the emotional status of the older adult. In cultures with close families, more respect and inclusion in the lives of their families, or maintenance of communication and relationships with their families, will encourage and maintain emotional competencies and enhance quality of life for older adults.

Depression

Depression should not be automatically expected to appear in the older adult. In some older adults, depression occurs as a continuation of a negative attitude from young adulthood. A young person who looks at life's events in a pessimistic way may be vulnerable to developing depression as an older adult. However, late-onset depression (or a change in personality) may be attributed to changes in the brain itself. The traditional symptoms of depression as listed in the *Diagnostic and Statistical Manual of Mental Disorders, Fourth Edition, Text Revision (DSM-IV-TR)* criteria for diagnosis of major depression may not be completely accurate for older adults (Barg, 2006). Older adults may be taking medications for various medical conditions that have side effects that mimic depression. Therefore depression can be overdiagnosed or underdiagnosed (Agronin, 2010). Several factors increase the vulnerability of the older adult to depression. Chronic poor health can lead to stress, decreased activity, and fewer social interactions, which can trigger depression. Prescribed treatment of the medical conditions can induce changes that result in a deepened depression. Depression itself in turn can also trigger physical illness.

Patient Teaching

Helping the older adult manage stressful life events, strengthening coping strategies, and providing social support can help avoid the development of depression for many older adults. Any person who first develops depression as an older adult usually has experiences and coping styles that can be used by a professional therapist in individual or group sessions to help treat the depressive symptoms. Providing access to mental health care and early screening for the presence of risk and depressive symptoms can empower older adults to be in control of their own emotions.

The American Psychiatric Association (APA) Division of Clinical Psychology and the American Association of Geriatric Psychiatry have developed evidence-based practice guidelines that recommend specific treatments for a variety of psychological problems. However, there is little research concerning the application of these guidelines to the older adult population.

Obstacles in accessing or using available mental health-care resources have led to the emergence of self-help techniques that are available to all at low cost. Self-help resources include books and support groups led by clergy, peer counselors, and others who advertise their successes. Many psychologists prescribe self-help resources to supplement their therapies (Smith, 2012). The combination of various types of interventions has been embraced by the interdisciplinary Society for the Exploration of Psychotherapy Integration (SEPI). This and other professional networks, such as the Association for Behavioral and Cognitive Therapies (ABCT) and Anxiety and Depression Association of America (ADAA) organizations, offer conferences and newsletters on effective mental health care. The American Association of Retired Persons (AARP) is also an advocate for the older adult regarding education for healthy living.

CLINICAL DISEASE

Good health in older people is often defined as the absence of disease or disability. However, normal body changes resulting from aging, such as ovarian failure or menopause, place a risk on the cardiovascular, bone, and metabolic systems. This occurs at a time when emotional stress may increase because of other life changes.

Lifespan Considerations

The combination of subclinical cardiovascular changes associated with aging and the response to stressful life events can affect the risk factors for the development of a clinical disease. Individuals who characteristically hid or suppressed their emotions in young adulthood and held a pessimistic view toward life events may be at a higher risk for clinical disease as they age. This may indicate that prevention of disease in the older adult lies partially in the development of positive attitudes and coping skills.

PHYSICAL ACTIVITY

Numerous changes occur with age including metabolic function, cardiac function, muscular strength, and bone structure. Many of these changes occur regardless of physical-activity levels, but exercise can significantly slow the aging process, essentially increasing life expectancy by 30-50% (Chodzko-Zajko, 2009).

Resting metabolic rate decreases with age, so fewer calories are burned during a resting state. Without adjustments in food intake and energy output (exercise), this metabolic shift is likely to result in weight gain. Regular aerobic exercise increases caloric expenditure, which helps maintain a caloric balance. Examples of light- to moderate-intensity aerobic activities for seniors include walking, swimming, dancing, bicycling, tennis, and various aerobic exercise classes.

Muscle strengthening exercises can increase the amount of metabolically active muscle tissue, or at least slow the decreases in muscle mass that often come with age and a sedentary lifestyle (Sundell, 2011). Decreases in muscle mass during aging impact daily functioning and eventually impede independence and reduce quality of life. Regardless of age or initial strength level, improvements can be achieved through regular muscle-strengthening activities. Muscle-strengthening exercises for seniors can include carrying groceries, yoga, tai chi, heavy gardening, and exercises with weights or exercise bands. Stronger muscles and joints also reduce the risk of falling, which is a significant danger for the elderly population. Regular balance exercises such as practicing walking backwards and sideways in a safe environment can also result in fewer falls.

There is evidence that physical activity has a protecive effect on cognitive function in the older population (Rolland, 2010). Habits of physical activity may be used in the future to aid in the battle of maladies such as Alzheimer's disease.

An active person entering late adulthood can and should continue his or her level of physical activity. Older adults should continue, when possible, to achieve the same guidelines as those in middle adulthood. A total of 2½ hours of moderate to vigorous physical aerobic activity spread throughout the course of a week is a baseline goal for adults of all ages. When that baseline is achieved, the guidelines shift to encourage 5 hours per week, with vigorous exercise counting as double (1 minute of vigorous exercise equals 2 minutes of moderate exercise). More benefits can be achieved with more vigorous activity levels.

Many people entering late adulthood have spent years or even decades being sedentary or nearly sedentary, and as a result have a very low level of fitness. As the aging process begins to threaten their independence, physical activity becomes an essential component for an elderly person to maintain cardiac and muscle function, balance, and range of motion. A combination of aerobic training and resistance traning can slow the aging process up to the age of about 80 years. Beyond the age of 80, physical fitness can maintain good health and quality of life until just before death (Nelson, 2007).

Seniors with very low levels of fitness can achieve a significant training response even from low-intensity training. Improvements can be seen even when the heart rates reach only 100 beats per minute during periodic 10-minute exercise sessions. Higher exercise heart rates will elicit stronger training responses.

TEACHING TECHNIQUES

Human growth and development occurs in a sequential pattern, and developmental tasks are often related to the phases or stages within these patterns. Therefore within any stage or phase of development there can be a wide variation of abilities that are mastered. A person's ability and readiness to learn depends on his or her stage of development; physical, psychological, and social health; support systems and environmental stress; and personal motivation. It must be noted, however, that chronological age is not a specific indicator of stage of development.

A *teaching moment* has been defined as the point at which the learner is most receptive to change or growth within a situation (Havighurst, 1974). The learner must be motivated to learn, and the teaching must be relevant to the learner and appropriate to the developmental stage and abilities of the learner. For the older adult, learning is enhanced if mutual respect exists between teacher and learner. The teacher should recognize and appreciate the lifelong accomplishments of the older adult, should be nonjudgmental, and should foster an environment conducive to learning. Visual aids should include large print in a bright color. Vision decline in the older adult often causes color distortions, so medications or pills should not be referred to by color.

Hearing loss in the older adult usually affects perception of high-pitched sounds or rapid speech. Therefore shouting or raising the volume is not helpful. Speaking clearly and slowly, making eye contact while speaking, wearing lipstick or lip gloss (to assist visual perception), and using an interactive style to obtain feedback from the older adult will confirm that the information conveyed was understood.

Scheduling short teaching sessions enables the older adult to concentrate and absorb all the information throughout the session without losing concentration because of fatigue or other interference, such as having to leave the room to go to the bathroom. During educational sessions, the teacher can counteract avoidance or denial of the need to change lifestyle practices by validating the older adult's experiences and needs and by limiting topics to those related to the here and now. Relating learning topics to autonomy, social acceptability, and strong coping skills can boost learning effectiveness. Repetition of information helps encode information into long-term memory, especially if memory skills are in decline. Presenting information in different ways, visually, verbally, and experientially (hands-on), can also be an important aid to learning. However, repetition of material already known by the older adult can discourage him or her from feeling motivated to learn.

Health Promotion

Important goals in managing the aging process include preventing illness and disability, maintaining cognitive functioning, and maintaining an active and healthy lifestyle. Assessment for cardiovascular risks; nutritional needs; bone density; visual, hearing, and memory loss; depression; and specific concerns of the individual are helpful in developing a meaningful teaching plan for the individual. Decreasing stress and maintaining a positive attitude are essential to successful living (Figure 13-2).

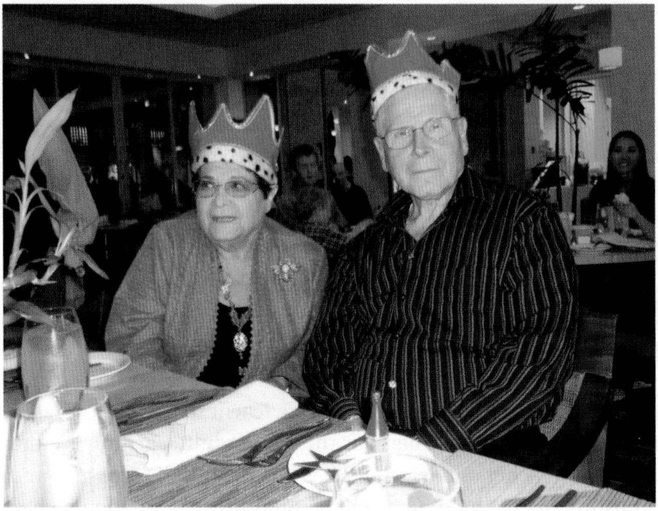

Figure 13-2 Older adults find pleasure in celebrating holidays and life events with others.

KEY POINTS

- A *Healthy People 2020* goal for the older adult is to increase the lifespan and quality of life by focusing on wellness and preventive care.
- Some health challenges for the older adult include managing on a reduced income, adjusting to changes in living arrangements, accessing preventive health care, maintaining nutrition, and preventing accidents.
- Elder abuse is the infliction of harm or neglect through actions or acts of omission.
- Menopause is not a disease; it is a natural occurrence in the life cycle.
- Health screenings for the older adult may include dental and vision checkups; screening for breast, cervical, and prostate cancer; checking blood glucose and lipid levels; weight and blood pressure monitoring; and alcohol and depression screening.
- The most common cause of sexual inactivity in the older adult is loss of a partner.
- Keeping an active mind and lifestyle can enhance memory performance in the older adult.
- Exercise prescriptions for older adults should include aerobic exercise, muscle strengthening exercise, flexibility exercise, and exercise to improve balance to prevent falls.

- Seniors with low levels of fitness can achieve a significant response from low intensity exercise. The frail elderly can achieve benefits of exercises performed in a chair.
- An older adult can benefit from the use of memory aids such as lists or calendar notes.
- Basic needs for autonomy, social competence, and relatedness in the older adult motivate continued social interactions and prevent isolation and disengagement.
- Several factors cause older adults to be vulnerable to developing depression.
- Providing access to mental health care, early screening, and a combination of social and psychological interventions can help avoid the development of depression in the older adult.
- Specific teaching techniques can enhance the learning process for the older adult.

Critical Thinking

Health-care teaching is important for older adults. What teaching techniques might be helpful for effectively teaching a group of older adults?

REVIEW QUESTIONS

1. Old age is defined by the U.S. government as the time when full Social Security benefits become available, which is when one reaches the age of:
   a. 55 to 57.
   b. 65 to 67.
   c. 75 to 77.
   d. 85 to 87.

2. The problem of polypharmacy involves:
   a. inaccessibility of drugstores.
   b. ingestion of multiple medications.
   c. online drug availability.
   d. use of prescription medications.

3. Complementary and alternative medicine involves the use of:
   a. herbs, biofeedback, or soy products.
   b. hormones to treat menopause.
   c. antibiotics to treat infections.
   d. contraceptive pills.

4. One method that will help prevent osteoporosis includes:
   a. sedentary activities.
   b. weight-bearing exercises.
   c. a diet high in potassium.
   d. bone density study.

5. A teaching moment occurs when the learner:
   a. is motivated and receptive.
   b. is quietly listening.
   c. is momentarily distracted.
   d. answers a question.

CHAPTER

14 Advanced Old Age and Geriatrics

http://evolve.elsevier.com/Leifer/growth

OBJECTIVES

1. Explain the concept of geriatrics.
2. Discuss the anticipated future increase in the advanced old-age population as related to the development of geriatrics as a specialty.
3. State four normal physiological changes that occur in the geriatric adult.
4. List the major developmental tasks of the geriatric adult.
5. Name three psychological changes or challenges that occur in the geriatric adult.
6. Discuss three specific psychosocial problems associated with aging.
7. List four specific health-promoting activities for the geriatric adult.
8. Discuss the role of diet, exercise, and stress management in achieving the goals of *Healthy People 2020* in relation to the older adult.
9. Discuss the sexuality needs of the geriatric adult.
10. Discuss six health-maintenance requirements for adults who are in advanced old age.
11. Discuss various modifications of the environment necessary for the geriatric adult.
12. State four factors to consider when helping to select a nursing home for placement.
13. Discuss alternatives to nursing-home care.
14. Define activities of daily living.
15. Discuss principles of elder care and the role of the health-care worker.
16. Discuss the teaching needs of the geriatric adult.

KEY TERMS

activities of daily living (ADLs)
ageism
Alzheimer's disease
apoptosis
atrophy
biological clock
disengagement
elder abuse
free radical
geriatrics
immune theory
osteoporosis
senescence
wear-and-tear theory

DEFINITION

Some define old age according to chronological age or physiological decline, such as the occurrence of menopause and skin or hair changes. Others define old age as a time when psychological changes occur. For the purposes of statistics, old age is defined as above the age of 65-67, and the term "seniors" is preferred to the term "elderly."

Senescence is described as a period in an older adult's life in which the body begins to age and weaken. It is considered a signal of the final stage or end of the lifespan. Senescence is a gradual process, and people age in different ways and at different rates. The health needs of advanced old age may differ slightly from those of late adulthood. For example, the incidence of chronic disease increases markedly after age 80. Social gerontologists have defined senescence in years and it had been categorized by Ebersole and Hess, in 1998 as:

- Young-old: 65 to 75
- Old: 76 to 84
- Old-old: 85 to 99
- Elite-old: 100 and older

Since aging is not a disease, the definition of old age varies as people live longer and health care improves. The ages in categories of old age are changing rapidly, and standard definitions no longer reflect reality. Modern gerontologists list old age as when the prospects of living less than 15 more years is evident (Sanderson, 2008). The term *advanced old age* as used in this chapter refers to people over the age of 75 years.

Geriatrics is the study of a rapidly expanding age group and has become a specialty in the health-care field. Geriatrics includes the biological, psychological, physiological, and sociological aspects of aging. The goal in the care of an advanced old-age adult is to maximize the ability to function and to live independently and to shorten the period of illness and disability. *Healthy People 2020* topic areas and goals for the aged adult are listed in Box 14-1.

A Census Bureau report describes the oldest Americans (CDC, 2010) and reports that in 1980 there were 720,000 Americans above the age of 90, and in 2008 there were 1.9 million people over the age of 90. One percent of the young elderly (65-69) lived in nursing or assisted-living homes, 3% of those aged 75-79 were in nursing/assisted-living homes; 11% of those 85-89 were in nursing/assisted-living homes, and 19% of those over 90 were in nursing homes or assisted-living facilities. There are many who make significant contributions and achievements in their old age, including Ethel Percy Andrus who founded the American Association of Retired Persons (AARP) at the age of 74 in 1958. Harry Bernstein published his first book *The Invisible Wall* at the age of 96 in 2007. Arthur Winston retired at the age of 100 from the Los Angeles Metro after 72 years of service (Young, 2007).

BOX 14-1 *Healthy People 2020* Topics and Goals for the Aged

The following *Healthy People 2020* goals are designed to increase the number of healthy, aged people who continue to enjoy life and to contribute to society:

- Provide access to preventive-health services
- Manage chronic illnesses such as diabetes, heart disease, and stroke
- Diagnose and manage dementias
- Encourage health-promotion activities
- Reduce pneumococcal infections and influenza
- Increase hearing and vision screening and care
- Train caregivers for the elderly
- Improve housing, transportation, and coordination of care

Data from United States Department of Health and Human Services: *Healthy People 2020*, Washington, DC, 2011, U.S. Government Printing Office.

THEORIES OF THE AGING PROCESS

The process of aging occurs as a result of multiple factors, including the genetic lifespan of cells. The past lifestyle, level of activity, dietary practices, and social support all play roles in the process of aging as well. Selected theories concerning the aging process follow.

Cellular Changes

Free Radicals

Ions travel in pairs within cells and are stable. For example, sodium and chloride are paired in the cell as sodium chloride (salt). When one ion breaks off and is no longer paired, it becomes a free radical. Free radicals are unstable. They attack other molecules in the body, which results in cell damage that cannot be repaired. The numbers of free radicals in people increase as they age.

Biological Clock (Programmed Cell Death)

Also known as apoptosis, the membrane surrounding a cell starts breaking down. As this process continues, the debris is phagocytized (eaten) by surrounding cellular materials. This biological clock process dictates the occurrence of menopause in women and contributes to the body changes that ultimately result in death. Interestingly, the ovary is the only organ that appears to have a "programmed senescence in adult life that leads to predictable complete loss of function during aging in all human populations" (Thibodeau & Patton, 2010).

Wear-and-Tear Theory

The wear-and-tear theory can be equated with a machine. Just as the parts in a machine begin to wear out or break down, so too does the human body. With humans, not all parts are so easily replaced or repaired. An example would be the ease and frequency of hip or knee replacement surgery versus heart transplantation.

Immune Theory

As one ages, the body finds it more difficult to tell the difference between healthy and defective cells, and the body responds by destroying both types. Immune theory states that the end result is that the body's immune response is impaired, which causes the aging person to be more susceptible to a variety of illnesses or infections. Decreased immune function of the thymus gland, lymph nodes, spleen, and possibly bone marrow are also thought to be contributing factors to immune-system impairment.

Cellular damage or decline during a number of years results in the activation of the stress responses in the body in an attempt to repair what it can. When the body is unable to repair itself as efficiently as it did in the past, changes occur in the various body systems.

PHYSIOLOGICAL CHANGES

Bones and Cartilage

The loss of body water and bone mass and the degeneration of spinal disks result in a decrease in height during the aging process. A decrease in body mass and a loss of body water occur after age 65. Collagen in the body becomes rigid, and elastin in the body becomes brittle. These substances transport material between cells, and the changes that occur during the aging process result in decreased function of the cells.

The loss of estrogen decreases the ability of the body to use calcium to maintain bone density. Loss of bone mass can result in osteoporosis, which is a thinning of the bone. This predisposes the geriatric adult to bone fractures. Posture and balance may change, and falls become a common problem.

Blood Vessels

Arterial walls thicken with fatty deposits and connective tissue resulting in a narrowing of the arteries. As a consequence, coronary arteries provide less oxygenated blood to the heart muscle. The heart muscles become less elastic. Oxygen exchange slows, and blood pressure may rise to compensate for the lowered oxygen supply. These processes predispose the geriatric adult to the development of high blood pressure, which can result in a stroke. It takes longer for the heart to beat faster in response to activity or stress, and therefore the observable response to pain, stress, or anxiety may be delayed. This means that the health-care worker cannot rely on observing changes in the vital signs to determine the presence of pain, stress, or anxiety.

Lungs

The ribs and cartilage become more rigid, and thus the respiratory muscles have to work harder. Lung tissue loses elasticity, so geriatric adults may not breathe as deeply or cough as effectively, making them more vulnerable to respiratory infections.

Kidneys and Bladder

The rate that the kidneys filter the blood slows, so medications and other substances take longer to leave the body. This can result in an accumulation of medication in the blood and a subsequent overdose reaction. Bladder capacity decreases, with urinary frequency a common result. In men, an enlarged prostate may block the urethra, resulting in urinary frequency or complete obstruction of urinary flow. This obstruction of urinary flow is known as urinary retention and requires prompt medical intervention.

Metabolism

A slowed metabolism can cause retention of glucose (sugars) and lipids (fats). Therefore the geriatric adult is at risk for developing elevated serum lipids. In the geriatric person, a fasting blood glucose level reading will be more accurate than a glucose level measured 2 hours after a meal has been consumed (Sieck, 2003).

Digestion

The decreased motility of the gastrointestinal system results in slower emptying of the stomach by digestion and elimination. Digestive enzymes also decrease, which can result in poor appetite and digestive disturbances. The replacement of taste buds with connective tissue leaves only about 40% of taste buds present by 75 years of age, which can also result in the loss of appetite (Thibodeau & Patton, 2010).

A slowed gag reflex increases the risk of choking, so the geriatric adult should eat slowly while sitting upright. A decrease in *peristalsis* (a wavelike motion that causes intestinal contents to be moved through the gastrointestinal tract) can cause constipation and discomfort from gas. This discomfort often leads the older person to use laxatives and antacids, which may decrease nutrient absorption and may cause other health problems.

Teeth

Tooth loss is common, and the remaining teeth often do not provide optimum cutting or chewing abilities. This influences nutritional intake and may also negatively affect self-image. As time passes, receding gums can lead to ill-fitting dentures and gum lesions (sores). Regular follow-up with a dentist is essential. Providing nutritious foods that are attractively prepared and easy to chew will help meet the nutritional needs of the geriatric adult.

Skin

As the body ages, the repair and replacement of skin cells takes longer. Because of the loss of subcutaneous fat and collagen, the skin becomes thinner, and *turgor* (elasticity) is poorer. This makes the geriatric person more vulnerable to skin injury, and healing of skin wounds is slower. The thin, dry skin develops wrinkles and spotty pigmentation. The ability to perceive cold and hot sensations also decreases, and geriatric adults are at an increased risk for burns. A decrease in the number and function of sweat glands in the skin results in difficulty adjusting to changes in environmental temperature. Chilling (hypothermia) and heat exhaustion occur more easily.

Eyes

A loss of cells in the optic nerve makes it more difficult to see details. Eyesight declines. The pupil of the eye opens and closes more slowly, so more time is needed to adapt visually to the surroundings when moving from light to dark areas. Cataracts develop in the lens of the eye, which further decrease vision in advanced old age. Fifty percent of persons older than 75 may develop cataracts because of the natural aging process. Cataract surgery is common for this age group and is successful in restoring vision in most cases.

Advancing age and diabetes are two of the risk factors for the development of glaucoma, which is atrophy of the optic nerve and increased intraocular pressure. Glaucoma is the leading cause of blindness, and the condition occurs in 15% of people more than 80 years of age. All adults should be periodically screened for the development of glaucoma. Age-related macular degeneration (AMD) is a retinal degeneration that causes the loss of central vision in the geriatric adult. Some peripheral vision may be retained, and total blindness is rare.

Ears

Degenerative changes in the bones of the middle ear result in a decrease in hearing ability, and a significant loss of hair cells in the organ of corti in the inner ear results in difficulty in hearing certain frequencies of sound (Thibodeau & Patton, 2010). There is therefore usually some difficulty in hearing that occurs in the older adult. Communication with geriatric persons is often a problem because they may not hear all the words in the sentence and may misinterpret what is said. Therefore when teaching geriatric patients, it is wise to ask them to repeat what was said to ensure that clear communication and understanding is taking place.

Nervous System

Neurons atrophy (decrease in size) during the aging process, and the transmission of impulses to the brain becomes sluggish. Because of the fatty deposits within the walls of the blood vessels, blood flow to the brain slows. Motor responses and reaction time to stimuli are delayed, and maintaining environmental safety is a challenge.

SEXUALITY

As people age, specific changes in sexual responses occur. However, it is a myth that the aged person ceases to desire or experience sexual intimacy or pleasure. Part of the reason for this myth is that the concept of love and romance, as portrayed in the media, focuses more on the young adult and the relationship of sex to having children. People of advanced age may even feel guilty or abnormal because they recognize that they continue to have sexual feelings. Some older women may believe that they are less sexually attractive than younger women, and they often choose to dress in a way that they think is more appropriate for their age. The media advertise surgery for facelifts, and cosmetic surgery is popular. Older men are also having more cosmetic surgery in an effort to maintain attractiveness to potential partners. For a variety of reasons, some men attempt to take partners who are decades younger than they are. Aging without protest is becoming more popular today, with the older woman taking pride in maintaining her physical and mental competencies while allowing her face and body to show the natural consequences of age and experience.

Health Promotion

Medications are often prescribed for the geriatric patient without considering or educating the person about potential effects on sexual performance. Many medications prescribed for conditions common to the aged have inhibitory effects on sexual interest, arousal, and performance. To ensure compliance with the medication regimen, appropriate education about these effects must be an integral part of the overall provision of health care in the aging population. It is also important to instruct the aging adult about the prevention of sexually transmitted diseases (STDs), including human immunodeficiency syndrome/acquired immunodeficiency syndrome (HIV/AIDS), because this age group is just as likely as their younger cohorts to receive or transmit a communicable disease. About 19% of persons identified as having HIV in America are older than 50 years of age (HRSA, 2011). Because pregnancy prevention is not a concern in the geriatric population, condoms may be considered unnecessary, and therefore the rate of STDs in this age group continues to increase. Some elderly persons might also attribute the signs and symptoms of HIV/AIDS as being "symptoms of old age," and thus they do not seek testing at an early stage.

Personality and behavior are important dimensions in sexuality. According to the World Health Organization (Lindau, 2007), there are three key elements to consider within the concept of sexuality: (1) the capacity to enhance and control sexual and reproductive behavior in accordance with a social and personal ethic; (2) freedom from fear, shame, guilt, false beliefs, and other psychological factors inhibiting sexual responses; and (3) freedom from organic disorder, disease, and deficiencies that interfere with sexual or reproductive function. When working with the geriatric adult, one must take into consideration these three primary elements of sexuality. Box 14-2 provides some details concerning the aging process and its effects on sexuality.

Sexual Responses in the Aging Woman

Menopause, or climacteric, in women does not decrease sexual response, because androgens are no longer inhibited by estrogens. Because of varying hormone levels, women will notice dryness in the vaginal mucosa, hot flashes, and other assorted hormone-related body changes. Frequent sexual activity, use of creams and water-soluble lubricants in the vagina, exercise, proper nutrition, and soy supplements can be alternatives to hormone replacement therapy (HRT); HRT may be contraindicated in some women. Although the erotic responses of the nipple and clitoris do not decrease, the intensity of vaginal lubrication and tissue expansion during sexual arousal does decrease with age and can make sexual activity uncomfortable. This is primarily because of decreased levels of estrogen. The ability to achieve multiple orgasms continues, although the intensity is decreased. As part of a health-maintenance plan, women should continue to obtain regular health screenings.

Sexual Responses in the Aging Man

Testosterone production decreases between the ages of 40 and 60 but remains stable thereafter. This leads to a decrease in the size and firmness of the penis and reduced production, motility, and lifespan of sperm. Men are often able to retain fertility into their eighth decade of life, despite the decline in actual sperm count and sperm activity by up to 30% (DeLamater, 2005).

BOX 14-2 Factors That Influence Sexuality in the Geriatric Adult

ATTITUDE/INTEREST

- Previous life experiences
- Body-image perception
- Mental function
- Self-expectations and image promotion
- Social contact/isolation
- Environment/privacy

SEXUAL HEALTH

- Incontinence, urinary/fecal devices
- Reduction in mobility
- Impotence and menopause
- Chronic or terminal illness
- Medications and their side effects

The ability to attain an erection may be delayed and requires increased physiological stimulation as men age. Anxiety may also contribute to increased delay or sexual dysfunction. However, men soon realize that after the erection is achieved it can be maintained for a longer period compared with earlier years. The intensity of orgasm may be decreased, but the pleasurable response is usually retained.

A decrease in men's sexual function is similar to that in women and is referred to as the male climacteric. Some men experience similar symptoms of hot flashes, feelings of suffocation, and depression. These symptoms can usually be treated with hormonal replacement, such as testosterone, synthetic androgens, and in some cases estrogen (Thibodeau & Patton, 2010). A consequence of decreased sexual activity is the increased risk of inflammation and enlargement of the prostate gland.

The Impact of Illness on Sexuality

Cancer of the prostate is a risk, and preventive screening via periodic examinations, which may include prostate-specific antigen (PSA) blood levels and professional guidance, are recommended in this age group. Hormone treatments for cancer of the prostate can interfere with achieving and maintaining penile erection. Some men who have had surgery of the prostate gland experience retrograde ejaculation into the urinary bladder rather than out through the urethra.

After a heart attack, the aged man is given extensive information about dietary changes he needs to follow, but rarely is he or his partner educated about possible alternatives that can be used to fulfill sexual needs. Hospitals and nursing homes are often insensitive to the sexual needs of the aged, and sexual opportunity, privacy, and programs are often absent from care plans. Postoperative instructions concerning surgery that involve reproductive organs should include an understanding of the effects on sexuality and the options available to cope with these effects.

Patient Teaching

Health-care workers have the opportunity to discuss with patients the discomforts or problems with sexual functioning in the aging patient, in the postoperative patient, and in the perimenopausal and postmenopausal woman. Patients should be taught that maintaining physical activity can help them to enjoy erotic activity. Studies by Masters and Johnson (1976) explain that regular sexual activity with a partner, or through masturbation, also contribute to maintaining the capacity for sexual pleasure. Overeating, drinking alcohol, and a sedentary lifestyle all negatively affect sexual vigor. The normal alterations of aging may decrease, but they do not eliminate the ability to enjoy a satisfactory sex life.

The health-care worker should help the aged understand the normal changes and responses in their bodies to avoid misinterpretations. Intimacy is a lifelong need. For some, cuddling and caressing is all that is needed, whereas others prefer to form an increased intellectual and emotional closeness with friends and to develop interests that will meet their intimacy needs. Sexual concerns in the geriatric adult can be discussed with the health-care provider for assessment and intervention.

PSYCHOLOGICAL CHANGES

Throughout the life cycle, attractiveness and personal appearance have a high value. The media and the marketplace offer makeup and clothing that emphasize appearing eternally young. A person's negative self-image may affect his or her ability to function. Fortunately the aging process is a gradual one that provides time for coping and adaptation to the physical changes that are evident as one grows older. Roles may change. The dependent wife may become the caregiver and decision maker if the husband becomes disabled. An older man may take on homemaking duties if the younger wife continues to work. These various role adjustments require adaptation and acceptance.

Cultural Considerations

Culture also affects the aging process. In cultures where people of advanced old age are valued and respected, the feeling of self-worth contributes to general health. In cultures where people of advanced old age are avoided (ageism), a feeling of usefulness declines and depression can set in. Geriatric persons usually fear loss of independence and fear disability that will make them a burden to their families.

The loss of peers, siblings, and even a spouse can result in loneliness. Disengagement is the process in which an older adult withdraws from social contacts and relinquishes independence and control to others. A decline in income may require relocation, and a new environment may intensify the feeling of loneliness. Some guidance may be needed to help the older person seek new relationships and activities that are enjoyable. Grandparenting can be a source of satisfaction if the children and grandchildren live nearby (Figure 14-1). People of advanced old age often are afraid to try new things and may be slow to learn, because concentration and memory decline with advancing age.

The development of dementias that involve cognitive impairments including memory loss, loss of ability to communicate, and decreased functioning in social situations (such as Alzheimer's disease) often leads to complete dependence on others. There

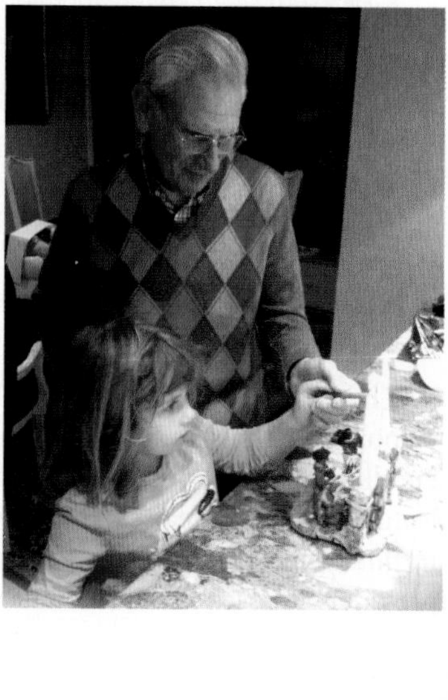

Figure 14-1 Grandparenting can be a source of satisfaction for the geriatric adult. The interactions benefit both the child and the grandparent.

are several organizations and resources that address the needs of older Americans and can aid with the diagnosis and management of persons with dementias, including the American Association of Homes and Services for aging and the Gerontological Society of America (GSA).

A study at Columbia University in New York developed a tool to predict the time from diagnosis, to nursing home, to death for Alzheimer's patients (Stern et al, 1997). The tool calculates predictions based on a questionnaire that evaluates extrapyramidal signs, psychological symptoms, age at onset, current age, gender, and the results of a mini mental test score. The tool may be useful in planning the care of some elderly persons diagnosed with dementia. A White House Conference on this topic, held in 2005, focused on the theme of "The Dynamics of Aging: From Awareness to Action," which suggested policies to Congress and the President concerning the needs of the aged population. A year later, the Older American Act of 2006, which supported national long-term care strategies for the country, was passed (IOM, 2008).

DEVELOPMENTAL TASKS

Mastering the crisis of ego integrity versus despair is the challenge of the older adult (see Chapter 5). Mastering the crisis of immortality versus extinction is the major task of advanced old age. Reflecting on their own accomplishments and legacies brings ego integrity and satisfaction to geriatric adults and implies successful mastery of the developmental tasks from previous stages of the life cycle.

Reminiscing about past experiences is therapeutic. If reflection about life's experiences brings feelings of unresolved conflicts and failures, then a feeling of despair will prevail, resulting in anxiety, bitterness, and perhaps even stress and illness. Ego integrity is achieved when reminiscing reveals satisfaction with past achievements and a sense of leaving a positive legacy or memories behind. If geriatric adults can focus on prioritizing activities that bring them pleasure, they can enjoy daily life.

A major developmental task of old age and sometimes advanced old age is adjusting to retirement. The work setting is no longer the center for maintaining a feeling of self-worth, so having a hobby or interest to pursue that offers a sense of fulfillment and satisfaction is essential in maintaining good mental health (Figure 14-2). Another developmental task

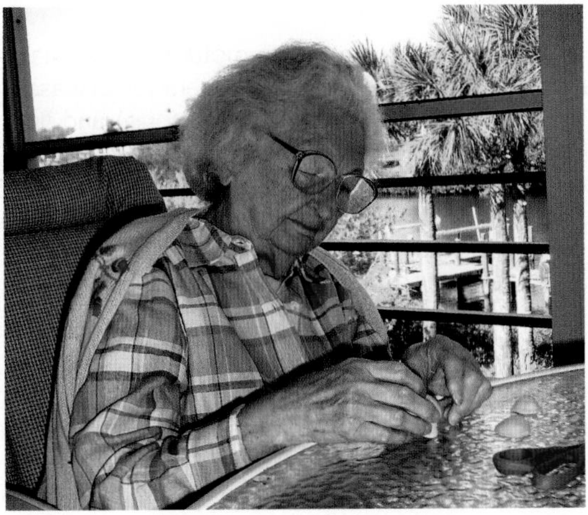

Figure 14-2 Older adults can engage in hobbies or activities that bring them pleasure and help maintain an active mind and body.

for the advanced old age group is adjusting to and accepting the frailties of aging and the accompanying changes in physical appearance and lifestyles.

Lifespan Considerations

Today better foods, safer surroundings, and high-tech medical care have extended lifespan expectations. However, lifestyle modifications that include exercise, a healthy diet, and stress management are essential to achieve this goal.

PHYSICAL EXERCISE

"Use it or lose it" is an old adage, and it is true. The losses in physiological functioning may be related to a lack of activity (Thibodeau & Patton, 2010). Regular exercise promotes mental and physical health. In accordance with *Healthy People 2020* goals, regular exercise should be maintained as long as possible. Natural activities such as walking, jogging, or swimming are appropriate and can provide pleasure. The frail elderly can achieve some benefits from exercises performed in a chair (Baumgardner, 2008). Guidelines for physical activity for older adults are discussed in Chapter 13.

HEALTHY PEOPLE 2020 GOALS

OCCUPATIONAL ACTIVITIES

Adjusting to retirement from the life's work, and finding fulfillment and self-worth from volunteer activities, hobbies, or travel, can help maintain an active mind and body. This is often referred to as the *activity theory* and is related to a positive transition in the aging adult.

NUTRITION

Maintaining adequate nutrition intake is important for health maintenance. There are challenges to overcome, such as dental loss, adaptation to dentures, slowed digestion, constipation, and a decline in the ability to buy or prepare nutritious meals. Many communities offer a Meals on Wheels service that delivers one meal a day to geriatric residents. Senior centers within the community often serve one meal a day as well, and this environment has the added advantage of providing socialization for older adults.

PREVENTION OF ILLNESS

Providing regular health checkups and follow-up for abnormal symptoms is essential for health maintenance. Immunizations recommended by the Centers for Disease Control and Prevention, such as the pneumococcal vaccine (pneumonia) and flu shots, are also advisable (see Appendix A). Close monitoring of chronic illnesses such as heart disease, high blood pressure, arthritis, and visual disturbances is important. Providing access to regular medical care is often a challenge due to immobility, lack of transportation, and other factors. The geriatric adult should be screened periodically for colon cancer, breast cancer, prostate cancer, and lipid disorders.

MENTAL HEALTH

Depression is the most common mental health problem in the geriatric age group. It is typically brought on by isolation from social contacts, change in environment, low self-esteem, and loss of loved ones. Suicide is also common in this age group. Psychological counseling, establishment of social contact and support, and engaging in pleasurable activities on a daily basis help avoid the development of depression. To maintain mental health, the person of advanced old age must be realistic, use strengths and coping strategies to handle physiological changes, and set new goals that are positive and attainable.

ENVIRONMENTAL CONTROLS

Reducing the risk of falls and fractures can be achieved by providing a safe environment. Avoiding the use of slippery area rugs, using handrails in bathrooms to assist with changes in body position, and maintaining effective lighting are environmental modifications that are easy to achieve.

ELDER ABUSE

Elder abuse is the intentional infliction of mental, emotional, or physical pain or the failure to provide the care necessary for optimal survival (i.e., neglect). In some cases the abuse may be economic, depriving geriatric adults of their life savings. Dependency, frailty, illness, and metal disability may make the geriatric adult more vulnerable to abuse. When the caregiver is a family member, the combined effect of fatigue and overwhelming responsibilities to spouse, children, job, and care of a geriatric adult may cause caregiver strain, which may result in some type of elder abuse. Healthcare workers can intervene by offering resources for caregiver support, such as respite care, support groups, education, and stress management.

Signs of abuse may include depression, social isolation, clusters of bruises, unexplained burns, contractures, undernutrition, dehydration, and missed follow-up healthcare appointments. All caregivers should be alert to elder abuse, because it may go unreported by the geriatric adult, whose self-esteem may have been destroyed. Referral to adult protective services may be necessary, or placement in another environment may be advisable.

POLYPHARMACY AND MEDICATION ERRORS

Polypharmacy is the use of many medications prescribed for different chronic illnesses. The medications taken may interact with one another and may produce unwanted side effects. The geriatric person also may forget to take one dose or may accidentally take a double dose, which can result in toxicity and illness. Monitoring of medications should be a priority in elder care. The decreased organ function found in advanced old age contributes to a delay in excretion of the drug from the body, and toxicity can also develop. Drug dosages and effects need to be carefully monitored and explained to patients and their caregivers.

PLACEMENT ALTERNATIVES

Sometimes geriatric adults suffer from multiple chronic illnesses. They also may have cognitive impairments such as Alzheimer's disease, which involves loss of memory, disorientation, and loss of the ability to communicate and function in social situations. The complete dependence on others for activities of daily living (ADLs) such as bathing, tooth-brushing, dressing, and eating may lead to the need for placement in a nursing home or long-term care facility (Box 14-3).

Some nursing homes offer basic nursing care; others offer physical and recreational activities as well. Entering a nursing home often requires relinquishing independence and control over one's life, and many geriatric patients decline rapidly in this type of less personal environment. Selection of a nursing home should include factors such as cost, insurance coverage, accessibility to medical services, philosophy of care, staffing, social

(Continued)

Lifespan Considerations—cont'd

services, and availability of occupational, physical, and speech therapy. Some facilities offer pet therapy, which is the use of pets as friends and dependents. Providing a clean homelike setting with open visiting hours, spiritual care, and pleasant visual surroundings is important (Box 14-4).

There are alternatives to nursing-home care for the adult in advanced old age. Long-term care insurance, if purchased before it is needed, can provide in-home care and assistance. Some facilities offer assisted living in a residential setting for the geriatric adult who needs minimal or moderate supervision and care. Some families buy larger homes or build additions for geriatric parents so that parents' independence is maintained even though they are close by. In some communities, visiting health-care workers can attend the homebound geriatric person and can provide supervision, care, and education.

ROLE OF THE HEALTH-CARE WORKER

Most geriatric adults develop coping strategies to handle the gradual aging process. Often, minor changes in the environment can enhance their ability to function. For example, the geriatric person with decreased lung capacity and high blood pressure may manage well in a ground-floor apartment but may have difficulty if walking up stairs is a required daily activity.

It is important to observe family interaction. An overprotective family who insists on restraining the geriatric person in a wheelchair or in a bed because of the fear of falling will foster dependency that can result in dysfunction and psychological decline. Changes in

BOX 14-3 Activities of Daily Living

Assisted-living facilities can help with cleaning, laundry, meals, and recreational activities. The ability to manage the following activities of daily living (ADLs) is essential for independent living:

- Eating
- Toileting, bathing, and grooming
- Cooking
- Shopping
- Taking medications

BOX 14-4 Concerns Related to Living Arrangements

- Access to health care and assessment
- Individual's perception of move as "dumping" or as assistance
- Control of patient's finances
- Personal space allowed
- Accommodation of special needs
- Privacy or shared room
- Providing pet care, allowing plants in room
- Peer-group activity
- Rehabilitation and therapies available

aging include physiological, psychological, social, economic, and cultural factors that influence the way one ages and the rate of the aging process.

There are many positive aspects of aging. Geriatric adults offer others a wealth of experience, expertise, and wisdom. They provide a grandchild with a relationship that cannot be equaled and that contributes to the development of the child and the well-being of the geriatric adult (Figure 14-3). Understanding the developmental tasks of advanced old age, knowing the physiological and psychological changes and challenges that geriatric persons face, and empowering those in advanced old age to maintain autonomy or control over their lives is the focus of geriatric care (Box 14-5).

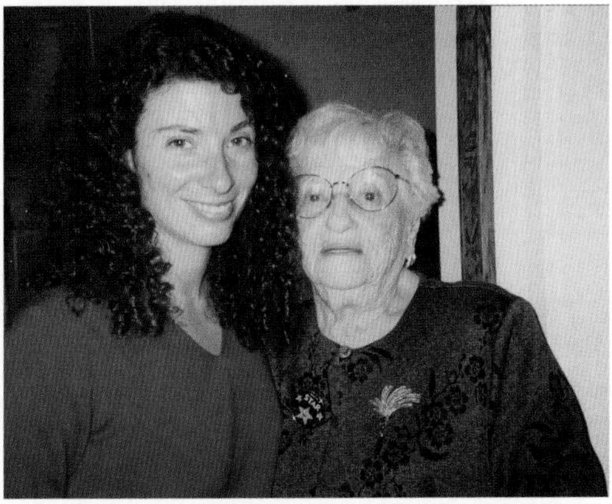

Figure 14-3 A relative visits a woman who has just celebrated her one-hundredth birthday. Adults in the geriatric age group can benefit from assisted-living facilities that enable the older adults to maintain personal independence. Friends, family, and visitors to their homes receive the benefits of the experience, the wisdom, and the expertise of geriatric adults.

BOX 14-5 Principles of Elder Care

- Encourage confidence
- Raise self-image
- Provide empowerment
- Demonstrate kind, caring manner
- Identify and include family and social-support systems
- Actively listen
- Integrate spirituality, hope, and faith
- Assist in setting personal goals
- Monitor exercise and nutrition
- Follow-up on health concerns

KEY POINTS

- Senescence is categorized as including the young-old, old, old-old, and elite-old.
- The physiological changes in advanced old age affect all body systems, but the degree is dependent on genetics, lifestyle, dietary practices, and social support.
- Immortality versus extinction is the major task or challenge that the advanced old age population must face.
- Some health-promotion activities in which the geriatric adult can participate are physical exercise, balanced nutrition, preventive health maintenance (such as receiving the flu vaccine),

(Continued)

KEY POINTS—cont'd

and controlling the safety of his or her environment.
- The need for a sense of being loved and valued continues throughout the lifespan and includes fulfilling the sexual needs of the geriatric adult.
- Lifestyle adjustments, including a healthful diet, exercise, and stress management, can aid modern medicine in extending the lifespan.
- Elder abuse is the physical, mental, social, or financial neglect or mistreatment of the geriatric adult.
- A variety of living options is available to geriatric adults, including living in their own homes, with other family members, living in assisted-living apartments, or living in skilled/long-term care facilities.
- Activities of daily living involve the ability to independently eat, dress, wash, toilet, and communicate.
- The health-care worker can provide education and guidance in meeting the life tasks of the geriatric adult.

Critical Thinking

Discuss some advantages and disadvantages of three different living arrangements available for geriatric patients. What factors should be considered when helping a geriatric patient select a living arrangement?

REVIEW QUESTIONS

1. **Osteoporosis is:**
   a. the loss of bone mass.
   b. the occurrence of bone fractures.
   c. the development of mental confusion.
   d. an inevitable part of the aging process.

2. **Senescence is a period in an adult's life when:**
   a. the body begins to age and weaken.
   b. sexual desires disappear.
   c. mental confusion occurs.
   d. death is imminent.

3. **In men, fertility may be retained until the:**
   a. age of 65.
   b. age of 70.
   c. age of 80.
   d. midlife crisis occurs.

4. **Preventative screening for the presence of cancer of the prostate includes:**
   a. periodic examinations and professional guidance.
   b. radiograph of the prostate.
   c. annual magnetic resonance imaging exam.
   d. annual Pap test.

5. **The major task of the advanced old age adult includes:**
   a. immortality versus extinction.
   b. identity versus role confusion.
   c. intimacy versus isolation.
   d. ego-integrity versus despair.

CHAPTER 15

Planning for the End of Life

http://evolve.elsevier.com/Leifer/growth

OBJECTIVES

1. Describe the grieving process for the patient who is facing death.
2. List the stages of the dying process.
3. Discuss behaviors related to the dying process.
4. Describe the philosophy of hospice and palliative care.
5. Define quality of life from a child's point of view.
6. Summarize the statements in the Dying Person's Bill of Rights.
7. Discuss the response and needs of the family of the dying patient.
8. Review ethical and legal issues involved in end-of-life care.
9. State the role of the health-care worker in end-of-life care.
10. State three cultural practices related to end-of-life care.
11. Describe the development of the concept of death and dying in young children.
12. Discuss similarities and differences in end-of-life care for adults and children.
13. List signs of impending death.

KEY TERMS

Advance health care directives (AHCDs)
assisted suicide
culturally competent
durable power of attorney for health care
euthanasia
hospice care
informed consent
palliative care
therapeutic communication
therapeutic presence

DEATH AS PART OF THE LIFE CYCLE

Death is a normal part of the life cycle. Many older people prepare for death by writing a last will and testament, by documenting in advance directives for health care, or by making advance funeral arrangements, which may include the purchase of a burial plot. Few people are really prepared for the actual event.

Most people who think about death associate it with the elderly, but death is not unique to the aged. The sudden, unexpected death of a young person causes different emotions and behaviors in the survivors. The process of death can occur in the acute-care hospital amid the surroundings of whirring machines, twisted tubes, and medical and nursing staff who are strangers, or it can occur in the peaceful home or hospice environment in a room with family and familiar caregivers surrounding the bed.

Cultural Considerations

The care of a dying person, called end-of-life (EOL) care, involves ethical and legal issues and religious and cultural responsibilities that need to be addressed by the health-care team.

Surveys have shown that the two most common fears associated with death are the fear of pain and the fear of being a burden to the family (Firestone, 2009). The biggest barrier to the patient accessing hospice or palliative-care facilities is the fear of letting go of all hope for survival.

Hospice is a concept of palliative care that offers comfort to patients and families who have limited life expectancy and are facing death. Although symptomatic relief is offered, hospice does not have curative goals. Emotional, spiritual, and physical support is given based on the needs of the patient and the belief that death is imminent and a normal process.

No specific technique or procedure can describe exactly what to do for a patient who is dying or for the family who is in anguish. A flexible approach is needed to meet the needs of the patient and family. Often the mere presence of a health-care worker provides the support that is needed. Remaining near the patient and family, or simply holding a hand, provides strength while facilitating the expression of emotions and grief. This is known as therapeutic presence.

Lifespan Considerations

Understanding the patient's and the family's wishes, religious and cultural needs, and legal and ethical protocols is essential for the health-care worker (see Chapter 3 for cultural considerations related to death). The physical, psychological, spiritual, and social needs of the family as a unit are part of the care of a dying patient. Most care plans focus on a positive outcome for the care provided, and few see any positive outcome when death occurs. However, providing death with dignity is a quality process in the closure of a life. Helping to decrease pain, promote comfort, and reduce stress are considered positive outcomes in the care of dying patients and the care of their families.

SIGNS AND SYMPTOMS OF DEATH

The family should be prepared for the symptoms that accompany death (Box 15-1), and the information should be communicated with sensitivity. Even when the death of a person is expected, the finality of the actual death still will come as a shock to most family members.

THE PROCESS OF DYING

The process of dying is psychological and physiological. *Psychological* death begins when a person is told that he or she has a terminal illness. Sometimes the death of a spouse or a peer causes a person to believe that his or her own death is near. For example, when an older person realizes he is the last of his generation living, he begins to face his own future death. *Physiological* death starts when the body processes decline in function.

BOX 15-1 Common Signs of Impending Death

- Increasing weakness, immobility
- Weight loss
- Decreased appetite
- Loss of bowel and bladder control
- Decreased awareness of surroundings*
- Diaphoresis (sweating)
- Lung congestion (loose gurgling sound, referred to as the death rattle)
- Altered breathing patterns (periods of apnea, often called Cheyne-Stokes respirations)
- Decreased urine output
- Slowed pulse
- Cold and mottled extremities
- Relaxed and open jaw

*Even though the person may appear to be asleep or in a coma, hearing is the last sense to be lost. Family and caregivers should continue to talk to the dying person.

Psychological Responses of the Dying Patient

As part of the life cycle, death is accompanied by tasks and responses. Most people who realize they are facing death go through a grieving process (Table 15-1). The process may start with disbelief (e.g., "This can't be happening to me"). This stage is often accompanied by periods of crying and mourning for what will be left behind, future events that will be missed, and unfulfilled opportunities in relationships and activities. This grief process may or may not proceed to clinical depression. The normal sadness of grieving the end of life may occur in spurts as assistance in the activities of daily living (ADLs) is increasingly required, and the deterioration resulting from a condition becomes real. This kind of decrease in independence may trigger a period of sadness.

Disability and increasing dependence on others may cause the patient to lose self-esteem and to be concerned with body image. The normal grief process can be interrupted by visits from close family or friends. Periods of pleasure can occur during the grief process if the patient is not clinically depressed. A glimmer of hope is often seen during the grief process, because there is always the thought that some last-minute reprieve or mistake in diagnosis will occur. However, this thought typically does not promote hope if the patient is clinically depressed.

TABLE 15-1 Behaviors and Stages of Dying

Stages	Behaviors
Denial: "This can't be real"	Shock, numbness
Anger: "Why me?"	Disruptive behaviors, turmoil
Bargaining: Making deals with a god	Anxiety, conflict, confusion
Depression: Feeling of loss	Withdrawal, guilt, grief
Acceptance: "My time has come"	Vulnerability

Data from Kübler-Ross E: *On death and dying*, New York, 1969, Macmillan; Kinney M, et al, editors: *AACN's clinical reference for critical care nursing*, ed 4, St Louis, 1996, Mosby; Stroebe H, Hansson R, Stroebe W, Schut H: *Handbook of bereavement research: consequences, coping and care*, Washington D.C., 2001, American Psychological Association.

A good social support system can assist the dying patient through the preparatory grief process. The health-care worker can help the person prepare for death by understanding and accepting the stages of grieving, mobilizing support systems, and using coping strategies. *Therapeutic presence* consists of being there and providing support and comfort for the patient and the family unit. Therapeutic communication involves accepting the patient's emotional outbursts and expressions of anger and encouraging venting and verbalization. The health-care worker should maintain communication with the family and should explain the stages of grief and the related behaviors. Talking with the patient about family, past achievements, and legacies can also be helpful.

Clinical depression can often be avoided by identifying common fears of patients who are facing death and making efforts to alleviate those fears. Therapeutic presence of family and staff can alleviate the fear of abandonment, and fear of the unknown can be reduced by educating the family and patient and by offering support to them. Simple relaxation techniques are often helpful. A spiritual history obtained as part of the care plan can enable assessment of spiritual or cultural needs and practices that would be helpful when providing individualized care. The multidisciplinary health-care team, working closely with the patient and family, can help provide a death with peace and dignity.

Some patients do not progress through the stages as outlined by Kübler-Ross and may never pass beyond the stage of denial (see Table 15-1). Some people regress to previous stages from time to time during their journey toward death. Hope need not be abandoned during any stage. It has long been understood that a terminally ill patient can sometimes willfully prolong his or her life when desiring to be present at an important family event, such as a birth or a wedding, and then the patient may die soon afterward. Some people faced with the diagnosis of a terminal illness lose the will to live, whereas others decide to live life to the fullest as long as they are able. There is no norm for the process of dying.

Family Behaviors Related to the Dying Process

Family members may show a variety of responses when a loved one is dying. In many ways these behaviors are similar to the dying person's responses and must be recognized and acknowledged. Health-care workers are able to help the family most by assessing their needs and informing them about what they may see when they enter the patient's room. Preparation and education are the keys to helping the family cope with whatever lies ahead.

Two specific behaviors, *helplessness* and *guilt*, should be quickly recognized, and appropriate interventions should be implemented as soon as possible. To minimize the sense of helplessness, the health-care worker needs to educate and inform family members of what is happening and allow the family to assist in providing care, which can include washing the patient's face, adjusting a pillow, or just sitting at the bedside so that they may hold hands with their loved one.

Guilt is a much more difficult behavior for the health-care worker to manage. The setting often determines the level of guilt a family member may experience. For example, if in an intensive-care unit, the family may feel not only overwhelmed with all the machinery, but may also feel additional secondary guilt related to the different types of invasive procedures that may be required to keep the patient alive. If the guilt of one family member is related to an interpersonal conflict with the patient that occurred before the dying process or death of the patient, this family member may be in direct conflict with the rest of the family regarding what type or extent of interventions they want to have performed for the patient. In many cases the guilt experience may cause the family member to insist on everything being done regardless of the outcome or level of suffering the dying person may have to endure. Therefore it is imperative to help the family member to resolve feelings of guilt, so that a more individualized and appropriate approach can be undertaken in the treatment and plan of care for the dying patient.

Pain related to dying appears to be a common fear that most people experience. Many state that they "hope it's quick and painless." A variety of pain-relieving techniques can be used to help make the dying person as comfortable as possible. These techniques range from back rubs, position changes, scented oils or candles, acupressure, acupuncture, herbs, and nonnarcotic or opioid pain relievers. The goal is to ensure that the pain is relieved as much as possible while also allowing the dying person to complete any unfinished tasks.

Family, friends, and sometimes even health-care workers may seek advice concerning what to say to a person who is dying. The fear of saying the wrong thing often keeps people away from the bedside of a person who is dying, which often means that the needs of the patient (as well as the needs of others related to or involved with the patient) may remain unmet. Table 15-2 offers some suggestions for what to say and what not to say, often referred to as *therapeutic communication.*

TABLE 15-2 Therapeutic Communication

What to Say (Therapeutic Comments)	What Not to Say (Nontherapeutic Comments)
"Tell me how you are feeling."	"You need to be strong for your family."
"It's okay to cry."	"Don't cry."
"It sounds as if you are dealing with painful memories."	"It is God's will."
"I'm here if you want to talk."	"You will be out of pain soon."

Cultural Considerations

The behaviors of the family related to the care of a terminally ill relative may be influenced in part by the family's cultural beliefs and practices. Health-care workers must be culturally competent; that is, they must be aware of the cultural practices of others and accept their practices in a nonjudgmental way. Cultural competence is developed through cultural awareness, knowledge of various cultural practices, skill in incorporating cultural beliefs into a patient care plan, and experience with persons from diverse cultures. Part of health-care education includes encounters with patients and coworkers from diverse settings. Understanding that culture influences thoughts, language, symbolic artifacts (such as bracelets or amulets), and actions that reflect specific traditions, customs, and rituals helps the health-care worker understand behaviors and practices common to specific cultural groups.

Culture and health-care are interrelated. Culture influences an individual's attitude toward illness, nutrition, health care, and health-care providers. A cultural assessment and history are important parts of a patient's care plan. A family-care plan facilitates a more comprehensive cultural assessment, especially when related to end-of-life care. Interpreters should be provided whenever necessary to ensure accurate communication. Table 15-3 describes the dying rituals of selected cultures.

TABLE 15-3 Dying Rituals of Various Cultures

	Preparation	Home vs. Hospital	Special Needs
Native American	May avoid contact with the dying person. Grieving is usually done in private, away from the person who is dying.	Concern for comfort and naturalness of the dying process.	May request shaman or healers to address spiritual health of the dying.
Arab American	Head of family to be informed privately of impending death. He will then determine how the rest of the family is to be informed.	Generally, prefer hospital to home setting in the hope that Western medicine may be able to hold off death.	Muslims do not need Imam in attendance until the process of dying begins or the patient has died. Have a private room available for the family, so that they may grieve together.
Cambodian (Khmer)	Parents or older children are to be notified, so that religious leader and other family members may be contacted.	Comfortable with death occurring at home or in hospital environment.	Incense is used. Family grieves quietly and wears white while mourning.
East Indian	Believes only the body dies and that the soul lives on. Hindus and Sikhs believe in the concept of reincarnation. Dying person is typically not told of impending death	Prefer death to occur in the privacy of the home so family and friends can visit. Religious ceremonies can also be conducted at home without interruption from hospital staff	Family must be notified if death is imminent and be allowed to remain at bedside until death has occurred. Those of Hindu faith will mourn for 40 days

Filipino	Prefer that the family tell the patient he or she is dying.	Prefer to die at home if terminal, because they want to die with dignity intact as much as possible.	Family prays at bedside. Patient usually has religious medallion of some kind on body or in hand. Will want a chaplain/priest at bedside to receive the Sacrament of the Sick or to have Last Rites performed.
Hispanic	May wish to protect ill person from knowledge of impending death. Family prefers to inform patient. Family may want time alone with person to say good-bye. May call clergy.	Prefer death at home to preserve dignity and location of spirit. Privacy is important to the family. Family usually stays with patient. Do not resuscitate (DNR) orders usually are not acceptable.	Pregnant women and children may be prohibited from contact with dying patient. Amulets, prayer beads at bedside are common. Eldest child may be responsible for health-care decisions.
West Indian	Prefer to see the body immediately after death. Surviving spouse is to be notified of death with children present.	Terminally ill may be taken home to be cared for as a sign of respect, loyalty, and obligation.	As death approaches, family and friends will want to be at the bedside to witness the death and to pray for the person's passing on.

Data from Smith SF, Duell DJ, Martin BC: *Clinical nursing skills: basic to advanced skills*, New York, 2000, Prentice-Hall; Leifer G: *Introduction to maternity & pediatric nursing*, ed 6, Philadelphia, 2011, Saunders; Lipson JG, Dibble SL, Minarik PA: *Culture & nursing care: a pocket guide*, San Francisco, 1996, UCSF Nursing Press.

OPTIONS FOR END-OF-LIFE CARE

Acute Care of the Dying Patient

Over the past several decades, the medical field has seen a number of positive changes in its ability to care for the sick, injured, or dying. With the advent of new technology, health-care workers are now able to resuscitate premature infants and help them to survive with the aid of machines until their own small bodies are able to take over the task. A gravely ill patient may be kept alive for an indefinite amount of time, which may allow the family to gather at the bedside to say their final good-byes. However, there are times when modern technology cannot keep someone alive. For whatever reason, the person's body has taken all it can and is unable to fight to survive. It is usually at this time when the physician speaks to the family to discuss the options and possible outcomes. These options can include continuation of full life support, such as a ventilator (breathing machine), intravenous medications to keep the heart beating and the blood pressure high enough to circulate blood throughout the body, and full cardiopulmonary resuscitation (CPR). The options can also include removing all life support or life-sustaining equipment and stopping all drugs except those that can provide sedation and relief of pain. The Dying Person's Bill of Rights is outlined in Box 15-2.

BOX 15-2 The Dying Person's Bill of Rights

I have the right to be treated as a living human being until I die.
I have the right to maintain a sense of hopefulness, however its focus may change.
I have the right to be cared for by those who can maintain a sense of hopefulness, however its focus may change.
I have the right to express my feelings and emotions about my approaching death in my own way.
I have the right to participate in decisions concerning my care.
I have the right to expect continuing medical and nursing attention even if "cure" goals must be changed to "comfort" goals.
I have the right not to die alone.
I have the right to be free from pain.
I have the right to have my questions answered honestly.
I have the right not to be deceived.
I have the right to have help from and for my family in accepting my death.
I have the right to die in peace and with dignity.
I have the right to retain my individuality and not to be judged for my decisions, which may be contrary to the beliefs of others.
I have the right to discuss and enlarge my religious and spiritual experiences, regardless of what they may mean to others.
I have the right to expect that the sanctity of the human body will be respected after death.
I have the right to be cared for by caring, sensitive, knowledgeable people who will try to understand my needs and will be able to gain some satisfaction in helping me face my death.

Created at the workshop "The Terminally Ill Patient and the Helping Person," sponsored by the Southwestern Michigan In-Service Education Council and conducted by Amelia J. Barbus, Associate Professor of Nursing, Wayne State University, 1975. From Barbus A: The dying patient's bill of rights, *Am J Nurs* 75:99, 1975.

Hospice Care

As mentioned earlier in this chapter, hospice care is a program that supports the patient and family through the dying process and helps the survivors through the period of bereavement. The program originated in England as a response to the growing awareness of the unmet needs of the dying patient. The hospice plan is based on the philosophy that death is a part of the normal life cycle. The physical, psychological, spiritual, and social needs of the dying patient are addressed. The hospice program of care started in the Eastern United States in 1974 and became a recognized Medicare benefit in 1982.

The hospice plan involves palliative care, which is defined by the World Health Organization (WHO) as the "active total care of patients whose disease is not responsive to curative therapy" (WHO, 1990). The goal is the best possible quality of life for patients and their families, and aggressive curative efforts are not pursued. The varied settings for hospice care can include the home, nursing facilities, or long-term care facilities. Medication is prescribed for relief of pain and discomfort rather than for curative reasons. The hospice palliative-care program provides comprehensive patient-centered care with a physician and nurse as the key links of a multidisciplinary team. Financing sources for hospice care are insurance companies, veteran's benefit services, Medicare/Medicaid, and private payments. The eligibility requirements for hospice care may be restricted by the rules of the funding source used.

ETHICAL AND LEGAL ISSUES

Ethical issues concerning death are influenced by values, culture, and religion, whereas legal issues are rooted in the law. The responsibilities of health-care workers are to be familiar with the laws, recognize the cultural needs of the patient and family, and make the family aware of options available and the consequences of each option. Informed consent is based on respect for the dignity and rights of individuals and their right to make decisions about themselves and their health care.

The Kennedy Institute of Ethics was established in 1971 in Washington, D.C. This group deals with laws (formal rules), ethics (informal rules), and bioethics (health-care regulations and research). The President's Commission for the Study of Ethical Problems in Medicine and Research was established in 1978, which reported on issues in the health-care system. Decisions concerning end-of-life care, such as terminating life support, consenting to organ donation, and protecting the rights of incompetent patients, were researched. As a result of the research findings, policies were developed that addressed informed consent, advance directives, and durable power of attorney for health care.

Advance Directives

Advance health care directives (AHCDs) are used to inform health-care providers and family members of the wishes of the patient as related to the level of lifesaving measures or heroics to be used when the patient is near death and is unable to communicate. The U.S. Congress passed, as part of the Omnibus Budget Reconciliation Act of 1990, the Patient Self-Determination Act. This act became law in December 1991 (U.S. Public Law 101-508). The Patient Self-Determination Act mandates that, at the time of admission to an acute-care or long-term care facility, all patients must be asked if they have executed an advance health care directive. If they have not, they must be given information defining AHCDs and should be told at the time of admission that they have the right to (1) state such directives and (2) accept or refuse any medical treatment.

There is a significant drawback to waiting for an illness or a hospital admission to draw up an AHCD. Many times, patients are admitted to a hospital with an acute illness or in a crisis. These types of situations typically involve a great deal of physical and emotional stress, and medications may dull the senses and prevent rational, clear thinking. Ultimately, advanced health care directives written and signed by the patient before he or she becomes critically ill will help lessen the burden of decisions that must be made by the family members in a time of crisis.

Durable Power of Attorney for Health Care

The durable power of attorney for health care is a type of advance directive that transfers the health-care decision-making power to a person designated by the patient. It is used when the patient cannot communicate, and it must be set up and signed before the person becomes incapacitated.

Living Will

A living will is usually drawn up before a patient is terminally ill or incapacitated. It describes the wishes of the person concerning end-of-life care. State laws vary concerning the recognition of living wills, but such documents are more valid as expressions of a person's wishes than casual statements made during family discussions, and the living will is usually respected and upheld by the courts.

Do Not Resuscitate Order

A do not resuscitate (DNR) order can be written only by a physician on the basis of the patient's living will or durable power of attorney for health care. DNR means that if a patient stops breathing or the heartbeat is incompatible with life (e.g., asystole or "flat line"), aggressive methods of resuscitation such as CPR will not be attempted.

Assisted Suicide and Euthanasia

Suicide is the taking of one's own life. Assisted suicide is the action of a person other than the patient to facilitate suicide. The word euthanasia comes from the Greek *eu* ("good") and *thanatos* ("death"). It is an intentional act (such as the lethal injection of a drug), which causes death. Both assisted suicide and euthanasia involve legal, moral, and ethical issues that have been tested in the courts through the years and remain controversial. The legality of assisted suicide in the United States varies by state. Oregon legalized assisted suicide in 1997, Washington state legalized assisted suicide in 2008, and Montana legalized assisted suicide in 2009 (Associated Press, 2011). The Netherlands, Belgium, and Luxembourg also permit euthanasia assisted by a physician.

Health-care professionals are often asked by the patient or family to participate in hastening the end of life. The core of the debate against assisted suicide and euthanasia is the premise that providing effective palliative, pain-free end-of-life care will eliminate the need for people to request such an action.

ROLE OF THE HEALTH-CARE WORKER IN END-OF-LIFE CARE

The health-care worker must understand the process of dying, offer support and empathy to the patient and family, and assist the family to recognize and manage options and supportive resources. Standards of professional practice in nursing have been developed jointly by the Hospice and Palliative Nurses Association, the American Nurses Association, and the National Hospice and Palliative Care Organization. The role of the nurse and health-care worker in end-of-life care is to perform the following:

- Ensure education of the patient and family concerning the diagnosis
- Ensure that informed consent is provided with a clear offer of all available options of care
- Ensure that the patient's and family's cultural and personal wishes are respected
- Communicate with the multidisciplinary health-care team when death is imminent or has occurred

DEATH OF A CHILD

An understanding of death is often first taught to children as they learn about the life cycle of plants and animals in school. Students in sociology classes discuss cultural and religious customs of funerals and burials. The media review the life and death of celebrities. High school students may receive an assignment to write an opinion paper concerning the right to die or the final destiny of death.

Health-care workers often help parents guide children in developing a positive attitude toward and a fuller understanding of death. Discussion of experiences with loss in everyday life using a plant, pet, or movie character creates opportunities to discuss death in a non-threatening manner. Many children's books are available to introduce the concept of death at age-appropriate levels.

Discussion of life and death should be a normal part of the growth and development experience to prepare a child to understand and handle death whenever it occurs. The concept of death is often influenced by exposure and discussion at home, in school, or at church, although the understanding of death is closely related to Piaget's stages of cognitive development (see Chapter 5). A child's first experience with death usually occurs when a pet dies. Telling a child that a pet is being put to sleep does not add to the understanding of death and in fact may cause the child to be afraid to go to sleep. Often the child's first experience with the death of a person occurs when a grandparent dies. The occurrence of death should not be hidden but should be openly discussed to enable effective coping strategies to be developed.

Children who have a terminal illness typically progress through specific stages as they prepare for death, and they are often more aware of their condition than their parents realize. Children as young as age 2 respond to their parents' emotions and nonverbal behavior. Therefore truthfulness, explained in age-appropriate terms in a supportive, nonthreatening manner, is the optimal approach in the care of a terminally ill child. Efforts at covering up or hiding the terminal nature of the condition merely obstruct vital communication between the parent and child, and communication could be more useful than false cheer.

The initial stage of awareness (Bluebond-Langner, 1996) involves the child adapting to an identity or niche in the family as being the sick child. Special privileges or attention may be given to the child, and siblings often do not understand the favored status. The dying child soon learns that there is a relationship among medications, treatments, and recovery and adapts to the need for daily medication. Eventually, as the condition deteriorates, the child begins to realize he or she is different from peers. As the illness progresses, the child sees the illness as a lifelong challenge and feels he or she will always be sick. In the final stage, the child develops an awareness of the terminal nature of the illness, often asks direct questions about death, and may express inner fears and fantasies. The focus of care may initially be on educating the child and family about the disease. Later, specific fears expressed by the child or family are an appropriate focus of care. Siblings should be included in the plan of care, so they do not feel abandoned or punished or do not develop an overwhelming sense of sibling rivalry and, later, guilt feelings.

The role of the health-care worker is to provide support for the patient, parents, siblings, family, and school contacts. The death of a child is not normally a part of the natural life cycle, and so the emotional impact on the family is often devastating. The dying child should be provided with age-appropriate routines and activities for as long as possible. Contact with all family members should be encouraged. Questions should be answered truthfully, and the health-care worker should try to empower the child as much as possible. The adolescent is most aware of the loss of expected life experiences when facing death. Outbursts of anger are common and should be accepted and understood. Caregivers also need a support system of peers to cope with the death of a child. Parents will need help with coping strategies and assistance with the care of other children and family members during the grief process. Community resources should be used to help the family through the difficult times.

Developmental Concepts of Death and Dying

Death and dying are understood in different ways by children of different ages and developmental stages (Table 15-4). It is important to recognize the ability of the child to understand what is happening and to help the family communicate with the dying child or the child who has lost a family member. In infants and young children, a separation anxiety disorder may occur that is evidenced by the stages of *protest* (crying), *despair* (sadness), and eventual *disengagement* with the deceased person.

Toddler

The toddler views separation as temporary, because he or she is just learning to separate from the parent and to understand object permanence. The toddler's behavior may reflect a response to changes in caregivers and routines.

Preschooler

The thinking of a preschooler is not logical in the way that an adult's is. The preschool-age child thinks of death as reversible. The preschooler employs magical thinking and may believe his or her own negative thoughts caused the ill sibling to go away. He or she may also fear abandonment.

School-Age Child

Concrete thinking enables the school-age child to realize death is permanent and the deceased sibling will be absent from family activities. The school-age child should attend the funeral or memorial service. The school-age child does not yet understand his or her own mortality.

TABLE 15-4 Developmental Concepts of Death and Dying*

Age	Concept	Response	Interventions
Infants	Not applicable.	React to separation and alteration of routine or stress behavior of caregiver.	Maintain a familiar daily routine if possible.
Toddlers	Perceive anxiety of those around them. Do not understand permanence of death or that they can die.	Take on the anxiety and emotions of those around them.	Maintain a familiar routine. Explain in simple terms what is happening.
Preschool-age children	Understand that death is feared by adults. View death as reversible and may see it as being similar to sleep. *Magical thinking* may distort reality of death.	Often ask why and how questions about death. May feel their thoughts or actions caused the death or caused their own illness as a punishment. May cling or withdraw.	Avoid explaining death as a type of sleep. Accept temporary regression. Reassure that they are not the cause of the death. Help facilitate the grieving process through play.
School-age children	Begin to understand death as permanent and inevitable but often feel it occurs in others or in the remote future. May believe in continuation of life in another form.	Curious about details of death. May fear separation from family or friends. May romanticize death according to TV experiences.	Emotional restraint of caregiver makes it more difficult for child to express emotions. Encourage active participation in grieving process. Encourage the asking of questions and the expression of feelings. Answer questions truthfully.
Adolescents	Understand death is permanent and inevitable. May begin to question the meaning of life.	Can relate death to cultural or religious beliefs or practices. Most feel immortal and may become defiant and rebellious when facing their own deaths. Faith can help adolescents cope.	Extra effort is needed to help parent maintain communication with adolescent. Listen to adolescents' thoughts and fears and answer questions truthfully. Include adolescents in family discussions and decisions.

*The ability of the child to understand the nature and consequences of death varies according to culture, experiences, cognitive development, and family stability. The child's external behavior often does not reflect the internal intensity of his or her feelings.

Adolescent

Adolescents can think abstractly. The adolescent mourns and understands the effect of death on others in the family and community. A dying teen usually resents his or her dependence on others. Comfort and pain relief are very important, and the adolescent should be involved in decision making. Adolescents may have difficulty coping with their own death and will often deny their own mortality by engaging in risky activities.

It is important to understand that quality of life for a child means participating in age-appropriate activities as normal, healthy children do. Visits from friends and attending school even part time, help the child and the family to cope with what is happening.

PHYSICAL CARE AFTER DEATH

The physical care of the patient is performed according to the culture of the patient and the protocols of the institution. The health-care worker should communicate with the family concerning policies and routines related to care and transport of the body, because cultural or religious practices may require flexibility in the procedure. The time of death may be the last opportunity for some family members to see or touch their loved one, so they may appreciate some private time with the deceased to help with closure. Often when a child dies the parents may wish to hold the child snugly wrapped in a blanket for a time.

Family members may need assistance in notifying extended family and friends; therefore helping to facilitate phone calls is valuable. Talking about the death is part of the healing process. Providing referral for the funeral arrangements and for the planning of the memorial service may also be helpful to the family. The use of community resources for bereavement support groups helps survivors realize that they are not alone. See Chapter 16 concerning the bereavement process.

KEY POINTS

- The grieving process of a patient facing death includes the stages of denial, anger, bargaining, depression, and acceptance.
- Hospice care is based on the philosophy that death is a normal part of the life cycle. The physical, psychological, spiritual, and social needs of the dying person are addressed in hospice care.
- Palliative care is the total care of patients without the use of aggressive curative efforts. Comfort is the core of this type of care.
- Some ethical and legal issues involved in end-of-life care include understanding of advanced directives, living wills, and DNR orders.
- Assisted suicide or euthanasia is the action of a person other than the patient to facilitate suicide. It is not legal in most states and remains a controversial legal, moral and ethical issue.
- Cultural practices of the family should be respected during end-of-life care.
- Family and friends should continue to talk to the dying person, because hearing is the last sense to be lost.
- An understanding of death is taught to children as they study the life cycle of plants and animals in school. Students and teachers in sociology classes discuss customs and cultures. The death of a family pet may be a common experience that children share concerning death.

- Death and dying are understood in different ways by children of different ages and developmental stages. Communication with children at their level of understanding is important.
- Quality of life for ill children involves inclusion in age-appropriate routines and activities for as long as possible.
- Some signs of impending death include weakness, immobility, altered breathing patterns, cold and mottled extremities, and decreased awareness of surroundings.
- The role of the health-care worker in end-of-life care is to educate the family and patient concerning options and resources, to provide support, and to maintain communication with the health-care team. The health-care worker can provide the family with strategies and resources to cope with end-of-life care.

Critical Thinking

An 84-year-old man states that he is afraid he may be dying. He further states that he does not want to be alone or to experience the pain of a slow death, and he asks the nurse to help him to die now with dignity. What ethical issues, legal issues, and alternative options should be discussed with this person?

REVIEW QUESTIONS

1. The biggest barrier to accessing hospice care is the:
   a. cost of care provided.
   b. required referral by health-care provider.
   c. loss of hope for a cure.
   d. lack of insurance coverage.

2. Hospice care involves:
   a. palliative measures.
   b. curative therapy.
   c. custodial measures.
   d. alternative therapies.

3. Advance directives are used to:
   a. determine end-of-life care measures.
   b. determine who will inherit property.
   c. provide consent for surgery.
   d. determine visitors allowed for the patient.

4. A durable power of attorney for health care is best set up:
   a. when illness strikes.
   b. before illness strikes.
   c. when death is imminent.
   d. after death occurs.

5. The preschool-age child views death as:
   a. a permanent loss.
   b. a temporary separation.
   c. abandonment of care.
   d. relief from pain.

CHAPTER

16 Loss, Grief, and Bereavement

http://evolve.elsevier.com/Leifer/growth

OBJECTIVES

1. List the normal losses that occur during the stages of the life cycle.
2. State how the response to normal losses influences responses to loss of life.
3. Explain the difference between grief, mourning, and bereavement.
4. List the stages and tasks of the grieving process.
5. Describe an emotional, cognitive, and behavioral response to grief.
6. State two religious and two cultural practices related to death.
7. List two components of an abnormal grief response.
8. State the response to loss and grief at different development stages within the lifespan.
9. Discuss the achievement of the letting-go phase of the grief process.
10. State four ways condolences can be expressed.

KEY TERMS

anticipatory grief
bereavement
condolence
culture
eulogy
funeral
grief
legacy
mourning

THE CONCEPT OF LOSS

Loss is a natural part of life, but it is often painful and requires difficult adjustments. The experience of loss occurs at almost every stage of life, not just at life's end.

NORMAL LOSSES DURING THE LIFE CYCLE

Perhaps the first experience of loss is the newborn's loss of the security of the womb. When the newborn later develops an attachment to the mother, the goal of the newborn is to prevent the loss of the mother, who is needed for survival. The very act of attachment of the infant to his or her mother or the husband to his wife makes the person vulnerable to the experience of loss.

The toddler endures the loss of being the exclusive focus of his or her parents when a sibling arrives who can be viewed as a rival in sharing the love of the parents. Puberty involves the loss of the perceived body image of adulthood. The boy who does not attain a height of 6 feet or the girl who never develops a 36C breast size both deal with the loss of what they thought was to be.

When the teen leaves home for college, the teen loses the securities of home and family, and the parents lose control over their child. We lose our dreams of what might be when we settle for more realistic life goals. As we age we lose our youth, our beauty, our energy, our sight, and our health, and we must learn to cope with all these losses.

The normal losses of each stage of the life cycle involve some form of letting go and adapting. How a person responds to the various losses during life contributes to the development of that person's personality and how bereavement is managed when loss of life occurs.

ABNORMAL OR ATYPICAL LOSSES

Families across the nation suffered a loss of national security when Pearl Harbor was bombed on December 7, 1941. Confidence in the safety and security of our country was again lost when the World Trade Center towers and the Pentagon were attacked on September 11, 2001. Families in the United States had felt protected by the moat-like surroundings of the oceans that seemed impenetrable, and the loss of that feeling of security affected everyone in the country.

RESPONSES TO LOSS

To adapt to the various normal losses in life, the individual must learn how to cope with disappointments, and this learning usually results in maturity and personal growth. The response to normal losses during each phase of the life cycle determines how losses in old age are perceived and managed. The attitude toward loss often determines the quality of life that is maintained. Those who deny aging may turn to techniques such as plastic surgery to restore youthful looks. Others seemingly dance through old age gracefully. When past losses are not resolved, the losses involved in later life stages may reactivate old, unresolved sorrows. Passing successfully through Erikson's stages of the life cycle determines whether the older person will enjoy life to its end with new strengths and goals or just spend time waiting to be claimed by death.

TASKS ASSOCIATED WITH DEATH

Death is the ultimate loss—the loss of life. It is important to establish communication with those who are dying, but many people avoid discussions of death. The experience of death is a stage in life with its own tasks. Some people wish not to be conscious of death as it occurs. They opt for sedation and yearn for death during sleep. The hospice movement has enabled the terminally ill to experience the task of dying with dignity (see Chapter 15). Being satisfied with the legacy or the family one has left to the world may give the person a feeling of immortality. The legacy can be a grandchild, property, a culture, an organization, or writings. Establishing a spiritual connection and belief that there is an afterlife, a final reunion of all, also can be a meaningful task to pursue during the death process.

Grief

Understanding the dynamics of loss, dying, and grief is essential to help the patient and family go through the process of bereavement. Verbal and nonverbal communication, therapeutic presence, and collaboration with the multidisciplinary health-care team are the core responsibilities of the health-care professional.

Grief Process

Grief is the emotional response to a loss and is a process through which a survivor accepts the loss. The grief process involves a series of stages, but travel through these stages is not always orderly. Grief can occur before the actual loss, when a terminal illness is diagnosed, or it may be initiated upon the actual death of the loved one. Grief that occurs before the loss is known as anticipatory grief (Lindeman, 1944). Mourning is the outward expression of grief. Mourning is often based on cultural practices and traditions. For example, in Jewish tradition, mirrors in the home are covered, and the immediate family sits on hard surfaces for a prescribed period after a loved one dies. Bereavement involves grief and mourning. It involves the time survivors first react to the reality of the loss, the adjustment to the loss, and the entering of a period where they can move on and continue with the fabric of life (Figure 16–1).

Culture, Religion, and Death

How individuals grieve is often directed by cultural and religious traditions and practices. Culture is a pattern of behavior, language, and practices that are transmitted through the generations (see Chapter 3). Within each culture, these practices may vary. Table 16-1 reviews the death rituals and practices of selected cultures, and Table 16-2 reviews common religious practices related to death. Understanding common religious and cultural practices enables health-care workers to individualize their approach to the grieving survivor and family following the death of a loved one.

Normal Grief Responses

Normal grief reactions often involve *physical symptoms* (e.g., lack of energy, weight gain, weight loss, or insomnia), *emotional symptoms* (e.g., anger, anxiety, relief, or despair), *cognitive reactions* (e.g., disbelief, confusion, or inability to concentrate), and *behavioral symptoms* (e.g., crying, impaired functioning, withdrawal, or changing of relationships).

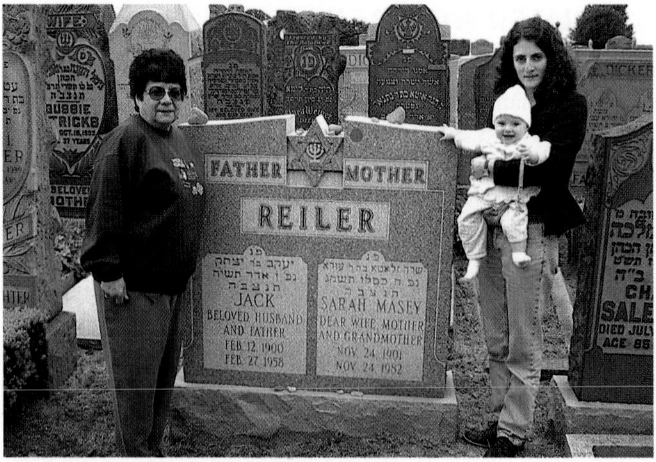

Figure 16–1 Most cultures include a ritual of memorializing family members who have died. Periodic visits to the cemetery to reflect, to offer respect, and to say prayers are healthy adaptations during the grieving process.

TABLE 16-1 Common Death Rituals of Selected Cultures

Culture	Preparation	Special Needs	Care of the Body	Organ Donations and Autopsy
Native American	Displays obvious signs of grief, such as crying, singing, or hugging of the deceased.		An open window with special position of the body may be preferred to allow for the spirit to leave the body.	Generally not desired.
Arab American	Family should be allowed to grieve together in privacy.	Grief tends to be open, loud, and unrestrained. After death has occurred, an Imam will read passages from the Koran over the body.	Special bathing of the body is required after death, and the body is turned toward Mecca.	Believe presenting the intact body to Allah preserves integrity.
Cambodian (Khmer)	Immediate family is responsible for notifying clergy and extended family.	Incense is used. Family grieves quietly and wears white while mourning.	Family members or monk cleanse the body. On night of death, prayers by monk are important.	Prefer body to be intact, even though it will be cremated. Believe in rebirth or reincarnation.
East Indian	Believe it is only the body that dies; the soul lives on. Hindus and Sikhs believe in the concept of reincarnation. Dying person is typically not told of impending death.	Family must be allowed to remain at bedside until death has occurred. Hindus will mourn for 40 days.	Body is washed and prepared by immediate family members, placed in new clothing, and prepared for the cremation ceremony. Ashes are typically saved until they can be taken and placed in the Ganges River in India.	Not allowed.

(Continued)

TABLE 16-1 Common Death Rituals of Selected Cultures—cont'd

Culture	Preparation	Special Needs	Care of the Body	Organ Donations and Autopsy
Filipino	Will want a chaplain or priest at bedside to receive the Sacrament of the Sick or Last Rites.	Family prays at bedside. Patient usually has religious medallion of some kind on body or in hand. Family tends to be somewhat vocal at time of death. Allow for privacy as much as possible.	Family will take part in washing/cleansing the body before it is taken away. Death is handled with dignity because it is a highly spiritual event in this culture.	Cremation not the norm. May allow organ donation in some cases.
Hispanic	Will have multiple family members at bedside. Prefer priest to provide Last Rites and pray over patient/body, usually with family present.	Pregnant women may not be present at bedside or at funeral.	No special treatment or ritualistic cleansing or preparation of the body is done.	Typically not permitted.
West Indian	Prefer to see the body immediately after death has occurred. Surviving spouse is to be notified of death while children are present.	As death approaches, family and friends want to be at bedside to witness the death and pray for the loved one's passing.	Prefer hospital personnel to prepare the body for transfer to the morgue.	Preserving the integrity of the body is very important; therefore organ donation unlikely.

Data from Smith SF, Duell DJ, Martin BC: *Clinical nursing skills: basic to advanced skills,* New York, 2000, Prentice-Hall; Leifer G: *Introduction to maternity & pediatric nursing*, ed 6, Philadelphia, 2011, Saunders; Lipson JG, Dibble SL, Minarik PA: *Culture & nursing care: a pocket guide,* San Francisco, 1996, UCSF Nursing Press.

TABLE 16-2 Common Religious Practices Related to Death

Religion	Common Practices
Adventist, Christian Scientist, Eastern orthodox, Jehovah's Witness, Methodist, Roman Catholic and others	Catholics include annointing by a priest. Funerals held within 2 to 3 days. Some religious practices include a memorial service held at 40-day anniversary. Adventist, Christian Scientist, Jehovah's Witness, and Methodist religions do not require Last Rites. Roman Catholic and Eastern Orthodox religions require Last Rites. Jehovah's witness discourage autopsy and organ donation. Greek Orthodox may place a religious icon on the body. Some religious practices include moving the body feet first. Specific religious leaders and family should be consulted for preferred practices and rites.
Muslim	Male cousins or uncles take leadership roles. The head is elevated above the body and faces Mecca. Rarely express fear of death because of belief in Allah. Ritual hitting of the body may be common.
Jewish	The body is ritually washed after death and must not be moved on a Saturday. The body should not be left alone. Casket is made of wood with no metal parts. Funeral is held within 24-hours. Family sits Shiva for 7 days with mirrors covered. Mourning continues for 30 days, with wearing of a cut black ribbon on the lapel.
Hindu	May tie a thread around the wrist of the dying or place a basil leaf on the tongue. These should not be removed after death.
Mormon	Baptism can be done by proxy if not done in early life.

Schulz (1978) and Bowlby (1980) outlined three stages of grief that involve (1) initial shock and disbelief; (2) numbness and overwhelming sadness, with yearning and protest; and (3) reflection in search of meaning and possibly eventual acceptance. Elisabeth Kübler-Ross (1969) suggested three stages or tasks of the grieving process. See Table 16-3 for a description of the tasks of the grieving process and suggested interventions.

The health-care worker should maintain a pleasant and nonjudgmental attitude while providing therapeutic presence and should help survivors identify and mobilize a strong support system. Referral to support groups or bereavement counselors for needed guidance is important. Hospice agencies can assist with accessing these resources.

Dysfunctional Grieving

Dysfunctional grieving is the failure to follow a predictable course of a normal grieving process to a resolution, resulting in the person resorting to abnormal or maladaptive coping strategies. Dysfunctional grieving is described as the expression of unresolved issues and

TABLE 16-3 Tasks of the Grief Process

Stage	Task	Interventions
Notification of death	Share event with extended family and friends	Assist with initial coping or refer to community resources as needed Assess support system
Recognition of reality of death	Share the response by expressing grief	Understand anger may be directed toward health-care professional Survivors may need help with feelings of guilt
Adjustment or reintegration	Reorganize family structure and life goals	Survivor may need help setting up memory book and also planning for future and reintegrating into society

Adapted from Kübler-Ross E: On death and dying, New York, 1969, Macmillan.

BOX 16-1 Signs and Symptoms of Dysfunctional Grief

- Guilt about things other than actions taken or not taken by the survivor at the time of death
- Thoughts of death or suicide
- Morbid preoccupation with worthlessness
- Marked decrease in ability to concentrate
- Prolonged or marked inability to function
- Excessive and uncontrolled crying
- Inability to accept the reality of the death

Data from Miller-Keane, Marie O'Toole (2005) *Encyclopedia and Dictionary of Medicine, Nursing and Allied Health* 7th ed. WB Saunders Phila. And Wolraich M, Dworkin P, Protar D, Perrin E (2008) *Developmental-Behavioral Pediatrics: Evidence and Practice.* Elsevier.

symptoms that result in interference with life's functioning (Miller-Keane & O'Toole, 2005). In some instances the signs and symptoms appear similar to a major depressive episode. These signs and symptoms include insomnia, emotional lability, changes in appetite, and withdrawal from friends or social support systems (Box 16-1).

It is important to note that some of the signs and symptoms may be normal for the first few months after the death of a loved one. Typically, bereaved individuals slowly begin to resume normal activities of daily living (ADLs), maintain contact with family and friends, and accept other forms of support. It is not normal, however, to continue to remain isolated or removed from the real world for prolonged periods. Some form of intervention, whether medical, psychological, or both, may be necessary if the bereavement process is prolonged. Suicidal ideas may occur when the survivor begins to feel that life is not worth living without the deceased person. Professional intervention may be necessary. The death of a loved one by suicide also affects the grief process of the survivors. Box 16-2 describes the typical grief response following a death by suicide.

BOX 16-2 Special Aspects of Grief Following a Suicide

- Event involves social stigma
- Blaming often occurs
- Police investigation increases guilt
- Survivors feel death could have been prevented
- Survivors may feel decreased self-esteem
- Survivors feel rejected and deserted
- Family may worry about inherited predisposition

Role of the Health-Care Worker

The responsibility of the health-care worker does not end at the death of the patient. Preparing the family for the grief process and referring the family to community resources for counseling and other assistance are important. The focus of care is on the patient and the family unit, as described in Chapter 4. Cultural competence is the key to successful communication and support (see Chapter 3). Some general advice that can be provided to the grieving survivors (Becvar, 2001) is to:

- Accept advice with caution
- Accept emotions
- Forgive others
- Express emotions
- Cry and release pressure
- Avoid alcohol and drugs
- Rest, do chores, and seek the support of others

See Table 16-4 (and Chapter 15) for some suggestions of what to say and not to say.

TABLE 16-4 Communicating with the Bereaved*

What to Say (Therapeutic Comments)	What Not to Say (Nontherapeutic Comments)
"I am sorry for your loss."	"I know how you feel."
"It is okay to be angry with God and everyone else."	"You must not blame God. You should not feel like that."
"Grieving takes time. Take your time. Don't feel pushed to do anything."	"You will be okay in a week or so."
"It is not easy for you. Tell me about the person you lost."	"He lived a long and full life."
"Would you like to talk? I will listen."	"Tell me what happened."
"You did the best you could. It is okay to cry."	"Do not feel guilty. Do not cry."

*The most important thing to do is to listen.

Tasks of the Family

Preparing for a funeral is often the first task facing the family of the deceased. A funeral is an activity shortly after death involving a meaningful ceremony to remember the life of the deceased. It may or may not involve religious rituals. For the deceased, it serves the purpose of respectful recognition and disposition of the remains. For the family, it serves the purpose of confirming the reality and finality of the death; provides a climate to express grief; provides an opportunity for the community to pay respects; and recognizes, remembers, and honors the life of the one who has passed into death.

The funeral can take place in the home or in a commercial funeral-home facility. In some cultures, the family prepares a eulogy, a speech usually presented at the funeral ceremony intended to memorialize the deceased by including a condensed life history, details of interests and achievements at home and at work, family memories, and a summary of what the deceased enjoyed in life. It can contain humorous moments to remember as well as serious comments that honor the life of the deceased.

Family tasks related to loss of a family member may also include the reorganization of roles. Decisions need to be made regarding who will do the laundry, cook, care for the young or disabled, or earn money to pay the bills. Often children are required to fill adult roles. Parents who suffer a loss of a loved one may not be able to respond to the needs of young children. The resources of the family need to be assessed and used appropriately. In the weeks, months, and years after the death, however, overt support wanes, especially if family members live many miles apart. Professional help may be needed if financial issues spark animosity among survivors. Survivors who have had the opportunity to anticipate the death of a loved one may be better prepared for the changes and challenges they will face. However, the actual event usually sets in motion the typical stages of the grief process.

GRIEF EARLY IN THE LIFE CYCLE

Pregnant Women

Because pregnant women experience movement of the fetus by the second trimester of pregnancy, a close relationship or attachment between the mother and fetus begins to evolve. Typically the mother and father join together in planning their future and the future of their unborn infant. When a stillbirth occurs, both parents respond, but often the mother suffers a more intense grief reaction, which may spark interpersonal problems. The health-care team must take the time to provide much needed support during this difficult time. Acknowledging the existence of the baby as a separate person is important and may include taking careful pictures or footprints or cutting and preserving a curl of hair as a memento. A "memory kit" may be assembled to include items of importance to the parents (Figure 16-2).

Some parents wish to hold their infants to say good-bye. Parents should be taught about the grieving process, so each will understand what behaviors to expect. Options for funeral arrangements should be offered, and parents should be referred to support groups that may be beneficial in the weeks and months following their loss. Providing empathetic listening, therapeutic touch, and nonverbal support to the parents is most helpful. Attention to siblings and extended family is also important, because other family members may not verbalize their feelings as readily as the parents.

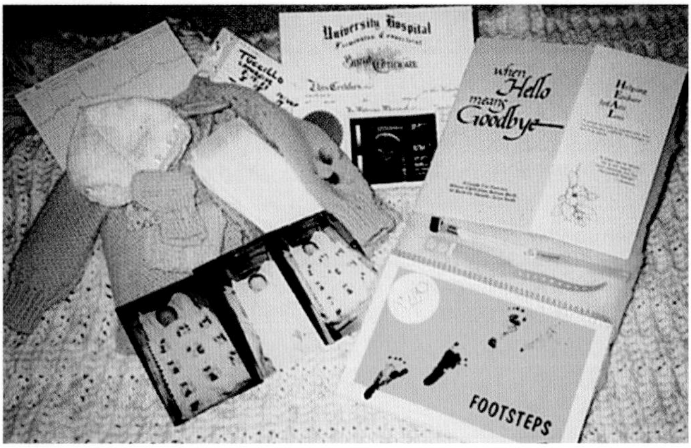

Figure 16–2 After pregnancy loss, the parents may take home a "memory kit." The kit can include pictures of the infant, the death certificate, footprints, identification bands, an ultrasound picture, or the first set of clothing, among other individual items that are important to the parents.

Clear information should be provided about the cause of death and any implications for future pregnancies. Women who become pregnant after experiencing a loss in a previous pregnancy need to be taught the positive milestones of the subsequent pregnancy to promote a positive attitude and to anticipate a positive outcome.

If the mother experiencing a pregnancy loss is an adolescent, the responses may be complicated by the thinking process of that level of development and the attitudes of the adults around her. Often the unmarried adolescent who experiences a miscarriage is not given permission to grieve, because some may feel the pregnancy was unwanted and would have complicated the adolescent's life. Therefore adolescents have a greater risk for developing depression, anger, or feelings of guilt that will affect their own growth and development process. Health-care workers need to offer to the adolescent information about the grief process, referral for counseling, and general empathy and support.

Infants

By the age of 10 months, when they have established an attachment, infants are capable of responding to loss. This response to loss may resurface in adulthood and may manifest as an inability to form attachments or as a more intense response to normal loss experiences. See Table 15-4 for the developmental concepts of death and dying and suggested interventions for infants and children.

Children

Young children may react to death in a manner reflecting their developmental stage. By age 6, children realize death is not reversible. Children may show anger at the person who left them, guilt because they blame themselves for the loved one's leaving, and fear that they will not be cared for and loved. Their immaturity prevents them from coping with these feelings and often prevents them from expressing these feelings. Young children need the support and guidance of understanding adults to help them through this stressful experience (Box 16-3).

BOX 16-3 Children Coping with Loss

Do not overload children with too much information because they are concrete thinkers.
Answers should be given in a simple and honest manner.
Play activities are a way children express grief.
Take the time to listen to children verbalize fears for the future and fears about their own mortality.
Allow children to remember, reminisce, and talk about the deceased.

Adapted from Mental Health America (2012): *Helping children cope with loss* (website): www.nmha.org/index.cfm?objectid=C7DF9628-1372-4D20-C884BF860DEF0A67. Accessed March 6, 2012.

Adolescents

Adolescents who lose a parent are usually at the point of moving into the adult role and may mourn the adult-to-adult relationship they had anticipated. The adolescent is establishing a sense of identity and may mourn the loss of sharing accomplishments with the parent who died. Adolescents may feel the need to take on the role of the deceased parent to help the surviving parent and family members, or they may slip back into a complete dependency role.

Young Adults

Young adults who are in a newly established marriage or family and are separated by death from the spouse may respond with rage at lost opportunities. Communicating with a grieving survivor is the responsibility of health care workers, because contact is often continued in the community setting. Helping the survivor through the grief process toward reintegration and adjustment is both challenging and rewarding.

THE HEALING PROCESS

Reintegration and Adjustment

Many people remain in emotional pain years after the loss of a loved one. Grief is considered to be a private emotion, and others may be glad not to intrude because they really do not know what to say or do. Some people say, "Don't feel bad," or "Don't cry." This type of response implies that the person who is grieving should not show the grief.

When a child loses a pet dog, parents may avoid having the child cope with grief by saying, "Don't worry—we will get you another dog." This implies that the loss can be replaced. Not showing the grief that is felt and trying to replace what is lost are not appropriate responses to grief, because they do not allow recovery to occur. There is no process or task to be mastered. The loss is covered up by burying and replacing it, leaving the child to grieve all alone.

Encouraging the cover-up of grief forces the person to act as if he or she has successfully managed the loss so that the person can be comfortably accepted back into his or her social group. These unresolved feelings may be buried, but their effects can last a lifetime. However, burying or hiding the grief may appear to be the better choice for the grieving person rather than being isolated from social contacts who may feel uncomfortable when he or she shows grief. Social isolation adds to emotional pain, and sleeplessness, confusion, and changes in behavior can result. Unresolved issues in the grieving process can lead to physical and mental illness. The health-care worker should try to help the grieving survivor master tasks that lead toward the healthy healing of grief.

Mastering Tasks Leading Toward Grief Healing

The health-care worker can help survivors in the task of grief healing by offering the following suggestions:

1. Find others who have experienced grief with whom feelings can be openly expressed—This can be a close friend, fellow survivor, or grief recovery group. Meet with these people on a regular basis.
2. Recognize that change has occurred and what has changed—Recognize that things cannot be the same as they were before the loss.
3. Accept change—Because nothing will be the same after a great loss, one must accept that change will occur. Change is beyond the person's control, so acceptance of change makes the task easier.
4. Make changes slowly—Most psychologists advise that drastic changes should not be made in the first year following the loss. Disposing of possessions or selling the house, for example, are decisions that need to be carefully thought out to avoid regrets.
5. Become aware of what was and recognize the good, the bad, the intense, and all other aspects of the relationship that were lost—This prevents placing the lost one on a pedestal and creating a shrine of honor to that person, which may really be a distortion of the reality. Selecting the memories that will become permanent is important. Recognize that you did the best you could in the relationship and what could have or should have been done was just not possible at that time.
6. Avoid thinking of what could have been, what should have been, and what might have been, and do not dwell on "if only" thoughts—Avoid blame—especially blaming God, which may adversely affect the spiritual side of life.
7. Let go of the past—This does not mean forgetting, it just means to let go and release the painful memories. Letting go and saying good-bye to a loved one need not mean saying good-bye to the loving memories. Letting go is saying good-bye to the pain, to the feeling of isolation, and to the physical nearness of the loved one. This type of letting go will enable one to move on. The health-care worker can assess the successful achievement of the letting-go stage, which is manifested by the ability of the survivor to express positive and negative memories of the deceased without feeling deep anguish.
8. Financial decisions will need inventory and review—New goals will have to be established and new strategies designed. Updating the last will and testament and other legal documents should reflect the changes incurred by the loss of a loved one.

HELPING GRIEVING SURVIVORS

Condolence

The word condolence means to express sympathy or to grieve together. To offer condolence to a survivor, one must elect to approach the grieving person. As one offers comfort and understanding to the survivor, profound perceptions about life and loss are sparked.

Disturbing questions arise, such as "What would I do if I was in this situation?" Often the person offering condolence does not know what to say and is concerned about saying the wrong thing. A feeling of helplessness follows, and the challenge of offering condolence may become overwhelming.

The health-care worker may offer condolences to the family after the death of a patient by sending a letter to the survivor or family. Friends of the deceased patient often look to the health-care worker for advice on how to offer condolences to the grieving survivors.

The grief experience is life changing. The goal is to move successfully into a new life that includes many changes and is not clouded by the unknown. The health-care worker is often called on to help support the bereaved. Supporting the bereaved means helping them preserve their dignity and understand the process they must journey through. The outcome of condolence is not meant to cure grieving persons of their feelings of loss. It is not meant to cheer them up. However, condolence may ease the emotional pain and help facilitate a healthy passage through the grieving process. A person providing condolence may receive the reward of strengthening his or her own coping strategies. Some ways to offer condolence include:

1. Writing a letter—A personal letter of condolence is more meaningful to a grieving survivor than a preprinted card from a store. Comments concerning the deceased person will be treasured, and sincere words of condolence will be a tribute to the deceased and will bring comfort to the grieving survivor. A favorite memory and a sincere offer to help when needed would be appropriate. The letter should not diminish the intensity of the grieving person's feelings with phrases such as, "I know exactly how you feel." It should not offer advice to bury the feelings by saying, "Don't cry." It should offer compassion and support, reminiscence of a memory, and assistance.
2. Visiting the survivor—A spoken word of comfort, a supporting hand on the shoulder, and face-to-face encounters are very meaningful to the grieving person. Touch breaks through the numbness stage of grief and may bring the grieving person out of isolation.
3. Helping with phone calls and arrangements for the funeral and receptions—Try to help with hotel accommodations for family members who must travel to attend the funeral.
4. Selecting a gift or service to provide—Cook a meal, babysit for younger children, or perform any other activity that will relieve the responsibilities of the grieving survivor.
5. Helping the adjustment of the household—Offer to assist with disposition of clothes or help to list the legal responsibilities and to set a list of priorities.
6. Including the survivor in occasional positive activities, especially during holiday times.
7. Remembering the anniversary of the death, offering support, and reinforcing coping strategies during any remembrance services.
8. Offering resources for coping—A book, website, or a community support group may help the grieving survivor to move through the grieving process.

The health-care worker has an important role in helping grieving survivors through the bereavement process. The end of a life is part of the life cycle, and coping with loss can be a developmental task in any stage.

KEY POINTS

- Loss is a part of life. Normal loss occurs in every stage of life, and coping strategies are developed in response to these losses.
- Understanding common religious and cultural rituals related to death (cultural competence) enables the health-care worker to meet the individual needs of the grieving survivor and family.
- Grief is the emotional response to loss.
- Anticipatory grief occurs before the death of a loved one, when death appears imminent. Some preparation for the grief process may occur, but the stages of the grief process remain the same.
- Mourning is the outward experience of grief.
- Bereavement involves grief and mourning.
- Stages of grieving generally involve shock, disbelief, and numbness; overwhelming sadness with yearning and protest; and reflection and search for meaning.
- The tasks of the grieving process include sharing the event, recognition of the reality of the loss, sharing the expression of grief, and reorganizing and reintegrating life goals.
- Alterations of the grieving process may occur in the case of sudden deaths, in unanticipated deaths, and in deaths involving children.
- When past losses are not resolved, handling the losses involved in retirement, aging, and the death of a spouse may be dysfunctional.
- Hiding the expression of grief or attempting to replace what is lost does not allow for healthy adaptation and recovery.
- Expressing grief, accepting changes, and establishing positive and negative memories help a person progress through the grieving process.
- The ability to express positive and negative memories of the deceased without suffering severe anguish may indicate that the survivor has successfully achieved the letting-go phase of the grieving process.
- Condolence is the sharing of grief with the survivors. There are many ways condolences can be expressed.

Critical Thinking

Plan a condolence visit to a neighbor whose husband died a week ago. Discuss how you would determine whether her grieving was normal or dysfunctional. How would you offer comfort to this person? What might you plan to say during the visit?

REVIEW QUESTIONS

1. **Normal losses that occur during the life cycle most often involve:**
   a. death of a loved one.
   b. any experience of letting go.
   c. wartime deaths.
   d. loss of property.
2. **Anticipatory grief is:**
   a. grief that occurs before a loss.
   b. grief that occurs after a person dies.
   c. mourning a loved one who dies.
   d. a fear of death.

3. Normal grief responses may include:
   a. inability to concentrate.
   b. rage.
   c. violence.
   d. inability to communicate.

4. A sign of dysfunctional grief may include:
   a. prolonged functional impairment.
   b. initial denial that death occurred.
   c. temporary social withdrawal.
   d. crying.

5. The role of the nurse or health-care worker after the patient's death involves:
   a. terminating professional responsibilities.
   b. preparing the family for the grieving process.
   c. referring the family to a psychiatrist.
   d. notifying the priest.

Child, Adolescent, and Adult Immunization Schedules

FIGURE 1: Recommended immunization schedule for persons aged 0 through 6 years—**United States, 2012** (for those who fall behind or start late, see the catch-up schedule [Figure 3])

Vaccine ▼ Age ▶	Birth	1 month	2 months	4 months	6 months	9 months	12 months	15 months	18 months	19–23 months	2–3 years	4–6 years
Hepatitis B[1]	**Hep B**	HepB					HepB					
Rotavirus[2]			RV	RV	RV[2]							
Diphtheria, tetanus, pertussis[3]			DTaP	DTaP	DTaP		see footnote[3]	DTaP				DTaP
Haemophilus influenzae type b[4]			Hib	Hib	Hib[4]		Hib					
Pneumococcal[5]			PCV	PCV	PCV		PCV				PPSV	
Inactivated poliovirus[6]			IPV	IPV			IPV					IPV
Influenza[7]								Influenza (Yearly)				
Measles, mumps, rubella[8]							MMR			see footnote[8]		MMR
Varicella[9]							Varicella			see footnote[9]		Varicella
Hepatitis A[10]								Dose 1[10]			HepA Series	
Meningococcal[11]									MCV4 — see footnote[11]			

Legend: Range of recommended ages for all children; Range of recommended ages for certain high-risk groups; Range of recommended ages for all children and certain high-risk groups

This schedule includes recommendations in effect as of December 23, 2011. Any dose not administered at the recommended age should be administered at a subsequent visit, when indicated and feasible. The use of a combination vaccine generally is preferred over separate injections of its equivalent component vaccines. Vaccination providers should consult the relevant Advisory Committee on Immunization Practices (ACIP) statement for detailed recommendations, available online at http://www.cdc.gov/vaccines/pubs/acip-list.htm. Clinically significant adverse events that follow vaccination should be reported to the Vaccine Adverse Event Reporting System (VAERS) online (http://www.vaers.hhs.gov) or by telephone (800-822-7967).

1. **Hepatitis B (HepB) vaccine.** (Minimum age: birth)
   At birth:
   - Administer monovalent HepB vaccine to all newborns before hospital discharge.
   - For infants born to hepatitis B surface antigen (HBsAg)–positive mothers, administer HepB vaccine and 0.5 mL of hepatitis B immune globulin (HBIG) within 12 hours of birth. These infants should be tested for HBsAg and antibody to HBsAg (anti-HBs) 1 to 2 months after completion of at least 3 doses of the HepB series, at age 9 through 18 months (generally at the next well-child visit).
   - If mother's HBsAg status is unknown, within 12 hours of birth administer HepB vaccine for infants weighing ≥2,000 grams, and HepB vaccine plus HBIG for infants weighing <2,000 grams. Determine mother's HBsAg status as soon as possible and, if she is HBsAg-positive, administer HBIG for infants weighing ≥2,000 grams (no later than age 1 week).

   Doses after the birth dose:
   - The second dose should be administered at age 1 to 2 months. Monovalent HepB vaccine should be used for doses administered before age 6 weeks.
   - Administration of a total of 4 doses of HepB vaccine is permissible when a combination vaccine containing HepB is administered after the birth dose.
   - Infants who did not receive a birth dose should receive 3 doses of a HepB-containing vaccine starting as soon as feasible (Figure 3).
   - The minimum interval between dose 1 and dose 2 is 4 weeks, and between dose 2 and 3 is 8 weeks. The final (third or fourth) dose in the HepB vaccine series should be administered no earlier than age 24 weeks and at least 16 weeks after the first dose.
2. **Rotavirus (RV) vaccines.** (Minimum age: 6 weeks for both RV-1 [Rotarix] and RV-5 [Rota Teq])
   - The maximum age for the first dose in the series is 14 weeks, 6 days; and 8 months, 0 days for the final dose in the series. Vaccination should not be initiated for infants aged 15 weeks, 0 days or older.
   - If RV-1 (Rotarix) is administered at ages 2 and 4 months, a dose at 6 months is not indicated.
3. **Diphtheria and tetanus toxoids and acellular pertussis (DTaP) vaccine.** (Minimum age: 6 weeks)
   - The fourth dose may be administered as early as age 12 months, provided at least 6 months have elapsed since the third dose.
4. ***Haemophilus influenzae* type b (Hib) conjugate vaccine.** (Minimum age: 6 weeks)
   - If PRP-OMP (PedvaxHIB or Comvax [HepB-Hib]) is administered at ages 2 and 4 months, a dose at age 6 months is not indicated.
   - Hiberix should only be used for the booster (final) dose in children aged 12 months through 4 years.
5. **Pneumococcal vaccines.** (Minimum age: 6 weeks for pneumococcal conjugate vaccine [PCV]; 2 years for pneumococcal polysaccharide vaccine [PPSV])
   - Administer 1 dose of PCV to all healthy children aged 24 through 59 months who are not completely vaccinated for their age.
   - For children who have received an age-appropriate series of 7-valent PCV (PCV7), a single supplemental dose of 13-valent PCV (PCV13) is recommended for:
     — All children aged 14 through 59 months
     — Children aged 60 through 71 months with underlying medical conditions.
   - Administer PPSV at least 8 weeks after last dose of PCV to children aged 2 years or older with certain underlying medical conditions, including a cochlear implant. See *MMWR* 2010:59(No. RR-11), available at http://www.cdc.gov/mmwr/pdf/rr/rr5911.pdf.
6. **Inactivated poliovirus vaccine (IPV).** (Minimum age: 6 weeks)
   - If 4 or more doses are administered before age 4 years, an additional dose should be administered at age 4 through 6 years.
   - The final dose in the series should be administered on or after the fourth birthday and at least 6 months after the previous dose.
7. **Influenza vaccines.** (Minimum age: 6 months for trivalent inactivated influenza vaccine [TIV]; 2 years for live, attenuated influenza vaccine [LAIV])
   - For most healthy children aged 2 years and older, either LAIV or TIV may be used. However, LAIV should not be administered to some children, including 1) children with asthma, 2) children 2 through 4 years who had wheezing in the past 12 months, or 3) children who have any other underlying medical conditions that predispose them to influenza complications. For all other contraindications to use of LAIV, see *MMWR* 2010;59(No. RR-8), available at http://www.cdc.gov/mmwr/pdf/rr/rr5908.pdf.
   - For children aged 6 months through 8 years:
     — For the 2011–12 season, administer 2 doses (separated by at least 4 weeks) to those who did not receive at least 1 dose of the 2010–11 vaccine. Those who received at least 1 dose of the 2010–11 vaccine require 1 dose for the 2011–12 season.
     — For the 2012–13 season, follow dosing guidelines in the 2012 ACIP influenza vaccine recommendations.
8. **Measles, mumps, and rubella (MMR) vaccine.** (Minimum age: 12 months)
   - The second dose may be administered before age 4 years, provided at least 4 weeks have elapsed since the first dose.
   - Administer MMR vaccine to infants aged 6 through 11 months who are traveling internationally. These children should be revaccinated with 2 doses of MMR vaccine, the first at ages 12 through 15 months and at least 4 weeks after the previous dose, and the second at ages 4 through 6 years.
9. **Varicella (VAR) vaccine.** (Minimum age: 12 months)
   - The second dose may be administered before age 4 years, provided at least 3 months have elapsed since the first dose.
   - For children aged 12 months through 12 years, the recommended minimum interval between doses is 3 months. However, if the second dose was administered at least 4 weeks after the first dose, it can be accepted as valid.
10. **Hepatitis A (HepA) vaccine.** (Minimum age: 12 months)
    - Administer the second (final) dose 6 to18 months after the first.
    - Unvaccinated children 24 months and older at high risk should be vaccinated. See *MMWR* 2006;55(No. RR-7), available at http://www.cdc.gov/mmwr/pdf/rr/rr5507.pdf.
    - A 2-dose HepA vaccine series is recommended for anyone aged 24 months and older, previously unvaccinated, for whom immunity against hepatitis A virus infection is desired.
11. **Meningococcal conjugate vaccines, quadrivalent (MCV4).** (Minimum age: 9 months for Menactra [MCV4-D], 2 years for Menveo [MCV4-CRM])
    - For children aged 9 through 23 months 1) with persistent complement component deficiency; 2) who are residents of or travelers to countries with hyperendemic or epidemic disease; or 3) who are present during outbreaks caused by a vaccine serogroup, administer 2 primary doses of MCV4-D, ideally at ages 9 months and 12 months or at least 8 weeks apart.
    - For children aged 24 months and older with 1) persistent complement component deficiency who have not been previously vaccinated; or 2) anatomic/functional asplenia, administer 2 primary doses of either MCV4 at least 8 weeks apart.
    - For children with anatomic/functional asplenia, if MCV4-D (Menactra) is used, administer at a minimum age of 2 years and at least 4 weeks after completion of all PCV doses.
    - See *MMWR* 2011;60:72–6, available at http://www.cdc.gov/mmwr/pdf/wk/mm6003. pdf, and Vaccines for Children Program resolution No. 6/11-1, available at http://www. cdc.gov/vaccines/programs/vfc/downloads/resolutions/06-11mening-mcv.pdf, and *MMWR* 2011;60:1391–2, available at http://www.cdc.gov/mmwr/pdf/wk/mm6040. pdf, for further guidance, including revaccination guidelines.

This schedule is approved by the Advisory Committee on Immunization Practices (http://www.cdc.gov/vaccines/recs/acip), the American Academy of Pediatrics (http://www.aap.org), and the American Academy of Family Physicians (http://www.aafp.org).
Department of Health and Human Services • Centers for Disease Control and Prevention

FIGURE 2: Recommended immunization schedule for persons aged 7 through 18 years—**United States, 2012** (for those who fall behind or start late, see the schedule below and the catch-up schedule [Figure 3])

Vaccine ▼ Age ►	7–10 years	11–12 years	13–18 years
Tetanus, diphtheria, pertussis[1]	1 dose (if indicated)	1 dose	1 dose (if indicated)
Human papillomavirus[2]	*see footnote*[2]	3 doses	Complete 3-dose series
Meningococcal[3]	See footnote[3]	Dose 1	Booster at 16 years old
Influenza[4]	Influenza (yearly)		
Pneumococcal[5]	See footnote [5]		
Hepatitis A[6]	Complete 2-dose series		
Hepatitis B[7]	Complete 3-dose series		
Inactivated poliovirus[8]	Complete 3-dose series		
Measles, mumps, rubella[9]	Complete 2-dose series		
Varicella[10]	Complete 2-dose series		

Range of recommended ages for all children

Range of recommended ages for catch-up immunization

Range of recommended ages for certain high-risk groups

This schedule includes recommendations in effect as of December 23, 2011. Any dose not administered at the recommended age should be administered at a subsequent visit, when indicated and feasible. The use of a combination vaccine generally is preferred over separate injections of its equivalent component vaccines. Vaccination providers should consult the relevant Advisory Committee on Immunization Practices (ACIP) statement for detailed recommendations, available online at http://www.cdc.gov/vaccines/pubs/acip-list.htm. Clinically significant adverse events that follow vaccination should be reported to the Vaccine Adverse Event Reporting System (VAERS) online (http://www.vaers.hhs.gov) or by telephone (800-822-7967).

1. **Tetanus and diphtheria toxoids and acellular pertussis (Tdap) vaccine.** (Minimum age: 10 years for Boostrix and 11 years for Adacel)
   - Persons aged 11 through 18 years who have not received Tdap vaccine should receive a dose followed by tetanus and diphtheria toxoids (Td) booster doses every 10 years thereafter.
   - Tdap vaccine should be substituted for a single dose of Td in the catch-up series for children aged 7 through 10 years. Refer to the catch-up schedule if additional doses of tetanus and diphtheria toxoid–containing vaccine are needed.
   - Tdap vaccine can be administered regardless of the interval since the last tetanus and diphtheria toxoid–containing vaccine.
2. **Human papillomavirus (HPV) vaccines (HPV4 [Gardasil] and HPV2 [Cervarix]).** (Minimum age: 9 years)
   - Either HPV4 or HPV2 is recommended in a 3-dose series for females aged 11 or 12 years. HPV4 is recommended in a 3-dose series for males aged 11 or 12 years.
   - The vaccine series can be started beginning at age 9 years.
   - Administer the second dose 1 to 2 months after the first dose and the third dose 6 months after the first dose (at least 24 weeks after the first dose).
   - See *MMWR* 2010;59:626–32, available at http://www.cdc.gov/mmwr/pdf/wk/mm5920.pdf.
3. **Meningococcal conjugate vaccines, quadrivalent (MCV4).**
   - Administer MCV4 at age 11 through 12 years with a booster dose at age 16 years.
   - Administer MCV4 at age 13 through 18 years if patient is not previously vaccinated.
   - If the first dose is administered at age 13 through 15 years, a booster dose should be administered at age 16 through 18 years with a minimum interval of at least 8 weeks after the preceding dose.
   - If the first dose is administered at age 16 years or older, a booster dose is not needed.
   - Administer 2 primary doses at least 8 weeks apart to previously unvaccinated persons with persistent complement component deficiency or anatomic/functional asplenia, and 1 dose every 5 years thereafter.
   - Adolescents aged 11 through 18 years with human immunodeficiency virus (HIV) infection should receive a 2-dose primary series of MCV4, at least 8 weeks apart.
   - See *MMWR* 2011;60:72–76, available at http://www.cdc.gov/mmwr/pdf/wk/mm6003.pdf, and Vaccines for Children Program resolution No. 6/11-1, available at http://www.cdc.gov/vaccines/programs/vfc/downloads/resolutions/06-11mening-mcv.pdf, for further guidelines.
4. **Influenza vaccines (trivalent inactivated influenza vaccine [TIV] and live, attenuated influenza vaccine [LAIV]).**
   - For most healthy, nonpregnant persons, either LAIV or TIV may be used, except LAIV should not be used for some persons, including those with asthma or any other underlying medical conditions that predispose them to influenza complications. For all other contraindications to use of LAIV, see *MMWR* 2010;59(No.RR-8), available at http://www.cdc.gov/mmwr/pdf/rr/rr5908.pdf.
   - Administer 1 dose to persons aged 9 years and older.
   - For children aged 6 months through 8 years:
     — For the 2011–12 season, administer 2 doses (separated by at least 4 weeks) to those who did not receive at least 1 dose of the 2010–11 vaccine. Those who received at least 1 dose of the 2010–11 vaccine require 1 dose for the 2011–12 season.
     — For the 2012–13 season, follow dosing guidelines in the 2012 ACIP influenza vaccine recommendations.
5. **Pneumococcal vaccines (pneumococcal conjugate vaccine [PCV] and pneumococcal polysaccharide vaccine [PPSV]).**
   - A single dose of PCV may be administered to children aged 6 through 18 years who have anatomic/functional asplenia, HIV infection or other immunocompromising condition, cochlear implant, or cerebral spinal fluid leak. See *MMWR* 2010:59(No. RR-11), available at http://www.cdc.gov/mmwr/pdf/rr/rr5911.pdf.
   - Administer PPSV at least 8 weeks after the last dose of PCV to children aged 2 years or older with certain underlying medical conditions, including a cochlear implant. A single revaccination should be administered after 5 years to children with anatomic/functional asplenia or an immunocompromising condition.
6. **Hepatitis A (HepA) vaccine.**
   - HepA vaccine is recommended for children older than 23 months who live in areas where vaccination programs target older children, who are at increased risk for infection, or for whom immunity against hepatitis A virus infection is desired. See *MMWR* 2006;55(No. RR-7), available at http://www.cdc.gov/mmwr/pdf/rr/rr5507.pdf.
   - Administer 2 doses at least 6 months apart to unvaccinated persons.
7. **Hepatitis B (HepB) vaccine.**
   - Administer the 3-dose series to those not previously vaccinated.
   - For those with incomplete vaccination, follow the catch-up recommendations (Figure 3).
   - A 2-dose series (doses separated by at least 4 months) of adult formulation Recombivax HB is licensed for use in children aged 11 through 15 years.
8. **Inactivated poliovirus vaccine (IPV).**
   - The final dose in the series should be administered at least 6 months after the previous dose.
   - If both OPV and IPV were administered as part of a series, a total of 4 doses should be administered, regardless of the child's current age.
   - IPV is not routinely recommended for U.S. residents aged18 years or older.
9. **Measles, mumps, and rubella (MMR) vaccine.**
   - The minimum interval between the 2 doses of MMR vaccine is 4 weeks.
10. **Varicella (VAR) vaccine.**
    - For persons without evidence of immunity (see *MMWR* 2007;56[No. RR-4], available at http://www.cdc.gov/mmwr/pdf/rr/rr5604.pdf), administer 2 doses if not previously vaccinated or the second dose if only 1 dose has been administered.
    - For persons aged 7 through 12 years, the recommended minimum interval between doses is 3 months. However, if the second dose was administered at least 4 weeks after the first dose, it can be accepted as valid.
    - For persons aged 13 years and older, the minimum interval between doses is 4 weeks.

This schedule is approved by the Advisory Committee on Immunization Practices (http://www.cdc.gov/vaccines/recs/acip), the American Academy of Pediatrics (http://www.aap.org), and the American Academy of Family Physicians (http://www.aafp.org).
Department of Health and Human Services • Centers for Disease Control and Prevention

FIGURE 3. Catch-up immunization schedule for persons aged 4 months through 18 years who start late or who are more than 1 month behind —**United States • 2012**
The figure below provides catch-up schedules and minimum intervals between doses for children whose vaccinations have been delayed. A vaccine series does not need to be restarted, regardless of the time that has elapsed between doses. Use the section appropriate for the child's age. **Always use this table in conjunction with the accompanying childhood and adolescent immunization schedules (Figures 1 and 2) and their respective footnotes.**

Persons aged 4 months through 6 years					
Vaccine	Minimum Age for Dose 1	Minimum Interval Between Doses			
		Dose 1 to dose 2	Dose 2 to dose 3	Dose 3 to dose 4	Dose 4 to dose 5
Hepatitis B	Birth	4 weeks	8 weeks and at least 16 weeks after first dose; minimum age for the final dose is 24 weeks		
Rotavirus[1]	6 weeks	4 weeks	4 weeks[1]		
Diphtheria, tetanus, pertussis[2]	6 weeks	4 weeks	4 weeks	6 months	6 months[2]
Haemophilus influenzae type b[3]	6 weeks	4 weeks if first dose administered at younger than age 12 months 8 weeks (as final dose) if first dose administered at age 12–14 months No further doses needed if first dose administered at age 15 months or older	4 weeks[3] if current age is younger than 12 months 8 weeks (as final dose)[3] if current age is 12 months or older and first dose administered at younger than age 12 months and second dose administered at younger than 15 months No further doses needed if previous dose administered at age 15 months or older	8 weeks (as final dose) This dose only necessary for children aged 12 months through 59 months who received 3 doses before age 12 months	
Pneumococcal[4]	6 weeks	4 weeks if first dose administered at younger than age 12 months 8 weeks (as final dose for healthy children) if first dose administered at age 12 months or older or current age 24 through 59 months No further doses needed for healthy children if first dose administered at age 24 months or older	4 weeks if current age is younger than 12 months 8 weeks (as final dose for healthy children) if current age is 12 months or older No further doses needed for healthy children if previous dose administered at age 24 months or older	8 weeks (as final dose) This dose only necessary for children aged 12 months through 59 months who received 3 doses before age 12 months or for children at high risk who received 3 doses at any age	
Inactivated poliovirus[5]	6 weeks	4 weeks	4 weeks	6 months[5] minimum age 4 years for final dose	
Meningococcal[6]	9 months	8 weeks[6]			
Measles, mumps, rubella[7]	12 months	4 weeks			
Varicella[8]	12 months	3 months			
Hepatitis A	12 months	6 months			
Persons aged 7 through 18 years					
Tetanus, diphtheria/ tetanus, diphtheria, pertussis[9]	7 years[9]	4 weeks	4 weeks if first dose administered at younger than age 12 months 6 months if first dose administered at 12 months or older	6 months if first dose administered at younger than age 12 months	
Human papillomavirus[10]	9 years	Routine dosing intervals are recommended[10]			
Hepatitis A	12 months	6 months			
Hepatitis B	Birth	4 weeks	8 weeks (and at least 16 weeks after first dose)		
Inactivated poliovirus[5]	6 weeks	4 weeks	4 weeks[5]	6 months[5]	
Meningococcal[6]	9 months	8 weeks[6]			
Measles, mumps, rubella[7]	12 months	4 weeks			
Varicella[8]	12 months	3 months if person is younger than age 13 years 4 weeks if person is aged 13 years or older			

1. **Rotavirus (RV) vaccines (RV-1 [Rotarix] and RV-5 [Rota Teq]).**
   - The maximum age for the first dose in the series is 14 weeks, 6 days; and 8 months, 0 days for the final dose in the series. Vaccination should not be initiated for infants aged 15 weeks, 0 days or older.
   - If RV-1 was administered for the first and second doses, a third dose is not indicated.
2. **Diphtheria and tetanus toxoids and acellular pertussis (DTaP) vaccine.**
   - The fifth dose is not necessary if the fourth dose was administered at age 4 years or older.
3. ***Haemophilus influenzae* type b (Hib) conjugate vaccine.**
   - Hib vaccine should be considered for unvaccinated persons aged 5 years or older who have sickle cell disease, leukemia, human immunodeficiency virus (HIV) infection, or anatomic/functional asplenia.
   - If the first 2 doses were PRP-OMP (PedvaxHIB or Comvax) and were administered at age 11 months or younger, the third (and final) dose should be administered at age 12 through 15 months and at least 8 weeks after the second dose.
   - If the first dose was administered at age 7 through 11 months, administer the second dose at least 4 weeks later and a final dose at age 12 through 15 months.
4. **Pneumococcal vaccines.** (Minimum age: 6 weeks for pneumococcal conjugate vaccine [PCV]; 2 years for pneumococcal polysaccharide vaccine [PPSV])
   - For children aged 24 through 71 months with underlying medical conditions, administer 1 dose of PCV if 3 doses of PCV were received previously, or administer 2 doses of PCV at least 8 weeks apart if fewer than 3 doses of PCV were received previously.
   - A single dose of PCV may be administered to certain children aged 6 through 18 years with underlying medical conditions. See age-specific schedules for details.
   - Administer PPSV to children aged 2 years or older with certain underlying medical conditions. See *MMWR* 2010:59(No. RR-11), available at http://www.cdc.gov/mmwr/pdf/rr/rr5911.pdf.
5. **Inactivated poliovirus vaccine (IPV).**
   - A fourth dose is not necessary if the third dose was administered at age 4 years or older and at least 6 months after the previous dose.
   - In the first 6 months of life, minimum age and minimum intervals are only recommended if the person is at risk for imminent exposure to circulating poliovirus (i.e., travel to a polio-endemic region or during an outbreak).
   - IPV is not routinely recommended for U.S. residents aged 18 years or older.
6. **Meningococcal conjugate vaccines, quadrivalent (MCV4).** (Minimum age: 9 months for Menactra [MCV4-D]; 2 years for Menveo [MCV4-CRM])
   - See Figure 1 ("Recommended immunization schedule for persons aged 0 through 6 years") and Figure 2 ("Recommended immunization schedule for persons aged 7 through 18 years") for further guidance.
7. **Measles, mumps, and rubella (MMR) vaccine.**
   - Administer the second dose routinely at age 4 through 6 years.
8. **Varicella (VAR) vaccine.**
   - Administer the second dose routinely at age 4 through 6 years. If the second dose was administered at least 4 weeks after the first dose, it can be accepted as valid.
9. **Tetanus and diphtheria toxoids (Td) and tetanus and diphtheria toxoids and acellular pertussis (Tdap) vaccines.**
   - For children aged 7 through 10 years who are not fully immunized with the childhood DTaP vaccine series, Tdap vaccine should be substituted for a single dose of Td vaccine in the catch-up series; if additional doses are needed, use Td vaccine. For these children, an adolescent Tdap vaccine dose should not be given.
   - An inadvertent dose of DTaP vaccine administered to children aged 7 through 10 years can count as part of the catch-up series. This dose can count as the adolescent Tdap dose, or the child can later receive a Tdap booster dose at age 11–12 years.
10. **Human papillomavirus (HPV) vaccines (HPV4 [Gardasil] and HPV2 [Cervarix]).**
    - Administer the vaccine series to females (either HPV2 or HPV4) and males (HPV4) at age 13 through 18 years if patient is not previously vaccinated.
    - Use recommended routine dosing intervals for vaccine series catch-up; see Figure 2 ("Recommended immunization schedule for persons aged 7 through 18 years").

Clinically significant adverse events that follow vaccination should be reported to the Vaccine Adverse Event Reporting System (VAERS) online (http://www.vaers.hhs.gov) or by telephone (800-822-7967). Suspected cases of vaccine-preventable diseases should be reported to the state or local health department. Additional information, including precautions and contraindications for vaccination, is available from CDC online (http://www.cdc.gov/vaccines) or by telephone (800-CDC-INFO [800-232-4636]).

Recommended Adult Immunization Schedule—United States - 2012

Note: These recommendations must be read with the footnotes that follow containing number of doses, intervals between doses, and other important information.

Figure 1. Recommended adult immunization schedule, by vaccine and age group[1]

VACCINE ▼ AGE GROUP ►	19-21 years	22-26 years	27-49 years	50-59 years	60-64 years	≥ 65 years
Influenza [2]	1 dose annually					
Tetanus, diphtheria, pertussis (Td/Tdap) [3,*]	Substitute 1-time dose of Tdap for Td booster; then boost with Td every 10 yrs					Td/Tdap[3]
Varicella [4,*]	2 Doses					
Human papillomavirus (HPV) Female [5,*]	3 doses					
Human papillomavirus (HPV) Male [5,*]	3 doses					
Zoster [6]					1 dose	
Measles, mumps, rubella (MMR) [7,*]	1 or 2 doses			1 dose		
Pneumococcal (polysaccharide) [8,9]	1 or 2 doses					1 dose
Meningococcal [10,*]	1 or more doses					
Hepatitis A [11,*]	2 doses					
Hepatitis B [12,*]	3 doses					

*Covered by the Vaccine Injury Compensation Program

- For all persons in this category who meet the age requirements and who lack documentation of vaccination or have no evidence of previous infection
- Recommended if some other risk factor is present (e.g., on the basis of medical, occupational, lifestyle, or other indications)
- Tdap recommended for ≥65 if contact with <12 month old child. Either Td or Tdap can be used if no infant contact
- No recommendation

Report all clinically significant postvaccination reactions to the Vaccine Adverse Event Reporting System (VAERS). Reporting forms and instructions on filing a VAERS report are available at www.vaers.hhs.gov or by telephone, 800-822-7967.

Information on how to file a Vaccine Injury Compensation Program claim is available at www.hrsa.gov/vaccinecompensation or by telephone, 800-338-2382. To file a claim for vaccine injury, contact the U.S. Court of Federal Claims, 717 Madison Place, N.W., Washington, D.C. 20005; telephone, 202-357-6400.

Additional information about the vaccines in this schedule, extent of available data, and contraindications for vaccination is also available at www.cdc.gov/vaccines or from the CDC-INFO Contact Center at 800-CDC-INFO (800-232-4636) in English and Spanish, 8:00 a.m. - 8:00 p.m. Eastern Time, Monday - Friday, excluding holidays.

Use of trade names and commercial sources is for identification only and does not imply endorsement by the U.S. Department of Health and Human Services.

Figure 2. Vaccines that might be indicated for adults based on medical and other indications[1]

VACCINE ▼ INDICATION ►	Pregnancy	Immunocompromising conditions (excluding human immunodeficiency virus [HIV])[4,6,7,14]	HIV infection[4,7,13,14] CD4+ T lymphocyte count <200 cells/μL	HIV infection CD4+ T lymphocyte count >200 cells/μL	Men who have sex with men (MSM)	Heart disease, chronic lung disease, chronic alcoholism	Asplenia[13] (including elective splenectomy and persistent complement component deficiencies)	Chronic liver disease	Diabetes, kidney failure, end-stage renal disease, receipt of hemodialysis	Health-care personnel
Influenza [2]	1 dose TIV annually				1 dose TIV or LAIV annually	1 dose TIV annually				1 dose TIV or LAIV annually
Tetanus, diphtheria, pertussis (Td/Tdap) [3,*]	Substitute 1-time dose of Tdap for Td booster; then boost with Td every 10 yrs									
Varicella [4,*]	Contraindicated			2 doses						
Human papillomavirus (HPV) Female [5,*]		3 doses through age 26 yrs				3 doses through age 26 yrs				
Human papillomavirus (HPV) Male [5,*]		3 doses through age 26 yrs				3 doses through age 21 yrs				
Zoster [6]	Contraindicated				1 dose					
Measles, mumps, rubella (MMR) [7,*]	Contraindicated			1 or 2 doses						
Pneumococcal (polysaccharide) [8,9]	1 or 2 doses									
Meningococcal [10,*]	1 or more doses									
Hepatitis A [11,*]	2 doses									
Hepatitis B [12,*]	3 doses									

*Covered by the Vaccine Injury Compensation Program

- For all persons in this category who meet the age requirements and who lack documentation of vaccination or have no evidence of previous infection
- Recommended if some other risk factor is present (e.g., on the basis of medical, occupational, lifestyle, or other indications)
- Contraindicated
- No recommendation

The recommendations in this schedule were approved by the Centers for Disease Control and Prevention's (CDC) Advisory Committee on Immunization Practices (ACIP), the American Academy of Family Physicians (AAFP), the American College of Physicians (ACP), American College of Obstetricians and Gynecologists (ACOG) and American College of Nurse-Midwives (ACNM).

These schedules indicate the recommended age groups and medical indications for which administration of currently licensed vaccines is commonly indicated for adults ages 19 years and older, as of January 1, 2012. For all vaccines being recommended on the Adult Immunization Schedule: a vaccine series does not need to be restarted, regardless of the time that has elapsed between doses. Licensed combination vaccines may be used whenever any components of the combination are indicated and when the vaccine's other components are not contraindicated. For detailed recommendations on all vaccines, including those used primarily for travelers or that are issued during the year, consult the manufacturers' package inserts and the complete statements from the Advisory Committee on Immunization Practices (www.cdc.gov/vaccines/pubs/acip-list.htm). Use of trade names and commercial sources is for identification only and does not imply endorsement by the U.S. Department of Health and Human Services.

CDC U.S. Department of Health and Human Services
Centers for Disease Control and Prevention

Footnotes — Recommended Adult Immunization Schedule—United States - 2012

1. **Additional information**
   - Advisory Committee on Immunization Practices (ACIP) vaccine recommendations and additional information are available at: http://www.cdc.gov/vaccines/pubs/acip-list.htm.
   - Information on travel vaccine requirements and recommendations (e.g., for hepatitis A and B, meningococcal, and other vaccines) available at http://wwwnc.cdc.gov/travel/page/vaccinations.htm.
2. **Influenza vaccination**
   - Annual vaccination against influenza is recommended for all persons 6 months of age and older.
   - Persons 6 months of age and older, including pregnant women, can receive the trivalent inactivated vaccine (TIV).
   - Healthy, nonpregnant adults younger than age 50 years without high-risk medical conditions can receive either intranasally administered live, attenuated influenza vaccine (LAIV) (FluMist), or TIV. Health-care personnel who care for severely immunocompromised persons (i.e., those who require care in a protected environment) should receive TIV rather than LAIV. Other persons should receive TIV.
   - The intramuscular or intradermal administered TIV are options for adults aged 18–64 years.
   - Adults aged 65 years and older can receive the standard dose TIV or the high-dose TIV (Fluzone High-Dose).
3. **Tetanus, diphtheria, and acellular pertussis (Td/Tdap) vaccination**
   - Administer a one-time dose of Tdap to adults younger than age 65 years who have not received Tdap previously or for whom vaccine status is unknown to replace one of the 10-year Td boosters.
   - Tdap is specifically recommended for the following persons:
     — pregnant women more than 20 weeks' gestation,
     — adults, regardless of age, who are close contacts of infants younger than age 12 months (e.g., parents, grandparents, or child care providers), and
     — health-care personnel.
   - Tdap can be administered regardless of interval since the most recent tetanus or diphtheria-containing vaccine.
   - Pregnant women not vaccinated during pregnancy should receive Tdap immediately postpartum.
   - Adults 65 years and older may receive Tdap.
   - Adults with unknown or incomplete history of completing a 3-dose primary vaccination series with Td-containing vaccines should begin or complete a primary vaccination series. Tdap should be substituted for a single dose of Td in the vaccination series with Tdap preferred as the first dose.
   - For unvaccinated adults, administer the first 2 doses at least 4 weeks apart and the third dose 6–12 months after the second.
   - If incompletely vaccinated (i.e., less than 3 doses), administer remaining doses.

   Refer to the ACIP statement for recommendations for administering Td/Tdap as prophylaxis in wound management (See footnote 1).
4. **Varicella vaccination**
   - All adults without evidence of immunity to varicella (as defined below) should receive 2 doses of single-antigen varicella vaccine or a second dose if they have received only 1 dose.
   - Special consideration for vaccination should be given to those who
     — have close contact with persons at high risk for severe disease (e.g., health-care personnel and family contacts of persons with immunocompromising conditions) or
     — are at high risk for exposure or transmission (e.g., teachers; child care employees; residents and staff members of institutional settings, including correctional institutions; college students; military personnel; adolescents and adults living in households with children; nonpregnant women of childbearing age; and international travelers).
   - Pregnant women should be assessed for evidence of varicella immunity. Women who do not have evidence of immunity should receive the first dose of varicella vaccine upon completion or termination of pregnancy and before discharge from the health-care facility. The second dose should be administered 4–8 weeks after the first dose.
   - Evidence of immunity to varicella in adults includes any of the following:
     — documentation of 2 doses of varicella vaccine at least 4 weeks apart;
     — U.S.-born before 1980 (although for health-care personnel and pregnant women, birth before 1980 should not be considered evidence of immunity);
     — history of varicella based on diagnosis or verification of varicella by a health-care provider (for a patient reporting a history of or having an atypical case, a mild case, or both, health-care providers should seek either an epidemiologic link to a typical varicella case or to a laboratory-confirmed case or evidence of laboratory confirmation, if it was performed at the time of acute disease);
     — history of herpes zoster based on diagnosis or verification of herpes zoster by a health-care provider; or
     — laboratory evidence of immunity or laboratory confirmation of disease.
5. **Human papillomavirus (HPV) vaccination**
   - Two vaccines are licensed for use in females, bivalent HPV vaccine (HPV2) and quadrivalent HPV vaccine (HPV4), and one HPV vaccine for use in males (HPV4).
   - For females, either HPV4 or HPV2 is recommended in a 3-dose series for routine vaccination at 11 or 12 years of age, and for those 13 through 26 years of age, if not previously vaccinated.
   - For males, HPV4 is recommended in a 3-dose series for routine vaccination at 11 or 12 years of age, and for those 13 through 21 years of age, if not previously vaccinated. Males 22 through 26 years of age may be vaccinated.
   - HPV vaccines are not live vaccines and can be administered to persons who are immunocompromised as a result of infection (including HIV infection), disease, or medications. Vaccine is recommended for immunocompromised persons through age 26 years who did not get any or all doses when they were younger. The immune response and vaccine efficacy might be less than that in immunocompetent persons.
   - Men who have sex with men (MSM) might especially benefit from vaccination to prevent condyloma and anal cancer. HPV4 is recommended for MSM through age 26 years who did not get any or all doses when they were younger.
   - Ideally, vaccine should be administered before potential exposure to HPV through sexual activity; however, persons who are sexually active should still be vaccinated consistent with age-based recommendations. HPV vaccine can be administered to persons with a history of genital warts, abnormal Papanicolaou test, or positive HPV DNA test.
   - A complete series for either HPV4 or HPV2 consists of 3 doses. The second dose should be administered 1–2 months after the first dose; the third dose should be administered 6 months after the first dose (at least 24 weeks after the first dose).
   - Although HPV vaccination is not specifically recommended for health-care personnel (HCP) based on their occupation, HCP should receive the HPV vaccine if they are in the recommended age group.
6. **Zoster vaccination**
   - A single dose of zoster vaccine is recommended for adults 60 years of age and older regardless of whether they report a prior episode of herpes zoster. Although the vaccine is licensed by the Food and Drug Administration (FDA) for use among and can be administered to persons 50 years and older, ACIP recommends that vaccination begins at 60 years of age.
   - Persons with chronic medical conditions may be vaccinated unless their condition constitutes a contraindication, such as pregnancy or severe immunodeficiency.
   - Although zoster vaccination is not specifically recommended for health-care personnel (HCP), HCP should receive the vaccine if they are in the recommended age group.
7. **Measles, mumps, rubella (MMR) vaccination**
   - Adults born before 1957 generally are considered immune to measles and mumps. All adults born in 1957 or later should have documentation of 1 or more doses of MMR vaccine unless they have a medical contraindication to the vaccine, laboratory evidence of immunity to each of the three diseases, or documentation of provider-diagnosed measles or mumps disease. For rubella, documentation of provider-diagnosed disease is not considered acceptable evidence of immunity.

   Measles component:
   - A routine second dose of MMR vaccine, administered a minimum of 28 days after the first dose, is recommended for adults who
     — are students in postsecondary educational institutions;
     — work in a health-care facility; or
     — plan to travel internationally.
   - Persons who received inactivated (killed) measles vaccine or measles vaccine of unknown type from 1963 to 1967 should be revaccinated with 2 doses of MMR vaccine.

   Mumps component:
   - A routine second dose of MMR vaccine, administered a minimum of 28 days after the first dose, is recommended for adults who
     — are students in postsecondary educational institutions;
     — work in a health-care facility; or
     — plan to travel internationally.
   - Persons vaccinated before 1979 with either killed mumps vaccine or mumps vaccine of unknown type who are at high risk for mumps infection (e.g., persons who are working in a health-care facility) should be considered for revaccination with 2 doses of MMR vaccine.

7. **Measles, mumps, rubella (MMR) vaccination (cont'd)**

   Rubella component:
   - For women of childbearing age, regardless of birth year, rubella immunity should be determined. If there is no evidence of immunity, women who are not pregnant should be vaccinated. Pregnant women who do not have evidence of immunity should receive MMR vaccine upon completion or termination of pregnancy and before discharge from the health-care facility.

   Health-care personnel born before 1957:
   - For unvaccinated health-care personnel born before 1957 who lack laboratory evidence of measles, mumps, and/or rubella immunity or laboratory confirmation of disease, health-care facilities should consider routinely vaccinating personnel with 2 doses of MMR vaccine at the appropriate interval for measles and mumps or 1 dose of MMR vaccine for rubella.
8. **Pneumococcal polysaccharide (PPSV) vaccination**
   - Vaccinate all persons with the following indications:
     — age 65 years and older without a history of PPSV vaccination;
     — adults younger than 65 years with chronic lung disease (including chronic obstructive pulmonary disease, emphysema, and asthma); chronic cardiovascular diseases; diabetes mellitus; chronic liver disease (including cirrhosis); alcoholism; cochlear implants; cerebrospinal fluid leaks; immunocompromising conditions; and functional or anatomic asplenia (e.g., sickle cell disease and other hemoglobinopathies, congenital or acquired asplenia, splenic dysfunction, or splenectomy [if elective splenectomy is planned, vaccinate at least 2 weeks before surgery]);
     — residents of nursing homes or long-term care facilities; and
     — adults who smoke cigarettes.
   - Persons with asymptomatic or symptomatic HIV infection should be vaccinated as soon as possible after their diagnosis.
   - When cancer chemotherapy or other immunosuppressive therapy is being considered, the interval between vaccination and initiation of immunosuppressive therapy should be at least 2 weeks. Vaccination during chemotherapy or radiation therapy should be avoided.
   - Routine use of PPSV is not recommended for American Indians/Alaska Natives or other persons younger than 65 years of age unless they have underlying medical conditions that are PPSV indications. However, public health authorities may consider recommending PPSV for American Indians/Alaska Natives who are living in areas where the risk for invasive pneumococcal disease is increased.
9. **Revaccination with PPSV**
   - One-time revaccination 5 years after the first dose is recommended for persons 19 through 64 years of age with chronic renal failure or nephrotic syndrome; functional or anatomic asplenia (e.g., sickle cell disease or splenectomy); and for persons with immunocompromising conditions.
   - Persons who received PPSV before age 65 years for any indication should receive another dose of the vaccine at age 65 years or later if at least 5 years have passed since their previous dose.
   - No further doses are needed for persons vaccinated with PPSV at or after age 65 years.
10. **Meningococcal vaccination**
    - Administer 2 doses of meningococcal conjugate vaccine quadrivalent (MCV4) at least 2 months apart to adults with functional asplenia or persistent complement component deficiencies.
    - HIV-infected persons who are vaccinated should also receive 2 doses.
    - Administer a single dose of meningococcal vaccine to microbiologists routinely exposed to isolates of *Neisseria meningitidis*, military recruits, and persons who travel to or live in countries in which meningococcal disease is hyperendemic or epidemic.
    - First-year college students up through age 21 years who are living in residence halls should be vaccinated if they have not received a dose on or after their 16th birthday.
    - MCV4 is preferred for adults with any of the preceding indications who are 55 years old and younger; meningococcal polysaccharide vaccine (MPSV4) is preferred for adults 56 years and older.
    - Revaccination with MCV4 every 5 years is recommended for adults previously vaccinated with MCV4 or MPSV4 who remain at increased risk for infection (e.g., adults with anatomic or functional asplenia or persistent complement component deficiencies).
11. **Hepatitis A vaccination**
    - Vaccinate any person seeking protection from hepatitis A virus (HAV) infection and persons with any of the following indications:
      — men who have sex with men and persons who use injection drugs;
      — persons working with HAV-infected primates or with HAV in a research laboratory setting;
      — persons with chronic liver disease and persons who receive clotting factor concentrates;
      — persons traveling to or working in countries that have high or intermediate endemicity of hepatitis A; and
      — unvaccinated persons who anticipate close personal contact (e.g., household or regular babysitting) with an international adoptee during the first 60 days after arrival in the United States from a country with high or intermediate endemicity. (See footnote 1 for more information on travel recommendations). The first dose of the 2-dose hepatitis A vaccine series should be administered as soon as adoption is planned, ideally 2 or more weeks before the arrival of the adoptee.
    - Single-antigen vaccine formulations should be administered in a 2-dose schedule at either 0 and 6–12 months (Havrix), or 0 and 6–18 months (Vaqta). If the combined hepatitis A and hepatitis B vaccine (Twinrix) is used, administer 3 doses at 0, 1, and 6 months; alternatively, a 4-dose schedule may be used, administered on days 0, 7, and 21–30 followed by a booster dose at month 12.
12. **Hepatitis B vaccination**
    - Vaccinate persons with any of the following indications and any person seeking protection from hepatitis B virus (HBV) infection:
      — sexually active persons who are not in a long-term, mutually monogamous relationship (e.g., persons with more than one sex partner during the previous 6 months); persons seeking evaluation or treatment for a sexually transmitted disease (STD); current or recent injection-drug users; and men who have sex with men;
      — health-care personnel and public-safety workers who are exposed to blood or other potentially infectious body fluids;
      — persons with diabetes younger than 60 years as soon as feasible after diagnosis; persons with diabetes who are 60 years or older at the discretion of the treating clinician based on increased need for assisted blood glucose monitoring in long-term care facilities, likelihood of acquiring hepatitis B infection, its complications or chronic sequelae, and likelihood of immune response to vaccination;
      — persons with end-stage renal disease, including patients receiving hemodialysis; persons with HIV infection; and persons with chronic liver disease;
      — household contacts and sex partners of persons with chronic HBV infection; clients and staff members of institutions for persons with developmental disabilities; and international travelers to countries with high or intermediate prevalence of chronic HBV infection; and
      — all adults in the following settings: STD treatment facilities; HIV testing and treatment facilities; facilities providing drug-abuse treatment and prevention services; health-care settings targeting services to injection-drug users or men who have sex with men; correctional facilities; end-stage renal disease programs and facilities for chronic hemodialysis patients; and institutions and nonresidential daycare facilities for persons with developmental disabilities.
    - Administer missing doses to complete a 3-dose series of hepatitis B vaccine to those persons not vaccinated or not completely vaccinated. The second dose should be administered 1 month after the first dose; the third dose should be given at least 2 months after the second dose (and at least 4 months after the first dose). If the combined hepatitis A and hepatitis B vaccine (Twinrix) is used, give 3 doses at 0, 1, and 6 months; alternatively, a 4-dose Twinrix schedule, administered on days 0, 7, and 21–30 followed by a booster dose at month 12 may be used.
    - Adult patients receiving hemodialysis or with other immunocompromising conditions should receive 1 dose of 40 μg/mL (Recombivax HB) administered on a 3-dose schedule or 2 doses of 20 μg/mL (Engerix-B) administered simultaneously on a 4-dose schedule at 0, 1, 2, and 6 months.
13. **Selected conditions for which *Haemophilus influenzae* type b (Hib) vaccine may be used**
    - 1 dose of Hib vaccine should be considered for persons who have sickle cell disease, leukemia, or HIV infection, or who have anatomic or functional asplenia if they have not previously received Hib vaccine.
14. **Immunocompromising conditions**
    - Inactivated vaccines generally are acceptable (e.g., pneumococcal, meningococcal, and influenza [inactivated influenza vaccine]), and live vaccines generally are avoided in persons with immune deficiencies or immunocompromising conditions. Information on specific conditions is available at http://www.cdc.gov/vaccines/pubs/acip-list.htm.

B Multilingual Glossary of Symptoms

glossary of Symptoms

Symptom	Definition
Abnormal Bleeding	Unusual loss of blood from stools, urine, bleeding gums, internal organs.
Chills	A feeling of being cold and shivering, usually with pale skin and a high temperature.
Cough	Rapid expulsion of air from the lungs in order to clear fluid, mucous, or phlegm.
Diarrhea	Having loose and watery stools (bowel movements) often.
Disorientation	To lose a sense of time, place, and one's personal identity.
Dizziness	A feeling of unsteadiness.
Dyspnea	Shortness of breath or difficulty breathing.
Fever	A rise in the temperature of the body above normal, usually when the body has an infection. (A temperature taken by mouth greater than 100.4° Fahrenheit means you have a fever.)
Headache	A pain located in the head, as over the eyes, at the temples, or at the bottom of the skull.
Hemoptysis	Coughing up blood (or bloody mucous).
Jaundice	Yellowing of eyes, skin.
Loss of Appetite	No desire to eat.
Loss of Consciousness (Unconscious)	Not responsive, not aware, not feeling, not thinking (sometimes as a result of fainting).
Malaise	Feeling generally weak and tired, and bodily discomfort.
Nausea	An unpleasant feeling in the stomach, with an urge to vomit (throw up).
Pain	An unpleasant feeling in the body that can range from being mild to extremely painful. The pain can be physical or emotional. Body pain is physical pain, usually due to tissue damage.
Rash	Red bumps (or flaky patches) on the body that are sometimes itchy.
Sore Throat	Pain or discomfort in swallowing.
Tremor	An uncontrollable trembling, shaking, or quivering from physical weakness, emotional stress, or disease.
Vomiting	To throw up what is inside the stomach through the mouth.

Division of Communicable Disease Control

IMM-835 (3/05)

glossary of Symptoms

Symptom	Spanish	Chinese	Korean
Abnormal Bleeding	Sangrado anormal	異常出血	비정상 출혈
Chills	Escalofrío	寒顫	오한
Cough	Tos	咳嗽	기침
Diarrhea	Diarrea, excrementos líquidos	腹瀉	설사
Disorientation	Desorientación, confusión mental	定向障礙	방향 감각 상실
Dizziness	Sentirese desmayado	頭暈	현기증
Dyspnea	Dificultad de respirar	呼吸困難	호흡 곤란
Fever	Fiebre	發燒	열
Headache	Dolor de cabeza intenso	頭痛	두통
Hemoptysis	Tos con sangre	咯血	객혈
Jaundice	Piel y ojos de color amarillo (ictericia)	黃疸	황달
Loss of Appetite	Pérdida del apetito	食欲不振	식욕 부진
Loss of Consciousness (Unconscious)	Desmayarse	失去知覺	무의식
Malaise	Indisposcición o malestar	不舒服	권태감
Nausea	Ganas de vomitar o náuseas	噁心	메스꺼움
Pain	Dolor	疼痛	통증
Rash	Erupción o sarpullido	皮疹	발진
Sore Throat	Dolor de garganta	喉嚨痛	목앓이
Tremor	Temblor continuo	震顫	떨림
Vomiting	Vómito	嘔吐	구토

Division of Communicable Disease Control IMM-835 (3/05)

glossary of Symptoms

Symptom	Japanese	Tagalog	Cambodian
Abnormal Bleeding	異常出血	Di-normal na Pagdugo	ឈាមហូរខុសធម្មតា
Chills	悪寒	Ginaw	ព្រឺរងារ
Cough	咳	Ubo	ក្អក
Diarrhea	下痢	Pagtatae	ជម្ងឺរាគ
Disorientation	方向感覚の喪失	Pagkalito	វង្វេងស្មារតី
Dizziness	めまい	Pagkahilo	វិលមុខ
Dyspnea	呼吸困難	Pangangapos ng Hininga	ពិបាកដកដង្ហើម
Fever	発熱	Lagnat	គ្រុន
Headache	頭痛	Sakit ng Ulo	ឈឺក្បាល
Hemoptysis	血を吐く	Pag-ubo ng Dugo	ក្អកធ្លាក់ឈាម
Jaundice	黄疸	Paninilaw ng Mata at Balat	ជម្ងឺខាន់លឿង
Loss of Appetite	食欲不振	Pagkawala ng Ganang Kumain	មិនឃ្លានអាហារ
Loss of Consciousness (Unconscious)	意識不明	Pagkawala ng Malay	ឥតដឹងខ្លួន
Malaise	倦怠感	Panlulupaypay	ល្ហិតល្ហៃ
Nausea	吐き気	Nasusuka	ចង់ក្អួត
Pain	痛み	Masakit	ឈឺ
Rash	発疹	Singaw sa Balat	កន្ទួលលើស្បែក
Sore Throat	喉の痛み	Masakit na Lalamunan	ឈឺបំពង់ក
Tremor	震え	Pangangatal	ញ័រញាក់
Vomiting	嘔吐	Pagsusuka	ក្អួត

Division of Communicable Disease Control IMM-835 (3/05)

glossary of Symptoms

Symptom	Hmong	Laotian	Vietnamese
Abnormal Bleeding	Los ntshav	ເລືອດອອກຜິດປົກກະຕິ	Chảy Máu Bất Thường
Chills	No	ໜາວໄຂ້ສັ່ນ	Ớn Lạnh
Cough	Hnoos	ອາການໄອ/ໄອ	Ho
Diarrhea	Thoj plab	ຖອກທ້ອງ	Tiêu Chảy
Disorientation	Feeb tsis meej	ສັບສົນ	Bối Rối Mất Định Hướng
Dizziness	Kiv taubhau	ູ້ສຶກວິນຫົວ	Chóng mặt
Dyspnea	Txog Siav	ຫາຍໃຈຝືດ	Hụt Hơi Khó Thở
Fever	Kub cev	ເປັນໄຂ້	Sốt
Headache	Mob taubhau	ເຈັບຫົວ	Nhức Đầu
Hemoptysis	Hnoos tau ntshav	ໄອອອກເລືອດ	Ho Khạc Ra Máu
Jaundice	Daj ntseg	ເປັນຂີ້ໝາກເຫລືອງ	Vàng Da
Loss of Appetite	Tsis qab los	ກິນເຂົ້າບໍ່ແຊບ	Biếng ăn
Loss of Consciousness (Unconscious)	Looj lawm	ໝົດສະຕິ (ສະຫລົບ)	Bất Tỉnh
Malaise	Nkees	ອາການບໍ່ສະບາຍ	Mệt Mỏi Uể Oải
Nausea	Xeev siab	ປວດຮາກ	Buồn Nôn
Pain	Mob	ເຈັບ/ປວດ	Đau Nhức
Rash	Ua xua	ຜື່ນແດງ	Da nổi mụn đỏ
Sore Throat	Mob cajpas	ເຈັບຄໍ	Đau Cổ Họng
Tremor	Tshee	ສັ່ນ	Run Rẩy
Vomiting	Ntuav	ຮາກ	Ói Mửa

Division of Communicable Disease Control IMM-835 (3/05)

glossary of Symptoms

Symptom	Arabic	Farsi	Armenian
Abnormal Bleeding	نزيف شديد غير طبيعي	خونریزی غیرعادی (آب نُرمال بلیدینگ)	Արտասովոր Արյունահոսություն
Chills	قشعريرة	لرز (چیلز)	Սարսռություն
Cough	سعال / كحة	سرفه (کاف)	Հազ
Diarrhea	إسهال	اسهال (دایِریا)	Լուծ
Disorientation	توهان	اختلال در جهت یابی (دیس اُرینتِیشِن)	Ապակողմնորոշում
Dizziness	دوخة/دوار	سرگیجه	Գլխապտույտ
Dyspnea	ضيقة نفس / صعوبة في التنفس	تنگی نفس (دیسپِنیا)	Անբավարար Շնչառություն
Fever	سخونة شديدة	تب (فیوِر)	Ջերմություն
Headache	صداع	سردرد (هِد اِک)	Գլխացավ
Hemoptysis	سعال مع بصق الدم / كحة مع بصق الدم	خلط خونی (هِمُپتا یسیس)	Արյունաբեր Հազ
Jaundice	الصفراء	یرقان . زردی (جاندیس)	Դեղնախտ
Loss of Appetite	فقدان الشهية/عدم الرغبة في الطعام	بی اشتهایی	Ախորժակի Կորուստ
Loss of Consciousness (Unconscious)	فقدان الوعي (فاقد الوعي)	ناهوشیاری (آنکانشِس نِس)	Ուշաթափություն (ուշակորույս լինել)
Malaise	تعب في الجسم كله	احساس بیحالی و ناخوشی، کوفتگی (مَلِیز)	Թուլություն
Nausea	ميل للتقيؤ/ غثيان	حال بهم خوردگی، تهوع (نازیا)	Սրտախառնություն
Pain	ألم	درد (پِین)	Ցավ
Rash	طفح	جوش و دانه های قرمز روی پوست (رَش)	Ցան
Sore Throat	ألم في الزور	گلو درد (سُرتُرت)	Կոկորդի Բորբոքում
Tremor	رعشة	لرزش و تکان غیر ارادی (ترِمُر)	Դող
Vomiting	تقيؤ	استفراغ (وامیتینگ)	Փսխումներ

Division of Communicable Disease Control IMM-835 (3/05)

Reproduced with permission from the California Department of Public Health, Immunization Branch

glossary of Symptoms

Symptom	Russian	Punjabi
Abnormal Bleeding	Кровотечение в брюшную полость	ਬਹੁਤ ਖ਼ੂਨ ਪੈਣਾ
Chills	Озноб	ਪਾਲਾ
Cough	Кашель	ਖੰਘ
Diarrhea	Понос	ਟੱਟੀਆਂ ਲੱਗਣਾ
Disorientation	Дезориентация	ਬੌਂਦਲਣਾ
Dizziness	Головокружение	ਚੱਕਰ ਆਉਣੇ
Dyspnea	Одышка	ਸਾਹ ਲੈਣ ਵਿਚ ਮੁਸ਼ਕਲ
Fever	Жар	ਬੁਖਾਰ
Headache	Головная боль	ਸਿਰਦਰਦ
Hemoptysis	Кровохарканье	ਖੰਘ ਨਾਲ ਖ਼ੂਨ ਆਉਣਾ
Jaundice	Желтуха	ਪੀਲੀਆ
Loss of Appetite	Потеря аппетита	ਭੁੱਖ ਨਾ ਲੱਗਣਾ
Loss of Consciousness (Unconscious)	Потеря сознания	ਬੇਹੋਸ਼ੀ
Malaise	Недомогание	ਕਮਜ਼ੋਰੀ
Nausea	Тошнота	ਜੀਅ ਕੱਚਾ ਹੋਣਾ
Pain	Боль	ਦਰਦ
Rash	Сыпь	ਧੱਫੜ
Sore Throat	Больное горло	ਗਲਾ ਦੁਖਣਾ
Tremor	Дрожь	ਕੰਬਣਾ
Vomiting	Рвота	ਉਲਟੀਆਂ

This glossary includes only the most common signs and symptoms of most communicable diseases. Disease investigators can use this as a supplement when interviewing non-English speaking clients. Languages included are the most common ones in California. A phonetic pronunciation supplement is available online for download at ***www.cdlhn.com.***

Division of Communicable Disease Control

IMM-835 (3/05)

Reproduced with permission from the California Department of Public Health, Immunization Branch

Glossary

Abstinence: Voluntarily refraining from indulging in practices such as sexual intercourse.

Accreditation: The process by which an institution is recognized as meeting specific predetermined standards of care.

Acculturation: The adjustment to a new culture.

Activities of daily living (ADL): Tasks that enable a person to meet his or her own basic needs, such as toileting, eating, and dressing.

Adolescence: The period between childhood and adulthood, which can be considered between the ages of 10 and 20.

Advance directive: A legal document that guides health-care personnel concerning a patient's wishes when that patient is no longer capable of making decisions.

Age-appropriate toys: Toys that are safe and promote the cognitive and motor development of a specific age group.

Ageism: Discrimination because of a person's age.

Alternative medicine: Therapies used *instead* of Western medical care.

Allele: A pairing of genes that contain specific inheritable characteristics.

Anticipatory grief: Grief that occurs before a loss.

Apgar score: A scoring system to evaluate the newborn at 1 and 5 minutes after birth.

Apoptosis: The programmed death of cells. Referred to as the biological clock, it leads to menopause and senescence.

Assisted suicide: An action of a person other than the patient to facilitate suicide.

Assistive devices: Items such as canes, walkers, and hearing aids that help a person maintain independent living.

Asynchronous: Not synchronous; Exhibiting asynchrony; not occurring at the same time, as when different parts of the body mature at different times causing an awkward appearance (e.g., during adolescence).

Atrophy: A decrease in the size of an organ or tissue.

Attachment: An affectionate bond that occurs over time as a result of interaction.

Autonomy: Functioning bond.

Behaviors: Individual responses or reactions to internal stimuli and external conditions.

Behavioral theories: Theories designed to explain the development of specific behaviors and suggest their relationships to other developing social skills.

Behaviorist theory: A theory that describes how and why behavioral learning alters behavior.

Beliefs: Cultural teachings of practices and values handed down for generations that determine how one behaves and responds to daily life and health-care practices.

Bereavement: A period of sadness and adjustment after the loss of a loved one.

Biology: An individual's genetic makeup (those factors with which he or she is born), family history (which may suggest risk for disease), and the physical and mental health problems acquired during life.

Biological clock: A programmed cell death that leads to menopause and deterioration associated with senescence.

Blended family: A family consisting of a mother or father, a stepparent, and children. One or both parents may bring children from a previous marriage or relationship to form a new, blended family.
Bonding: The development of a strong emotional attachment between individuals, such as a mother and her infant.
Cephalocaudal: The progression of the growth pattern that proceeds from head to toe.
Chromosome: A thread of protein and DNA contained in the nucleus of every cell.
Classical conditioning: Relates a positive or negative event to a specific behavior to promote or prevent that behavior from recurring.
Climacteric: The change of life in which hormonal shifts result in cessation of the reproductive ability in women and a corresponding decrease in sexual drive in men.
Clique: A social group with a fixed exclusive membership that shares similar interests, values, and tastes.
Cognitive style: A pattern of thought and reasoning.
Cognitive theories: Theories that focus on advancement of the development of thinking.
Coitus: Sexual intercourse.
Complementary medicine: Therapies used *together with* Western therapies.
Competence: Effective interactions; ability.
Conception: The union of the male sperm and female ovum; fertilization.
Condolence: The expression of sympathy or grieving together.
Cooperative play: A group of two or more children who cooperate by playing together.
Coping skill: A behavior that helps an individual adapt to or manage a stressful situation.
Corporal punishment: Spanking; focuses on the pain of the punishment and can role model aggression, in which case it will not accomplish the true goal of discipline.
Cultural assimilation: A process by which members of a specific cultural group lose some of the characteristics of that group and adapt to the practices of another group.
Cultural awareness: Recognizing the history of patients' ancestry or culture and how their customs influence the handling of problems, issues, or teachings.
Cultural care: Health-promotion activities initiated by a culturally competent health-care worker who enables a patient to modify health behaviors toward beneficial outcomes while respecting the patient's cultural values, beliefs, and practices.
Cultural competence: Involves cultural awareness, acceptance, and respect toward behaviors and practices that are different from one's own.
Cultural interventions: Interventions achieved when health-care information is presented in a way that includes specific cultural styles, colors, pictures, symbols, and so forth, that add credibility to the content by reflecting cultural values.
Cultural relativism: The concept that normalcy comes from the standard social practices of a specific culture.
Cultural sensitivity: Observing, using, and showing knowledge of culturally appropriate verbal language, body language, use of personal space, and gestures of respect toward family members while providing health care or teaching.
Cultural stereotyping: The assumption that all the people of one culture behave the same way and believe the same thing.
Culture: A set of learned values, beliefs, customs, and behaviors that is shared by interacting individuals, such as a family.
Culture shock: The effect of a sudden, drastic change in the cultural environment of an individual or family.

Defense mechanism: A reaction that is protective to the individual or helps conceal conflicts or anxieties.

Dental caries: Tooth decay.

Determinants of health: Genetic makeup, lifestyle behaviors, social and physical environment, and general policies and interventions that affect the health of the population.

Development: Indicates an increase in function and mastery of tasks for the specific phase in the lifespan.

Developmental stage: Patterns of development related to perception and response to environment.

Developmental task: A competency or skill that helps a person cope with the environment or advance personal development.

Discipline: A technique used to guide, teach, or correct behavior; it may include consequences but is not punishment.

Disengagement: Implies removing of emotional attachments to people, places, and objects.

Dizygotic: A type of twin that occurs when two ova are released at ovulation and each ovum is fertilized by a separate sperm.

Dominant gene: A gene that overpowers other genes so that its characteristics will be inherited.

Durable power of attorney for health care: A type of advance directive that gives decision-making power concerning health care to a person designated by the patient, to be used when the patient cannot speak for himself or herself.

Dysfunctional family: A family unit that does not offer consistency of membership or rules, may exhibit poor interpersonal relationships among its members, handles conflicts and problems poorly, and often cannot reach out to the community for help.

Early childhood: A period that includes children between the ages of 1 and 6. Early childhood is typically separated into two phases; ages 1 to 2 is the toddler phase, and ages 2 to 6 is the preschool phase.

Ectopic pregnancy: A pregnancy that occurs outside the uterus, usually in the fallopian tube.

Ejaculation: Release of sperm during orgasm.

Elder abuse: The infliction of harm or neglect through actions or acts of omission on an older person. The abuse can be physical, emotional, or financial and can include neglect or obstruction of personal rights.

Electra anxiety: Occurs when little girls compete with their mothers for love and attention from their fathers.

Empathy: Understanding how others feel.

Empowerment: Providing tools and knowledge to the family to enable informed participation in decision making.

Empty nest syndrome: When grown children start to leave home for the first time, causing parents to feel lonely or isolated.

En face: Face to face.

Engrossment: When fathers or significant others develop an intense focus on a newborn.

Ethnicity: A cultural pattern shared by people with the same cultural heritage. Language, preferred diet, specific customs, family roles, and religious beliefs are often shared among those with the same ethnicity.

Ethnocentrism: The belief that one's own culture is the standard of behavior and is better than other cultures.

Eulogy: A speech usually presented at the funeral ceremony intended to memorialize the deceased.

Euthanasia: An intentional act that causes death for the purpose of relieving pain and suffering.

Exercise: Specifically planned and structured repetitive activities designed for a level of calorie burning that increases endurance, balance, strength, or flexibility.

Expressive language: The ability to express thoughts in the words of a language.

Extrovert: An outgoing person who focuses on others in the environment.

Facebook depression: Depression that affects the teen who overuses social networking to the point of altering sleep and eating habits and isolating himself from peers and family, eventually succumbing to general depression.

Family: A basic human social system that involves commitment and interaction among its members.

Family systems theory: Theories that explain interconnected family functions and responses.

Federal Register: Federal legislation concerning health care is recorded and published in this document.

Fetal alcohol syndrome: A group of symptoms present in a newborn infant resulting from maternal ingestion of alcohol during pregnancy.

Fetus: An unborn infant from the ninth week of conception to birth.

Free radicals: When one ion of a molecule breaks off and is no longer paired. Free radicals produce a harmful effect on body tissues.

Funeral: An activity shortly after death involving a meaningful ceremony to remember the life of the deceased.

Gene therapy: Involves placing a therapeutic gene on the back of a virus vector, which will then carry the new gene into the cell that has a missing or defective gene.

Generativity: Contributing in a positive way to family or community. This contribution improves self-image and promotes subjective well-being.

Genetic code: The code contained in the genes of living cells that will determine what characteristics will be inherited.

Genetic counseling: The communication between a geneticist (a specialist in inherited conditions) and the parents regarding the risk of their infant inheriting genes that can result in an abnormality.

Genome: A complete set of chromosomes and DNA that contain all the genetic information in the human cell.

Geriatrics: The study of old age, including the biological, psychological, physiological, and sociological aspects of aging.

Gestation: The period between conception and birth.

Gestational diabetes: Diabetes that occurs during pregnancy.

Grief: The emotional response to a loss and is a process through which a survivor accepts the loss.

Growth: Indicates an increase in size.

Gonads: A term used to refer to ovaries in females and testicles in males.

Health indicators: The public health issues and concerns linked to the objectives of *Healthy People 2020*.

Health maintenance organization (HMO): A group medical practice that offers prepaid care for members.

Health status: Details concerning illness and other factors that affect health, which are measured by factors such as birth and death rates, life expectancy, and accessibility to health care.

Healthy People 2020: An evidence-based 10-year report card describing health-care accomplishments within the United States from the years 2000 to 2010 and a prescription for what needs to be done between now and the year 2020.

Homeopathy: The use of minute portions of chemicals for their healing power.
Hospice: A plan of terminal care that is based on the philosophy that death is a normal part of the life cycle. Hospice involves palliative care that meets the physical, psychological, spiritual, and social needs of the dying patient.
Hot flashes: A sensation caused by blood rushing to the surface of the skin as a result of dilation of capillaries.
Humanist theories: Theories that describe the influence of human experiences such as love and attachment on behavior and personality development.
Hysterectomy: Removal of the uterus.
Identity accommodation: Changing the concept of one's own identity to fit what is real, rather than what was dreamed or imagined.
Immune theory: A theory of aging that involves the concept that as one ages, the body finds it more difficult to tell the difference between healthy and defective cells.
Immunity: The body's resistance to disease-causing organisms.
Infant: The period between ages 4 weeks and 1 year.
Infant mortality rate: The number of deaths that occur before age 1 per 1000 live births.
Information processing: An input of information followed by a thought mechanism resulting in an output of judgment or decision making.
Informed consent: Providing the patient with information, in a language that the patient can understand, regarding the risks of, advantages to, and possible alternatives available for a medical or surgical procedure.
Initiative: The ability to take the first step or the leading movement.
Intimacy: Not only involving sexuality, intimacy involves developing a warm, trusting, honest relationship with another person with whom it is safe to be open and to express and share private thoughts.
Intimate partner violence: A term related to domestic violence, which can include psychological, physical, sexual, financial, and social abuses between intimate partners.
Introvert: A quiet person who focuses inwardly on himself or herself.
Latchkey children: Children who are allowed to remain without direct supervision, usually during the hours after school, because both parents work and extended family are not available to care for the children.
Late adulthood: The ages between 65 and 74 years.
Leading Health Indicators: Selected high-priority issues within *Healthy People 2020* for the current 10-year period.
Legacy: What one leaves to the world that may give a person a feeling of immortality; can be a child, grandchild, property, a culture, an organization, or writings.
Life expectancy: The average number of years a person born in a particular year is expected to live.
Looking-glass self: The development of a self-image by combining the way we portray ourselves to others and the way others evaluate us.
Managed care organization: An organization that standardizes medical practice guidelines to maintain the quality of care provided at the same time as it controls the costs of health care.
Medicaid: A type of federal welfare program in which benefits are provided on a basis of need or level of poverty.
Medicare: A type of a government-provided insurance program in which benefits are received after contributions are made through payroll deductions.
Menarche: The very first menstrual period.
Menopause: The cessation of the menstrual period as a result of hormonal changes in the body.

Menstrual cycle: Consists of (1) maturing of the egg in the ovary, (2) formation of blood and mucus in the lining of the uterus, (3) ovulation, and (4) expulsion of the unfertilized egg with the blood and mucous lining from the uterus. This cycle lasts approximately 28 days and repeats until menopause.
Middle adulthood: The ages between 40 and 60 years.
Middle childhood: The ages of children between 6 and 12 years.
Midlife crisis: A stressful period when an adult tries to make up for lost opportunities of the past or challenge the inevitability of the future.
Mnemonic technique: The use of rhymes for remembering certain things, such as the number of days in each month.
Monozygotic: A type of twin that develops when one single fertilized ovum separates into two separate embryos.
Moral behavior: Actions based on moral reasoning.
Moral reasoning: A capacity that develops in a child as he or she learns to understand rules and determine if an action is right or wrong.
Mourning: The outward expression of grief.
Multifetal: More than one fetus—that is, twins, triplets, quadruplets, septuplets.
Mutated: Malformed.
Neonatal: The first 30 days of life after birth.
Nocturnal emission: Ejaculation of semen during sleep.
Nonverbal language: The language of the motions, postures, and gestures of the body that is learned as part of communication.
Norms: Averages that can be used as guidelines for comparison concerning, for example, the age that specific abilities or skills are achieved or disappear.
Nurse practice acts: The scope of practice for each level of professional practice in nursing.
Nursing caries: Tooth decay that occurs when the infant is put to bed while sucking on a bottle of milk or juice. The milk or juice pools in the mouth, allowing bacterial organisms to grow.
Nursing Licensure Compact: A multistate licensing arrangement that enables traveling nurses to function in multiple states.
Object permanence: Knowing an object is there even though it is not within sight.
Occupational Health and Safety Act (OSHA): Standards of safety that must be maintained by employers to protect the health and safety of employees; mandates reporting of injuries sustained by workers.
Oedipus complex: Arises during the phallic stage of development. Freud suggested that little boys compete with their father for the mother's love and attention.
Operant conditioning: Involves behavioral consequences such as reward or punishment.
Ordinal position: Birth order; whether the infant is an only child, older child, youngest child, or middle child may influence the age and rapidity of mastering developmental tasks.
Oropharynx: The part of the anatomy that includes the mouth and throat.
Osteoporosis: The loss of bone mass.
Ovulation: Release of a matured egg from the ovary into the fallopian tube that leads to the uterus.
Palliative care: Total care of patients whose disease is not responsive to curative therapy.
Parallel play: When a young child plays next to a friend but does not interact with the friend during play.
Pelvic inflammatory disease: A serious complication of some sexually transmitted diseases (STDs), especially chlamydia and gonorrhea, that infects the uterus, fallopian tubes, and other reproductive organs.

Personality: A unique combination of characteristics that results in the individual's recurrent pattern of behavior.
Physical activity: Daily actions that use energy, such as dog walking or gardening.
Physical environment: Things that can be seen, touched, heard, smelled, and tasted and less tangible elements, such as radiation and ozone.
Pincer grasp: The ability to pick up small objects with the thumb and forefinger.
Plan of care: A tool for communication among multidisciplinary health care team members.
Plaque: A sticky, transparent mass of bacteria that grows on the surface and spreads to the roots of teeth.
Political action committees (PACs): Groups that influence governmental legislation by offering monetary contributions to legislators who support their needs and that provide lobbying efforts to create an awareness of needed legislation.
Polypharmacy: The ingestion of multiple medications in 1 day.
Postformal operational thought: The process of integrating various points of view to develop knowledge and understanding.
Posttraumatic stress disorder (PTSD): The development of characteristic symptoms following an extreme traumatic stressor.
Preferred provider organization (PPO): An organization that contracts with professionals in the medical field to provide care to a specific group of patients at an agreed-on fee-for-service rate.
Preschool phase: Age between 2 and 6 years.
Preverbal: Body language before the ability to speak.
Psychodynamic theories: Theories that focus on personality trait development and psychological challenges at different ages.
Proximodistal: From the midline of the body to the periphery.
Puberty: The age at which sexual maturity occurs; having the functional ability to reproduce. Puberty involves physical and psychological changes.
Receptive language: Ability to understand words.
Relatedness: A sense of belonging.
Reproductive health: A term used to describe the health of the reproductive organs in males and females.
Sandwich generation: A period in middle adulthood when persons must deal with increased financial and emotional responsibilities related to their children and increased demands placed on them by their older and possibly dependent parents.
Scope of practice: "The identification of and legal limitations to the usual and customary skill practices of a professional. The usual and customary practices are determined by the educational preparation for that profession" (from Nurse Practice Act, Business and Professional Code).
Secondary sex characteristics: The development of pubic, facial, and body hair; also, in boys the enlargement and darkening of the scrotum and an increase in penis size; in girls the enlargement of breasts and darkening around the areola.
Senescence: A period in an adult's life in which the body begins to age and weaken more noticeably.
Separation anxiety: When an infant cries or protests when the parent leaves the room or when a stranger approaches. Separation anxiety usually emerges after 6 months of age.

Sexuality: Beliefs and behaviors that surround physiological responses, emotions, and sociocultural values. Involves communication, a sense of closeness, and mutual comfort.
Sexually transmitted disease (STD): Disease that is transmitted through sexual intercourse and in some cases through oral copulation (oral sex).
Sexting: The sending or receiving of sexually explicit text messages and pictures.
Sibling rivalry: The competition between brothers and sisters, usually for parental attention and love.
SIDS: Sudden infant death syndrome.
Social cognition: An awareness and understanding of how a person's actions may affect other people. When children begin to understand social cognition, it enables them to cooperate better with peers, and it can enhance the child's self-concept.
Social environment: Interactions with family, friends, coworkers, and others in the community and social institutions, such as law enforcement, the workplace, places of worship, and schools.
Sociocultural theories: Theories that describe how culture influences behavior.
Social learning theory: Involves exposure to and imitation of a behavior.
Somatic: Pertaining to the body.
Spermatogenesis: The production of sperm.
Stagnation: The failure to achieve generativity.
Standards of practice: Guidelines used to determine type and quality of care provided to patients.
Stereotyping: Assuming that all people from a specific cultural or ethnic group behave or believe the same way.
Syndrome: A group of symptoms or signs of an abnormal condition.
Testicular self-examination (TSE): Self-examination of the testicles.
Theory: A group of concepts that forms the basis for understanding observations. An accepted theory is logical, consistent, and integrates past and current research.
Therapeutic communication: A form of communication that involves accepting the patient's emotional outbursts and expressions and encouraging venting and verbalization.
Therapeutic presence: Remaining near the patient and family, or simply holding a hand, thus providing strength while facilitating emotional expressions in patients and families during times of grief or stress.
Time-out: A form of discipline implemented as a response to unacceptable behavior. Effective discipline technique for children between the ages of 1 and 6 years.
Toddler phase: Period between the ages of 1 and 2 years.
Transitional phase: A period of young adulthood during which life choices are reviewed and reevaluated, and changes may be made.
Values: Deep feelings about what is right or wrong, good or bad.
Vaginal birth after cesarean (VBAC): A controversial practice in which a woman who previously had a cesarean section attempts to delivery a subsequent baby vaginally.
Viable: Able to survive outside the uterus.
Vigorous exercise: At least 20 minutes of exercise that causes sweating or breathing hard.
Virus vector: A virus that has the ability to enter specific cells in the body and act as a vehicle to carry substances to that cell.
Wear-and-tear theory: Like machinery, parts of the human body begin to wear out or break down over time.
Young adult: Person between the ages of 20 and 39 years.

Bibliography and Online Resources

CHAPTER 1 *HEALTHY PEOPLE 2020*

Anglin T: *Making Healthy People 2020 come alive for promoting adolescent health*, City Maternal Child Annual Conference, September 2010, Washington, DC, 2011, DHHS Maternal Child Bureau.

Berlinguer G: Globalization and global health, *Int J Health* 29 (3): 579-595, 1999.

Brundtland G: *Fifth Global Conference on Health Promotion*, Mexico City, June 5, 2000, from www.who.int/director-general/speeches/200/20000605_mexico.html.

Center for Disease Control and Prevention: Recent trends in infant mortality. In: *US: The Measure of America*, Washington DC, 2008, CDC.

Centers for Disease Control and Prevention (CDC): National Center for Health Statistics, Healthy People 2000 renew—review 1998–99, Atlanta, GA, 2000, CDC.

Davis L, Okuboye S, Ferguson S: Healthy People 2010: examining a decade of maternal-infant health, *Lifelines* 4 (3), 26-33, 2000.

U.S. Department of Health and Human Services (USDHHS): *Health: United States, 1989, and prevention profile*, Pub No (PHS) 90–1232. Hyattsville, MD, 1990, DHHS.

U.S. Department of Health and Human Services (USDHHS): *Healthy people 2010: national health promotion and disease prevention objectives*, Pub No 91–50213, Washington, DC, 1990, U.S. Government Printing Office.

U.S. Department of Health and Human Services Center for Medicare and Medicaid Services: Medicare Claims Data, Baltimore, MD, Feb 22, 2010, CMS, from www.CMS.Gov/preventiongeninfo/20_prevserv.asp. Accessed November 11, 2011.

Department of Health, Education and Welfare (DHEW): *Healthy people: the Surgeon General's report on health promotion and disease prevention*, PHS Pub No 79–55071, Washington, DC, 1979, DHEW.

Halton N: *Life course health development: a new approach for addressing upstream determinants of health and spending*, Washington, DC, 2009, Expert Voices, NIH Care Management Foundation.

Inman D, Van Bahergem K, La Rosa A, Garr D: Evidence based health promotion programs for schools and communities, *Prev Med* 40 (2): 207-219, 2011.

Institute of Medicine: *Commission of future health care workforce for older Americans: retooling for an aging America*. Washington, DC, 2008, National Academies Press.

Kubiszewski I: *The UN Millinium Declaration Summit of 2005*, Encyclopedia of Earth, New York, 2008, UN, from www.eoearth.org/article/united_nations_millenium_declaration. Accessed December 1, 2011.

U.S. Department of Health and Human Services (USDHHS): *Healthy people 2000: national health promotion and disease prevention objectives*, PHS Pub No 91–50213. Washington, DC, 1990, U.S. Government Printing Office.

Messias DH: Globalization, nursing and health for all, *J Nurs Scholarship: An Official Publication of Sigma Theta Tau International Honor Society of Nursing*, 33 (1):9, 2001.

MMWR Weekly Quickstats: Adolescent Death Rates 15-19 years of age in US 1985-2006, *Nov 7, 2008* 57 (44):1207, 2008.

National Center for Health Statistics: *Healthy people renew 1998–1999*, Hyattsville, MD, Washington, DC, 1999, U.S. Government Printing Office.

Obama B: *Issues in education: the race to the top*. Commencement Address, Memphis, TN, 2011, Booker T. Washington High School.

U.S. Department of Health and Human Services (USDHHS) Centers for Disease Control and Prevention: *Healthy people 2010: national vital statistics system*. McClean, VA, 1999, International Medical Publisher.

United Nations: *United Nations millinium declaration 6th Plenary meeting of the UN*, September 8, 2000, New York, 2000, Encyclopedia of Earth.

Quinton S: HHS releases leading health indicators for the next decade, *National J* 2011.

U.S. Department of Health and Human Services (USDHHS): *Healthy people 2010*, ed 2, Washington, DC, 2000, U.S. Government Printing Office.

WHO First International Conference on Health Promotion: Ottawa, Canada, Nov 21, 1986, from www.who.int/hpr/archive/docs/ottowa.html.

WHO: *WHO report on global public health security in the 21st century*, Geneva, Switzerland, 2007, from www.who.int/whr/2007/en/index.htm. Accessed November 11, 2011.

WHO: World *health statistics: progress in the health related millenium development goals fact sheet 290*, New York, 2010, WHO Information System.

Online Resources

www.health.gov/healthypeople
www.cdc.gov/nchs/hphome.htm
www.who.int/director-general/speeches/200/20000605/mexico.html

CHAPTER 2 GOVERNMENT INFLUENCES ON HEALTH CARE

Advisory Commission on Consumer Protection and Quality in Health Care Industry: *Quality first: better health care for all Americans*, Washington, DC, 1999, U.S. Government Printing Office.

American Hospital Association: *The patient care partnership: hospitals in pursuit of excellence*, from www.HPOE.org, 2009. Accessed November 11, 2011.

American Hospital Association: *Hospital care and systems of the future*, Chicago, 2011, AHA, TheInaugural Report of AHA Committee on Performance Improvement, from www.AHA.org/AHA/issues/communicating-with-patients/pt-care-partnership.html. Accessed November 1,2011.

Burcham M: Credentialing alternative medicine: a challenge for managed care organizations, *Manag Care Q* 7 (2):39, 1999.

Census Bureau: *Families and living arrangements*, Washington, DC, 2011, U.S. Census Bureau, Housing and Economic Statistics Division.

Chen I, Richter P, Miner L: FDA's new role in tobacco control, *Contemp Pediatr* 28 (11):39-45, 2011.

Danziger S, Oltmans K, Ananat E, Browning K: Childcare subsidies and transition from welfare to work. *Fam Relat* 52 (2):25-27, 2004.

Ewen D: *The Senate's 6 billion child care provision: a critical but modest investment*, Washington, DC, 2005, CLASP Center for Law and Social Policy.

Gordon S: Social media has good and bad effects on kids. *Healthy Day News*, March 28, 2011.

Hollenberg D: How do CAM therapies affect integrative care in a publicly funded health care system? *J Compliment Alternat Integrative Med* 14 (1):5-15, 2007.
Institute of Medicine: *Informing the future: critical issues in health care*, ed 6, Washington, DC, 2011a, National Academies Press.
Institute of Medicine: *The future of nursing: leading change, advancing health*, Washington, DC, 2011b, National Academies Press.
Knight W: *Managed care: what it is and how it works*, Gaithersburg, MD, 1998, Aspen Publishers.
Levy D, editor: *State by state guide to managed care law*. Gaithersburg, MD, 1999, Aspen Publishers.
Matthews H, Ewen D: *Presidential budget projects 300,000 low income children to lose child care by 2010*. Washington, DC, 2004, CLASP (Center for Law and Social Policy).
National Council of State Boards of Nursing: *Revised model of NPA and nursing administrative rules accepted by delegate assembly of NCSBN*. Article XViii and Chapter 18, 2008, from www.ncsbn.org. Accessed November 2011.
NCSBN: *Nursing licensure compact act fact sheet*, 2011, from www.ncsbn.org. Accessed December 2011.
Needell B: *Child Welfare Services Reports For California*, 2011, University Of California at Berkley Center for Social Services Research accesses 11/11 at http://CSSR.Berkley.EDU/254376childrenenteredfostercare/UCB/childwelfare.
U.S. Department of Health and Human Services (USDHHS): *Healthy People 2010*, ed 2, Washington, DC, 2000, U.S. Government Printing Office.
USDHHS: *Adoption and Foster Care Analysis and Report System (AFLARS) 2010 Data*, USDHHS Children and Family Services Bureau, 2011, from www.ACF.HHS.gov/programs/CB.
President's Advisory Committee on Consumer Protection and Quality in the Health Care Industry: *Consumer bill of rights and responsibilities*, 2009, from www.healthcarequality-commission.gov/final/append_a.html. Accessed October 20, 2011.
Reinhard S: *Consumer directed care and nurse practice acts*. Center for State Health Policy, 2001, from http://aspe.hhs.gov/daltcp/reports/2001/nursprac.pdf. Accessed November 2011.
Steinbrook R: Health care and the American Recovery and Reinvestment Act of 2009. *New Engl J Med* 360:1057-1061, 2010, from www.NIM.NIH.gov/medlineplus/patientrights.html.
United States Office of Personnel Management: *Patient's bill of rights*, 2009, from www.opm.gov/insure/health/billrights.asp#. Accessed October 20, 2011.

Online Resources

http://www.aha.org/about/org/hospitals-care-systems-future.shtml
www.dranonymous.com/dranon.html
www.healthcarelawnet.com/
www.bt.cdc.gov
www.NCSL.org
www.hpts.org
WWW.FDA.gov/tobaccoproducts/default.htm
Http://smokefree.gov
HTTP://teens.drugabuse.gov

CHAPTER 3 CULTURAL CONSIDERATIONS ACROSS THE LIFESPAN AND IN HEALTH AND ILLNESS

Agency for Health Care Research and Quality: Planning culturally and linguistically appropriate services: a guide for managed care plans. Rockville, MD, 2003, Agency for Health Care Research and Quality, from www.AHRQ.GOV/populations/planclas.htm. Accessed January 2012.

Callister L, Eads M, Diehl J: Perceptions of giving birth and adherence to cultural practices in Chinese women. *MCN* 36 (6):387-394, 2011.

Catalano J: *Nursing now*, ed 4, Philadelphia, 2006, FA Davis.

Cherry B, Jacob S: *Contemporary nursing issues trends and management*, ed 5, Philadelphia, 2011, Mosby Elsevier.

Flin R: Measuring safety, culture and behavior change in health care, *Safety Sci* 45 (6): 101-104, 2007.

Giger J, Davidhizer R: *Transcultural nursing*, ed 4, Philadelphia, 2004, Mosby.

Gupta V: Impact of culture on health care, *J Cult Diver* 17 (1):13-17, 2010.

Halligan M: Safety culture in health care: a review of concepts, dimensions, measures and progress, *Brit Med J* 20:338-343, 2011.

Huang A, Subak L, Thom D: Sexual function and aging in racially and ethnically diverse women, *J Am Geriatr Soc* 57:1362-1368, 2009.

Kavanaugh K, Knowlden V: *Many voices: toward a caring culture in healthcare and healing*, vol 3, Madison, WI, 2004, University of Wisconsin Press.

Kavanaugh K, Kennedy P: *Promoting cultural diversity strategies for health care*, LA California, 1992, Sage Publications.

Nash D: National priorities partnership: national priorities and goals-aligning our efforts to transform America's health care (Washington, DC), *Pharm Therapeutics* 34 (2):1-61, 2009.

Pender N, Murdaugh C, Parsons M: *Health promotion in nursing practice*, New York, 2011, Pearson.

Spector R: *Cultural diversity in health and illness*, Englewood Cliffs, NJ, 2000, Prentice Hall.

Taylor O: *Nature of communication disorders in culturally and linguistically diverse population*, California, 1986, College Hill Press.

USDHHS: *Culturally and linguistically appropriate services: standards of care*, Office of Minority Health and Resources for Health Care, 2011, from www.OMHRC.Gov/clas/po.htm. Accessed January 2012.

Watson A: *The art and science of human caring*, Los Angeles California, 1999, Sage Publications.

Wold G: *Basic geriatric care*, ed 4, Philadelphia, 2008, Mosby/Elsevier.

Online Resources

www.hrsa.gov/culturalcompetence/index.html
www.amsa.org/AMSA/homepage/about/committees/reach.aspx
www.ncbi.nim.nih.gov/books/nbk44249
www.culturediversity.org/provc.htm
www.OMHRC.gov/CLAS/po.HTM
www.AHRQ.gov/populations/planclas.htm

CHAPTER 4 THE INFLUENCE OF FAMILY ON DEVELOPING A LIFESTYLE

American Psychiatric Association: *Diagnostic and statistical manual of mental disorders*, ed 4, text rev, Washington, DC, 2000, American Psychiatric Association.

APA: *Diagnostic and statistical manual of mental disorders*, DSM5, Washington, DC, 2012, APA 2013 (5th edition).

Baronowski T, Nader P: Family health behavior. In Turk D, Kerns R, editors: *Health, illness and family*, New York, 1985, Wiley [classic].

Blackwell D, Blackwell J: Building alternative families, *Lifelines AWHONN* 3 (5):45-48, 2000.

Bowlby J: *Maternal care and mental health*, New York, 1951, Columbia University Press [classic].

Bucher L, Klemm P, Adepoju J: Fostering cultural competence: a multicultural care plan. *J Nurs Ed* 35 (7):334, 1996.

Chartrand M, Frank D, White L, Shope T: Effects of parents' wartime deployment on behavior of young children in military families, *Arch Ped/Adolesc Med* 162 (11):1009-1114, 2008.

Duvall E, Miller B: *Marriage and family development*, ed 6, New York, 1985, Harper and Row [classic].

Elhai J, Palmieri P: The factor structure of PTSD: a literature update. *J Anxiety Disord* 25:849-854, 2011.

Eth S, Pynoos R, editors: *PTSD in children*, Washington, DC, 1985, American Psychiatric Press [classic].

Gordon S: Social media has good and bad effects on kids; Healthy Days News, *U.S. News and World Report*, March 28, 2011.

Graham J, Forstadt L: *Child development and screen time: bulletin #4100*, University of Maine, 2010, Cooperative Extension Publications, from www.HTTP://UofMaine.EDU/publications/4100e. Accessed 2011.

Hae-Jung Song E, Anderson J: How violent videogames may violate children's health, *Contemp Pediatr* 18 (5):102, 2001.

Havighurst R: *Developmental tasks and education*, New York, 1974, David McKay [classic].

Jensen P, Shaw J: Children as victims of war: current knowledge and future research needs, *J Am Acad Child Adolesc Psychiatr* 32:697, 1993.

Kaiser Family Foundation: *Generation M2: media in the lives of 8-18 year olds*, 2010, from www.KFF.org/entmedia. Accessed November 2011.

Kim H: Children of divorced parents often fall behind classmates in math and social skills, *Am Soc Rev* 78 (3):487-511, 2011.

Koepp M, Gunn RN, Lawrence AD, et al: Evidence for striatal dopamine release during a video game, *Nature*, 393:266, 1998.

Levine M, Carey W, Crocker A: *Developmental-behavioral pediatrics*, ed 3, Philadelphia, 1999, WB Saunders. Also found at Carey W, Crocker A, Elias E, Feldman H, Coleman W: *Developmental and behavioral pediatrics*, ed 5, Philadelphia, 2008, Elsevier.

Meijer A: Child psychiatric sequelae of maternal war stress, *Acta Psychiatr Scand* 75:205, 1985.

Monahon C: *Children and trauma: a guide for parents and professionals*, San Francisco, 1997, Jossey Bass.

Needell B: *Child welfare services reports for California*, University of California at Berkley, 2011, Center for Social Services Research, from http://kidsdata.org/childwelfare. Accessed November 2011.

Needell B: *Child Welfare Services Reports For California,* 2011, University Of California at Berkley Center for Social Services Research accesses 11/11 at http://CSSR.Berkley.EDU/254376 childrenenteredfostercare/UCB/childwelfare.
Pagani L, Fitzpatrick C, Barnett T, Dubow E: Prospective association between early childhood TV exposure and academic, psychosocial, and physical well-being by middle childhood. *Arch Ped/Adolesc Med* 64 (5):425-431, 2010.
Pender N, Murdaugh C, Parsons M: *Health promotion in nursing practice*, ed 6, New York, 2011, Pearson.
Pfefferbaum B, Seale TW, McDonald NB, et al: Post-traumatic stress 2 years after the Oklahoma City bombing in youths geographically distant from the explosion, *Psychiatry* 63:358, 2000.
Popenoe D: The family transformed, *Fam Affairs* 2:1, 1989 [classic].
Rupured M, Smith P, Qiuck S: TV: Friend or Foe? *Res Fam Childr Newsletter* 6 (2):10-13, 2007.
Shaefer R: *Sociology: a brief introduction*, ed 4, Boston, 2002, McGraw-Hill.
Smilkstein G, Ashworth C, Montano D: The validity and reliability of the family Apgar as a test of family function, *J Fam Pract* 15:303, 1982.
Smilkstein G: The family Apgar: a proposal for a family function test and its use by physicians, *J Fam Pract* 6 (6):1231 [classic].
Sugar M: Toddlers' traumatic memories, *J Ment Health* 13:245, 1992.
Swerdlow J: Global cultures, *Natl Geogr* 196 (2):110-127, 1999.
U.S. Department of Health and Human Services (USDHHS): *Psychosocial issues for children and families in disasters,* Washington, DC, 1995, U.S. Government Printing Office.
White J: *Dynamics of family development: a theoretical perspective*, New York, 1991, Guilford Press.

Online Resources

www.NMHA.org
www.act.hhs.gov/prams/cb/dis/table/entryexit.htm
www.urban.org

CHAPTER 5 THEORIES OF DEVELOPMENT

Arlin P: Cognitive development in adulthood: a 5th stage? *Dev Psychol* 11:602, 1975 [classic].
Bandura A: *Social learning theory*, Englewood Cliffs, NJ, 1977, Prentice-Hall [classic].
Brofenbrenner U: *The ecology of human development*, Cambridge, MA, 1979, Harvard University Press [classic].
DuVall E: *Marriage and family development*, Philadelphia, 1977, JB Lippincott [classic].
Funder D: *Studying lives through time: personality and development*, Washington, DC, 1993, American Psychology Association.
Gormly A, Brodzinsky D: *Lifespan human development*, Philadelphia, 1989, Harcourt Brace [classic].
Havighurst R: *Developmental tasks and education*, New York, 1974, D. McKay [classic].
Kohlberg L: Development of moral character and moral ideology. In Hoffman H, Hoffman L, editors: *Review of child development research*, New York, 1964, Russell Sage [classic].
Kegan R: *The evolving of self: a theory of human development*, Cambridge, MA, 1982, Howard Press [classic].

Levinson DJ, Darrow CN, Klein EB: *The seasons of a man's life*, New York, 1978, Knopf [classic].
Loevinger J: *Scientific ways in the study of ego development*, Worchester, MA, 1979, Clark University Press [classic].
Piaget J: *The language of the child*, Philadelphia, 1926, Harcourt Brace [classic].
Skinner B: *Verbal behavior*, New York, 1987, Appleton-Century-Croft [classic].
Vygotsky L: *Thoughts and language*, Cambridge, MA: 1962, MIT Press [classic].

CHAPTER 6 PRENATAL INFLUENCES ON HEALTHY DEVELOPMENT

Barker D: *Mothers, babies and health in later life*, Philadelphia, 1998, Churchill-Livingstone.
Barker D, et al: Relationship of small head circumference and thinness at birth to death from cardiovascular disease in adult life, *Br Med J* 306:422, 1993.
Boake C: From Binet-Simon to Wechsler-Bellevue: tracing the history of intelligence testing, *J Clin Experimental Neuropsy* 24:383-405, 2002.
Brazelton T: *The neonatal behavioral assessment scale*, Philadelphia, 1973, JB Lippincott [classic].
Bronfenbrenner U, Ceci S: Heredity and environment and the question of "how?" In Plomin R, McLearn G, editors: *Nature, nurture and psychology*, Washington DC, 1993, American Psychological Association.
Burton G, Barker D, Moffitt A, Thornberg K: *The placenta and developmental programming*, Cambridge, 2011, Cambridge University Press.
Carey W, Crocker A, Elias E, Feldman H, Coleman W: *Developmental-behavioral pediatrics*, ed 4, Philadelphia, 2008, Elsevier.
Curhan G, Willet WC, Rimm EB, et al: Birth weight and adult hypertension and obesity in women, *Circulation* 94:1310, 1996.
Fall C: Fetal and early life origins of adult disease, *India J Pediatrics* 40 (5):480-502, 2003, on Pubmed 12768060. Accessed November 2011.
Flynn J: Massive IQ gains in 14 nations: what IQ tests really measure, *Psychol Bull* 101:171, 1987 [classic].
Gale C, O'Callaghan J, Bredow M, Christopher M: The influence of head growth in fetal life, infancy and childhood on later intelligence at 4-8 years, *J Ped* 118 (4):1486-1492, 2006.
Gluckman P, Hanson M, Spencer H, Bateson P: Environmental influence during pregnancy and their later consequences for health and disease later in life: implication for interpretation of empirical studies, *J Prac Biological Sci* 272 (1564):671-677, 2005.
Godfrey K, Barker D: Fetal nutrition and adult disease, *Amer J Clinical Nutrition* 71 (5):13445-13528, 2000.
Gopnik A, Meltzoff A, Kuhl P: *The scientist in the crib*, New York, 1999, Harper Collins.
Goldberg G, Prentice A: Maternal and fetal determinants of adult diseases, *Nutrit Rev* 52:191, 1994.
Goodwin S: Advances in genetics, New York, 2011, Academic Press.
Leifer G: *Introduction to maternity and pediatric nursing*, ed 6, Philadelphia, 2011, WB Saunders, an imprint of Elsevier.
NioLon R: *Are IQ tests biased?* 2005, from www.Psychpage.com. Accessed November 2011.
Petra R: Undernutrition during childhood leads to greater risk of heart disease in later life, *Medical World News Today,* 2011, from www.medicalnewstoday.com/articles/233354.php. Accessed November 2011.

Plomin R, McClearn GE, Smith DL, et al: DNA markers associated with high versus low IQ: the IQ quantitive trait loci project (QTL), *Behav Genet* 24:107, 1994.

Rich-Edwards J, et al: Birth weight and the risk of cardiovascular disease in a cohort of women followed up since 1976, *Br Med J* 315:396, 1997.

Rines K, Romundstad P, Nilsen T, Eskild A, Vatten L: Placental weight relative to birthweight and long term cardiovascular mortality, *Am J Epidemiol* 170 (5):622-631, 2009.

Rubin R: Maternal touch at first contact with the newborn infant, *Nurs Outlook* 11:828, 1963 [classic].

Shaheen S, et al: Relationship between pneumonia in early childhood and impaired lung function in late adult life, *Am J Resp Crit Care Med* 149:616, 1994.

Shenkin S, Bastin M, Macgillivray T, Deary I, Starr J, Wordlaw J: Birth parameters are associated with late-life white matter integrity in community-dwelling older people, *Stroke* 40:1225-1228, 2009, from at http://stroke.altajournals.org. Accessed November 2011.

Spahis J: Human genetics: constructing a family pedigree, *Am J Nurs* 102 (7):44-50, 2002.

Stein C, Kiemaran K, Shaheen S: Relationship of fetal growth to adult lung function in South India, *Thorax* 52:895, 1997.

Thompson J: Fetal nutrition and adult hypertension, diabetes, obesity and coronary artery disease, *Neonatal Network* 26 (4):235-240, 2007.

Tinkle M, Cheek D: Human genomics: challenges and opportunities, *J Obstet Gynecol Neonatal Nurs* 31 (2):188, 2002.

Weiss L, Sakiofski D, Prifitera A, Holfnak J: *WISC-IV: advanced clinical interpretation*, New York, 2006, Academic Press, Elsevier.

Williams J: Impact of genome research on children and their families, *J Pediatr Nurs* 15 (4):207-211, 2000.

Online Resources

www.jjpi.com/portal/jnj/jjpi

www.NHGRI.nih.gov/

www.ORNL.GOV/TechResources/human_genome/resource/elsi.hml

www.genesage.com

WWW.surgeongeneral.gov/initiatives/healthy-fit-nation/obesityvision2010.pdf

CHAPTER 7 THE INFANT

American Heart Association (AHA): Dietary guidelines revised for the new millennium, *Clinician Rev* 11 (8):58, 2001.

Atkinson W, et al: General recommendations immunizations: recommendations of the advisory committee on immunization practices, *MMWR* 51 (RR2):1-34, 2002.

Betz C: Healthy children 2010: implications for pediatric nursing practice, *J Pediatr Nurs* 17 (3):153, 2002.

Biagroll F: Proper use of child safety seats, *Am Fam Physician* 65 (10):2085, 2002.

Cahill J, Wagner C: Challenges in breastfeeding, *Contemp Pediatr* 19 (5):94, 2002.

Carey W, Crocker A, Elias E, Feldman H, Coleman W: *Developmental-behavioral pediatrics*, ed 4, Philadelphia, 2008, Elsevier.

Cordon I, Pipe M, Sayfan L, Melinder A, Goodman G: Memory for traumatic experiences in early childhood, *Dev Rev* 24:101-132, 2003, from www.ScienceDirect.com. Accessed November 2011.

Erikson E: *The life cycle completed: a review*, New York, 1994, WW Norton.

Evers D: Teaching mothers about childhood immunizations, *MCN: Am J Mater Child Nurs* 25 (5):253, 2001.

Fowles E: Brazelton neonatal behavior scale, *MCN: Am J Mater Child Nurs* 24 (6):287, 1999.

Gaensbauer T: Trauma in the preverbal period: symptoms, memories, and developmental impact, *Psychoanal Study Child* 50, 122, 1995.

Gainsbauer T: Representation of trauma in infancy: clinical and theoretical implications for understanding early memory, *J Inf Mental Health* 23 (3):259-277, 2002.

Howe J: *The fate of early memories: developmental science and retention of early memories*, Washington, DC, 2000, American Psychological Association.

Kleigman R, Stanton B, St. Geme J, Schor N, Behrman R: *Nelson's textbook of pediatrics*, St Louis, 2011, Elsevier.

Leifer G: *Introduction to maternity and pediatric nursing*, ed 6, Philadelphia, 2011, WB Saunders.

Lund C, Kuller J, et al: Neonatal skin care, *J Obstet, Gynecol Neonatal Nurs* 30 (1):30, 2001.

Medoff-Cooper B, et al: Nutritive sucking and neurobehavioral development in preterm infants, *MCN: Am J Mater Child Nurs* 25 (2):64, 2000.

Monastersky R: Look who's listening: new research shows babies employ many tricks to pick up language, *Chron Higher Ed* July 6:14, 2001.

Moon R: Are you talking to your parents about SIDS? *Contemp Pediatr* 18 (3):94, 2001.

National Association for Sports and Physical Education (NASPE): *Active start: a statement of physical activity guidelines for children: birth to age 5*, ed 2, Reston, Va, 2009, NASPE.

Olsen R, Barbaresi W: Development in the first year of life, *Contemp Pediatr* 15 (7):49, 1998.

Page-Geortz S, McCammon S, Westdahl C: Breastfeeding promotion, *Lifelines* 5 (1):41, 2001.

Paley J, Alpert J: Memory of infant trauma, *J Psychoanal Psychol* 20:329-347, 2003.

Roberts S, Dallal G: New childhood growth charts, *Nutrition Rev* 59 (2):31, 2001.

USDA: *Infant nutrition and feeding: a guide for use in the WIC and CSF programs*, Washington, DC, 2009, U.S. Department of Agriculture, Food and Nutrition Service, Special supplemental nutrition program for women, infants and children (WIC), Chapter 7: Physical activity in infancy, from www.nal.usda.gov/wicworks/topics/fg/chapter7_physicalactivity.pdf. Accessed November 2011.

U.S. Department of Agriculture, Food and Nutrition Service: *Physical activity in children special supplement*, Chapter 7: Infant nutrition and feeding: a guide for use in the WIC and CSF programs, Washington, DC, 2011, U.S. Department of Food and Nutrition, from www.nal.usda.gov/wicworks//topics/fg/chapter7_PhysicalActivity.pdf. Accessed November 2010.

Velsor-Fredrich B: Healthy people 2010: health appraisal of the nation and future objectives. *J Pediatr Nurs* 15 (1):47, 2000.

Wallerstedt C, Fletcher B: Teaching with toys, *Lifelines* 4 (4):45, 2000.

Online Resources

www.brightfutures.org/mentalhealth/index.HTML

www.jppi.com/portal/jnj/jjp

WWW.surgeongeneral.gov/initiatives/healthy-fit-nation/obesityvision2010.pdf

CHAPTER 8 EARLY CHILDHOOD

American Academy of Pediatric Dentistry: Guideline on infant oral health care, *AAPD Ref Manual* 33 (6):11-12, 2011.

American Academy of Pediatrics: Communication on psychological aspects of child and family health: guidance for effective discipline, *Pediatrics* 101:723, 1998.

American Academy of Pediatrics: Child passenger safety, *Pediatrics* 127 (4):788-793, 2012.

Banks JB: Childhood discipline: challenges for clinicians and parents, *Am Fam Physician* 66 (8):1447-1452, 2002.

Behrman R, Kliegman R, Jenson H: *Nelson's textbook on pediatrics*, ed 17, Philadelphia, 2004, WB Saunders.

Behrman R, Kliegman R: *Nelson's essentials of pediatrics*, ed 4, Philadelphia, 2002, WB Saunders.

Burr H: Modern theories of development, *Yale J Biolog Dev* 6 (2):201-203, December 1933 [classic].

Calkins S: Does adverse behavior during toddlerhood matter? the results of difficult temperament on maternal perception of behavior. *Infant Ment Health J* 23 (4):381, 2002.

Carey W, Crocker A, Elias E, Feldman H, Coleman W: *Developmental-behavioral medicine*, ed 4, St Louis, 2008, Elsevier.

Choy M: Children, sports injuries and mouthguards, *J Hawaii Dentistry* 37 (5):11-13, 2006.

Cech D, Marten S: *Functional movement development across the lifespan*, ed 2, Philadelphia, 2002, WB Saunders.

Chabner D: *The language of medicine*, ed 7, Philadelphia, 2004, WB Saunders.

Fournier R: Early clinical assessment for harsh childhood discipline strategies, *MCN: Am J Mater Child Nurs* 27 (1):34, 2002.

Fox S: *Human physiology*, New York, 2009, McGraw Hill.

Gluckman P, Hanson M, Spencer H, Bateson P: Environmental influences during development and later consequences for health and disease later in life, *Prac Biol Sci* 272:671-677, 2005.

Gottfried A, Bathurst L: Hand preference across time is related to intelligence in young girls, not boys. *Science* 221:1074, 1983 [classic].

Greenspan S: Assessing the emotional and social functioning of infants and young children. In Meisels S, Fenichel E, editors: *New visions for the developmental assessment of infants and young children*, Washington, DC, 1996, Zero to Three.

Guyton A, Hall J: *Textbook of medical physiology*, ed 12, Philadelphia, 2011, WB Saunders.

Kavey R, Daniels S, Lauer R, Atkins D, Hayman L, Taubert K: American Heart Association guidelines for primary prevention of atherosclerotic cardiovascular disease beginning in childhood, *Circulation* 107:1562-1566, 2003.

Kinsey A, Pomeroy W, Martin C: *Sexual behavior in the human male*, Philadelphia, 1948, WB Saunders [classic].

Kleigman R, Stanton B, St. Geme J, Schor N, Behrman R: *Nelson's textbook of pediatrics*, St Louis, 2011, Elsevier.

Lee J, Ramos-Gomez F, Quinonez R, Wilson A, Ng M, Elliott R, Molina J: Integrating infant oral health in clinical practice: challenges and practical solutions, *American Academy of Pediatric Dentistry Conference*, San Diego Ca, May 28, 2011.

Leifer G: *Introduction to maternity and pediatric nursing*, ed 6, Philadelphia, 2011, WB Saunders.

Levine M, Carey W, Crocker A: *Developmental-behavioral pediatrics*, ed 3, Philadelphia, 1999, WB Saunders.

Littleboy L, Reed M, Thompson J: *Special educational needs in early years: care and education*, London, 2000, Bailliere-Tindall/Elsevier Science.

Monastersky R: Look who's listening: new research shows babies employ many tricks to pick up language, *Chron Higher Ed* 14-16, July 6, 2001.

National Association for Sports and Physical Education: *Active start: physical activity in children: a statement of guidelines for children 5-12 years*, ed 2, Reston, VA, 2009, NASPE.

Olson S, Bates J, Sindy J, Shilling E: Early developmental precursors of impulsive and inattentive behavior in infancy through middle childhood, *J Child Psychol Psyc* 3 (4):435-448, 2002.

Petra R: *Medical news today*, 2011, from www.mednewstoday.com. Accessed November 2011.

Sherbondy R, Hertel J, Sebastianelli W: Effect of protective equipment on cervical spine alignment in collegiate lacross players, *Am J Sports Med* 34 (10):1675-1679, 2006.

U.S. Department of Health and Human Services: *Physical activity guidelines for Americans*, Washington, DC, 2011, DHHS, from www.health.gov/paguidelines. Accessed November 2011.

Zimmerman M: *Diagnosing DSM-IV psychiatric disorder in primary care*, East Greenwood, RI, 1994, Psychiatric Press.

Online Resources

www.aap.org
www.allergicchild.com
www.nfer.ac.uk/pubs/special.htm
WWW.surgeongeneral.gov/initiatives/healthy-fit-nation/obesityvision2010.pdf

CHAPTER 9 MIDDLE CHILDHOOD

American Academy of Pediatric Dentistry: Guideline on infant oral health care, *AAPD Ref Manual* 33 (6):11-12, 2011.

American Academy of Pediatrics Committee on Psychosocial Aspects of Child and Family Health: Guidance for effective discipline, *Pediatrics* 101:723, 1998.

American Academy of Pediatrics: *Disciplining your children.* Washington, DC, 2009, AAP. Accessed at www.AAP.org/discipline.

Banks JB: Childhood discipline: challenges for clinicians and parents, *Am Fam Physician* 66 (8):1447, 2002.

Betz C, Hunsberger M, Wright S: *Family-centered nursing care of children*, ed 2, Philadelphia, 1994, WB Saunders.

Behrman R, Kleigman R, Jenson H: *Nelson's textbook of pediatrics*, ed 17, Philadelphia, 2004, WB Saunders.

Brazelton T: *Touchpoints: your child's emotional and behavioral development*, Boston, 1992, Addison-Wesley.

Carey W, Crocker A, Elias E, Feldman H, Coleman W: *Developmental-behavioral pediatrics*, ed 4, St Louis, 2009, Elsevier.

Coe D, Pivarnik J, Womak C, Reeves M, Malina R: Effect of physical education and activity levels on academic achievement in children, *Med Sci Sport Exer* 38 (8):1515-1519, 2006.

Disckstein D: Oppositional defiant disorder, *J Amer Acad Child Adolesc Psyc* 49 (5):435-436, 2011.

Erath S, Bierman K: Aggressive marital conflict, maternal harsh punishment, and child-aggressive discipline behavior, *J Fam Psychol* 20 (2):217-226, 2006.

Elkind D: *The hurried child: growing up too fast, too soon*, Cambridge, MD, 2001, Perseus Publishers.

Herrenkohl R, Russo M: Abusive early child rearing and early childhood aggression, *Child Maltreatment* 6:3, 2001.

Kleigman R, Stanton B, St. Geme J, Schor N, Behrmann R: *Nelson's textbook of pediatrics*, ed 19, Philadelphia, 2011, Saunders.

Leifer G: *Introduction to maternity and pediatric nursing*, ed 6, Philadelphia, 2011, WB Saunders.

Levine M, Carey W, Crocker A, editors: *Developmental-behavioral pediatrics*, ed 3, Philadelphia, 1999, WB Saunders.

Monsen R: The child in the community: nursing makes a difference, *J Pediatr Nurs* 17 (6):439-441, 2002.

Pinderhughes E: Discipline responses: influence of parents, socioeconomic status, ethnicity, beliefs about parenting, stress and cognitive emotional processes, *J Fam Psychol* 14:380-400, 1998.

Rowe R, Costello E, Angold A, Copeland W, Maughan B: Developmental pathways in oppositional-defiant disorder, *J Abnorm Psychol* 119 (4):726-738, 1998.

U.S. Department of Health and Human Services: Physical activity guidelines for Americans, Washington, DC, 2011, USDHHS, from www.Health.gov/paguidelines. Accessed November 2011.

Online Resource

www.SIECUS.org

CHAPTER 10 ADOLESCENCE

American College of Sports Medicine: Current comment: youth strength training, Indiannapolis, 2010, ACSM, from www.acsm.org/docs/current-comments/youthstrength-training.pdf. Accessed November 2011.

American Psychiatric Association (APA): *Diagnostic and statistical manual of mental disorders*, ed 4, text rev. (DSM-IVTR), Washington, DC, 2000, APA.

Arner H, Burgess A, Asher J: Caring for pregnant teens: medico-legal issues for nurses, *JOGNN* 30 (2):230, 2001.

Behrman R, Kleigman R, Jenson H: *Nelson's textbook of pediatrics*, ed 17, Philadelphia, 2004, WB Saunders.

Carey W, Crocker A, Elias E, Feldman H, Coleman W: *Developmental-behavioral pediatrics*, ed 4, Elsevier, 2008, St Louis.

CDC: *Definition of vigorous activity*, 2006, from CDC.Gov/nccd/php/dnpa/physical/stats/definitions.htm. Accessed November 2011.

CDC: *Violence arrest rates for persons age 10-24 from 2005-2009*, 2010, from www.cdc.gov/violenceprevention/youthviolence/statistics_at-a_glance/vca_temp-trends.htm. Accessed November 2011.

CDC: *Teen pregnancy rate at record low*, CDC Reuters News, April 5, 2011, from www.CDC.gov.

Faigenbaum A: Resistance training for children and adolescents: are there health outcomes? *Am J Lifestyle Med* 1:190-200, 2007.

Faigenbaum A: Youth resistance training, *Sports Med Bull* 32 (2):28, 2003.

Guttmacher A: *Teen pregnancy: overall trends and state by state information*, New York, 1999, Allen Guttmacher Institute.

Jackson S, Jacob M, Landman-Peters K, Lonting A: Cognitive strategies employed in trying to arrange a first date, *J Adolesc* 24 (3):267-279, 2001.

Juang L, Silbereisen R: The relationship between adolescence academic capabilities, beliefs and parenting and school grades, *J Adolesc* 25 (1):3-18, 2002.

Kelland K: *Reuters reports adolescent death rate outpaces child mortality rate*, Reuters report of *Lancet* article, March 11, 2011, Reuters News Agency.

Kleigman R, Stanton B, St. Geme J, Schor N, Behrman R: *Nelson's textbook of pediatrics*, St Louis, 2011, Elsevier.

Larsen-Meyer D, Redman L, Heilbronn L, Martin C, Ravussen E: Caloric restriction with or without exercise, *J Med Sci Sport Exerc* 42 (1):152-159, 2010.

Leifer G: *Introduction to maternity and pediatric nursing*, ed 6, Philadelphia, 2011, WB Saunders.

Leifer R: *Vinegar into honey: seven steps to understanding and transforming anger, aggression and violence*, New York, 2008, Snow Lion Publications.

Levine M, Carey W, Crocker A: *Developmental-behavioral pediatrics*, ed 3, Philadelphia, 1999, WB Saunders.

Kracke B: Role of personality and peers in adolescents' career exploration, *J Adolesc* 25 (1):19-30, 2002.

Meeks W, Oosterwegel A, Volleberg H: Parental and peer attachment and identity development in adolescence, *J Adolesc* 25 (1):93-106, 2002.

National Adolescent Health Information Center (NAHIC): *Factsheet on mortality of adolescents*, 2006, from http://NAHIC.UCSF.EDU/downloads/mortality.pdf. Accessed November 2011.

Nieder T, Sieffge-Krenke I: Coping with stress in different phases of a romantic relationship, *J Adolesc* 24 (3):297-310, 2001.

Roth M, Parker J: Affective behavioral responses to friends who neglect their friends for a date partner, *J Adolesc* 24 (3):281, 2001.

Rowe D, Welch G, Heil D: Stride rate recommendations for moderate intensity walking, *J Med Sci Sports Exerc* 43 (2):312-318, 2011.

Shulman S, Kipnis O: Adolescents' romantic relationships, *J Adolesc* 24 (3):336, 2001.

Tarrant M, North AC, Edridge MD, et al: Social identity in adolescence, *J Adolesc* 24 (5):596, 2001.

Tilton-Weaver L, Bitunski E, Galambos N: Five images of maturity in adolescence: what does "grown-up mean?" *J Adolesc* 24 (2):143-158, 2001.

U.S. Department of Health and Human Services (USDHHS): *Healthy people 2010*, Washington, DC, McLean, VA, 2000, International Medical Publishing.

U.S. Department of Health and Human Services: *Physical activity guidelines for Americans, USHHS*, 2011, from www.health.gov/paguidelines. Accessed November 2011.

Veerman J, Healy G, Cobiac L, Vos T, Winkler E, Owen N, Dunstan D: TV viewing time and reduced life expectancy, *Br J Sports Med* doii 10:1136/bjsm.2011-0852662.

Zimmer-Gembeck M, Siebenbruner C, Collins W: Diverse aspects of dating, *J Adolesc* 24 (3):313-333, 2001.

Online Resources

www.itsyoursexife.com
www.aap.org/policy/0103.html
www.plannedparenthood.org
www.seventeen.com/sexsmarts

CHAPTER 11 YOUNG ADULTHOOD

American College of Obstetricians and Gynecologists: ACOG committee opinion no. 267: exercise during pregnancy and the postpartum period, *J Ob/Gyn* 99:171-173, 2009.
American College of Obstetricians and Gynecologists: *Getting in shape after your baby is born*, 2011, from www.acog.org/~/media/for%20patients/faq131.ashx. Accessed November 2011.
Benson V, Marano M: *Current estimates from the national health interview survey*, Atlanta, 1994, Centers for Disease Control and Prevention.
Commons M, Richards F, Armon C: *Beyond formal operations: late adolescent and adult cognitive development*, New York, 1982, Praeger [classic].
Gerber C, Blissmer B, Deschenes M, Franklyn B, LaMonte M, Lee I, Nieman D, Swain D: Quantity and quality of exercise for developing and maintaining cardiorespiratory musculoskeletal and neuromotor fitness in apparently healthy adults: guidance for prescribing exercise, *Med Sci Sports Exerc* 43 (7):1334-1359, 2011.
Gotchman D, editor: *Handbook of health behaviors research*, New York, 1997, Plenum Press.
Hatcher R,Trussel J, Nelson A, Cates W, Stewart F, Kowal D: *Contraceptive technology*, ed 19, New York, 2007, Ardent Media.
Leifer G: *Introduction to maternity and pediatric nursing*, ed 6, Philadelphia, 2011, WB Saunders.
Lewis B, Avery M, Jennings E, Sherwood N, Martinson B, Crain L: The effect of exercise during pregnancy on maternal outcomes: practical implications for practice, *Am J Lifestyle Med* 2 (5):441-455, 2008.
Levinson D, Darrow C, Klein EB: *The seasons of a man's life*, New York, 1978, Knopf [classic].
Murstein B: Marital choices. In Wolman B, editor: *Handbook of developmental psychology*, Englewood Cliffs, NJ, 1982, Prentice Hall [classic].
Rowe D, Welch D, Heil D: Stride rate recommendations for moderate intensity walking, *J Med Sci Sports Exerc* 43:312-318, 2011.
USDHHS: *Physical activity guidelines for Americans, USDHHS*, 2011, from www.health.gov/paguidelines. Accessed November 2011.

Online Resources

www.cdc.gov/ncipc/dvp/youpt/datviol.htm
www.oclc.org

CHAPTER 12 MIDDLE ADULTHOOD

Addis I, Vand Den Eiden S, Wassel-Fyr C: Sexual activity and function in middle age and older women, *J Ob/Gyn* 107:755-764, 2006.
Avis N, Blackwell S, Randolph J: Longitudinal changes in sexual functioning as women transition through menopause: results of a study on women's health across the nation, *Menopause* 16:442-452, 2009.
Boulis A, Jacobs J: *Women doctors and the evolution of health care in America*, Ithaca, NY, 2010, Cornell University Press.
Calandra J, Petterson R: Midlife sexuality, *Nurseweek* 14 (20):17-20, 2001.
Carr D: The older adult driver, *Am Fam Physician* 61 (1):141-146, 2000.
Cherry B, Jacob S: *Contemporary nursing, issues, trends, management*, ed 5, Philadelphia, 2011, Mosby, Elsevier.

Erikson E: *The life cycle completed: a review*, New York, 1994, WW Norton.
George S: The menopause experience: a woman's perspective, *J Obstet Gynecol Neonatal Nurs*, 31 (1):77-85, 2002.
Gerber C, Blissmer B, Deschenes M, Franklyn B, LaMonte M, Lee I, Nieman D, Swain D: Quantity and quality of exercise for developing and maintaining cardiorespiratory, musculoskeletal and neuromotor fitness in apparently healthy adults: guidance for prescribing exercise, *J Med Sci Sports Exerc* 43 (7):1334-1359, 2011.
Goldman L, Schafer A: *Cecil's textbook of medicine*, ed 24, Philadelphia, 2011, Saunders.
Graham H: *Understanding gender inequalities in health*, ed 2, Maidenhead, 2009, Open University Press.
Katz A: Sexuality after hysterectomy, *J Obstet Gynecol Neonatal Nurs* 31 (3):236, 2002.
Leifer R: *The happiness project*, New York, 1997, Snow Lion Publications.
Levinson D, Darrow C, Klein E: *The seasons of a man's life*, New York, 1978, Knopf.
MacClean A, Sweeting H, Hunt K: Gender differences in symptom reporting during childhood and adolescence, *J Soc Sci Med* 70:597-604, 2010.
Masters W, Johnson V, Kolodny R: *Masters and Johnson on sex and human loving*, Boston, 1986, Little Brown [classic].
Renucci A: *From past to present: the changing demographics of women in medicine*, San Francisco, CA, 2008, The American Academy of Opthalmology, Feb 2008, Opthalmology Times, from www.YO_info@AAO.org.
Rowe D, Welch G, Heil D: Stride rate recommendations for moderate intensity walking, *J Med Sci Sports Exerc* 43 (2):312-318, 2011.
Schwartz M, Klein A, McLucas B: Uterine artery embolization in treatment of fibroids, *Contemp Obstet Gynecol* 46 (8):14, 2001.
Scheick D: Mastering group leadership, *Psychosoc Nurs Mental Health Serv* 40 (9):35-36, 2002.
Skolnick A: *Embattled paradise: the American family in an age of uncertainty*, New York, 1991, Basic Books.
USDHHS: *Physical activity guidelines for Americans, USDHHS*, 2011, from www.health.gov/paguidelines. Accessed November 2011.
Vlassoff C: Gender differences in determinants and consequences of health and illness. *J Health Popul Nutr* 25 (1):47-61, 2007.
Waldron I: Changing gender roles and gender differences in health behavior. In Gochman D, editor: *Handbook of health behavior research*, New York, 1997, Plenum Press.
Willis S, Reed J: *Life in the middle*, San Diego, 1997, Academic Press.

Online Resources

www.mayohealth.org/mayo/9906/htm/screenings_men.htm
www.cdc.gov/nccdphp/hrt.htm
www.nlm.nih.gov/medlineplus/hormonereplacementtherapy.html

CHAPTER 13 LATE ADULTHOOD

Addis I, Van Den Eiden S, Wassel-Fyr C: Sexual activity and function in middle-age and older women, *J Ob/Gyn* 107:755-764, 2006.
Agronin M, Roose S: Managing depression in older adults: practice approaches to complex patients, *Primary Psychiatr* 16(9 suppl):1, 2010, American Association of Geratric Psychiatry.

Avis N, Blackwell S, Randolph J: Longitudinal changes in sexual functioning as women transition through menopause: results of a study of women's health across the nation, *Menopause* 16:442-452, 2009.

American Association for Geriatric Psychiatry (AAGP): *Position statement: psychotherapeutic medications in nursing homes*, Bethesda, MD, 2002, AAGP.

American Association of Geriatric Psychiatry (AAGP): *Geriatrics and mental health: the facts association of geriatric psychiatry*, Bethesda, MD, 2003, AAGP.

American Hospital Association: *First consulting group: when I am 64: how boomers will change health care*, Chicago, 2007, AHA.

Barg F, Huss-Ashmore R, Murray G, Bagner H, Gallo J: A mixed-method approach to understanding loneliness and depression in older adults. *J Gerontol Soc Sci* 61(6):S329-S339, 2006.

Baumeister R, Leary M: The need to belong: desire for interpersonal attachments as a fundamental human motivation, *Psychol Bull* 117:497, 1995.

Baumgardner W: Exercise slows the aging process, *Arch Int Med* 68(2):154-158, 2008.

Berliner H: Abuse of older adults, *Clin Ref Syst*, August 1, 1999.

Binstock R, George L: *Handbook of aging and social science*, New York, 1999, Academic Press/Elsevier.

Burr H: Modern theories of development, *Yale J Biol Med* 6 (2):201-203, December 2008.

Carr D: The older adult driver, *Am Fam Physician* 61 (1):141, 2002.

Carstensen L, Charles S, et al: Emotions in the second half of life: current directions in psychological science, *Psychol Sci* 7:144-149, 1998.

Catalano J: *Nursing now*, ed 4, Philadelphia, 2006, FA Davis.

Cherry B, Jacob S: *Contemporary nursing, issues, trends, management*, ed 5, Philadelphia, 2011, Elsevier, Mosby.

Chodzko-Zajko W, Proctor D, Singh M, Minson C, Nigg C, Salem G, Skinner J: American College of Sports Medicine position stand: exercise and physical activity for older adults, *Med Sci Sports Exerc* 41(7):1510-1530, 2009.

Cohen C: Guiding seniors, *RN* 64 (2):50, 2001.

Doughty S: The postmenopausal woman, *Adv Nurse Pract* 9 (7):35, 2001.

Ewing J: Detecting alcoholism: the CAGE questionnaire, *JAMA* 252:1905-1907, 1984 [classic].

Havighurst R: *Developmental tasks and education*, New York, 1974, David McKay [classic].

Huang A, Subak L, Thom D: Sexual function and aging in racially and ethnically diverse women, *J Am Geriatr Soc* 57:1362-1368, 2009.

Institute of Medicine: Committee on future health care workforce for older Americas: retooling for an aging America. Washington, DC, 2008, National Academy Press.

Kramarow E, Lubitz J, Lentzner H: Trends in health care of older Americans, 1970-2005, *Health Aff (Millwood)* 26 (5):1417-1425, September/October 2007.

Kumar S: WHO sets agenda for care of elderly, *Lancet* 353 (91):161, 353-361, 1999.

Leifer G: *Introduction to maternity and pediatric nursing*, ed 6, Philadelphia, 2011, WB Saunders.

Leifer R: *Vinegar into honey: seven steps to understanding and transforming anger, aggression and violence*, Ithaca, NY, 2008, Snow Lion Press.

Leuchter A: Brain structure and functional correlates of late life depression. In Schneider C, et al, editors: *Diagnosis and treatment of depression in later life*, Washington, DC, 1994, American Psychological Press.

Lindau S, Shumm L, Laumann E, Levinson W, Omuircheartaigh C, Eaite L: A study of sexuality among older adults in the US, *New Engl J Med* 357:762-774, 2007.

Longley R: *Census offers stats for older Americans*, Washington, DC, 2010, U.S. Government Census Bureau, from www.about.com. Accessed November 2011.

Lyon L: *Scientists are changing the definition of old age*, U.S. News and World Report, December 23, 2009.

Morley J: *The aging male: an issue of clinics in geriatric medicine*, Philadelphia, 2010, WB Saunders.

Morrow D, Leirer B, Altieri P, Fitzsimmons C: When expertise reduces age differences in performance, *Psychol Aging* 9:134, 1994.

Nelson M, Rejeski W, Blair S: Physical activity and physical health in older adults: recommendations of American College of Sports Medicine and American Heart Association, *Circulation* 116(9):1094-2005, 2007.

Newman B, Newman P: *Development through life: a psychosocial approach*, ed 10, Independence KY, 2008, Wadsworth.

Norcross J, Santrock JW, Smith TP, et al: *Authoritative guide to self help resources in mental health*, New York, 2000, Guilford Press.

O'Brien C: CAGE questionnaire for detection of alcoholism: a remarkably useful but simple tool, *JAMA* 300(17):2054-2056, 2008.

Ojta C, Fraga P, Forciea M: Antiaging therapy, *Hosp Pract* 36 (6):43, 2001.

Porter S, Hanley E: The musculoskeletal effects of smoking, *J Am Acad Orthoped Surg* 9, 9-17, 2001.

Qualls S, Beles A, editors: *Psychology and the aging revolution*, Washington, DC, 2000, American Psychological Association.

Rolland Y, Abellan Van Kan G, Vellas B: Healthy brain aging: role of exercise and physical activity, *Clin Geriatr Med* 26 (1):75-87, 2010.

Salthouse T, Coon V: Interpretation of differential deficits: the case of aging and mental arithmetic, *J Exp Pychol Learn* 20 (5):1172-1182, 1999.

Salthouse T: Mental exercise and aging: evaluating the use it or lose it hypothesis, *Prospectives Psychol Sci* 1(1):68-87, 2006.

Shephard R: Aging and exercise. In Fahey TD, editor: *Encyclopedia of Sports Medicine and Science*, Emerald Group Publishing Limited, 1998, Bingley, United Kingdom.

Smith M, Robinson L, Segal J: Depression self-help & treatment. Cambridge, MA, 2012, The Harvard Health Guide, Harvard Publications, from www.helpguide.org.

Sundell J: Resistance training is an effective tool against metabolic and frailty syndrome, *Adv Prevent Med* 98 (4):683, 2011.

Trompeter S, Bettencourt R, Barrett-Connor E: Sexual activity and satisfaction in healthy community dwelling older women, *AJM* 125 (1):37-43, 2012.

U.S. Department of Health and Human Services (USDHHS): *Healthy people 2020*, ed 3, Washington, DC, 2010, U.S. Government Printing Office.

USDHHS: *Physical activity guidelines for Americans*, Washington, DC, 2008, USDHHS, from www.health.gov/paguidelines. Accessed November 2011.

U.S. Department of Health and Human Services Center for Medicare and Medicaid Services: *Medicare claims 2010*, from www.CMS.gov/preventiongeninfo/20_prevserv.asp. Accessed November 2010.

USDHHS: *A profile of older Americans*: Washington, DC, 2010, USDHHS Administration on Aging.

Watson M: *Theories of human development*, Waltham, Mass, 2009, Brandeis University, The Great Courses.

Wold G: *Basic geriatric nursing*, ed 4, Philadelphia, 2008, Mosby/Elsevier.

World Health Organization (WHO): The Heidelberg guidelines for promoting physical activity among older persons, *J Aging Phys Act* 5 (1):8, 1997.
New definition of old age proposed, *Science Mag* 2010, United Press International, from www.UPI.com. Accessed November 2010.

Online Resources

www.aoa.gov/aoa/stats/profile/6.html
www.agingstats.gov
www.DHHS.gov/aging
www.infoaging.org
www.census.gov/prod/pubs
www.aagponline.org/proffacts_mh.asp

CHAPTER 14 ADVANCED OLD AGE AND GERIATRICS

Addis I, Van Den Eiden S, Wassel-Fyr C: Sexual activity and function in middle age and older women, *J Ob/Gyn* 107:755-764, 2006.
American Hospital Association (AHA): *First consulting group: when I am 64: how boomers will change health care*, Chicago, 2007, AHA, pp 1-23.
Baldwin K, Shaul M: When your patient can no longer live independently, *J Gerontol Nurs* 27 (11):10, 2001.
Barzilain N: New twist on becoming a centenarian: it's all in the genes, *J Am Geriatr Soc* 12:201-207, 2011.
Berlinger J: Domestic violence, *Nursing* 31 (8):58, 2001.
Binstock R, George L: Handbook of aging and social science, San Diego, 2011, Academic Press/Elsevier.
Burr H: Modern theories of development, *J Biolog Dev* 6 (2):201-203, 2010.
Butler R: A disease called ageism [editorial], *J Am Geriatr Soc* 38 (2):178-180, 1990.
Butler R: Age-ism: another form of bigotry, *Gerontologist* 9 (4):243-246, 1969 [classic].
Catalano J: *Nursing now*, ed 4, Philadelphia, 2006, FA Davis.
Catania JA: Older Americans and AIDS: transmission risks and primary prevention research needs, *Gerontologist* 29:373, 1989.
Cherry B, Jacob S: *Contemporary nursing, issues, trends and management*, ed 5, Philadelphia, 2011, Mosby/Elsevier.
Cohen C: Guiding seniors, *RN* 64 (2):50, 2001.
Cummings E, Henry W: *Growing old*, New York, 1961, Basic Books [classic].
DeLamater J, Sill M: Sexual desire in later life. *J Sex Res* 42(2):138-149, 2005.
Domrose C: Seasons of change, *Nurseweek* 15 (12):15, 2002.
Ebersole P, Hess P: *Toward healthy aging*, St Louis, 1998, Mosby.
Encyclopaedia Britannica: *Definition of senescence*, from http://dictionary.reference.com/browse/senescence. Accessed January 2012.
Friedman H: *Health psychology*, New York, 2002, Prentice-Hall.
Fuller G: Falls in the elder, *Am Fam Physician* 61 (7):2159-2168, 2000.
Goldman L, Schafer A: *Cecil textbook of medicine*, ed 24, Philadelphia, 2011, WB Saunders.
Guyton AC, Hall JE: *Textbook of medical physiology*, ed 12, Philadelphia, 2011, WB Saunders.

Huang A: Sexual function and aging in racially and ethnically diverse women, *J Am Geriatr Soc* 57:1362-1368, 2009.

HRSA: *HIV diseases in individuals age 50 and above.* CDC Division of HIV Prevention, 2011, from http://hab.hrsa.gov. Accessed January 2012.

Ivey J: Somebody's grandma and grandpa: children's responses to contact with elders, *MCN: Am J Mater Child Nurs* 26 (1):23, 2001.

Institute Of Medicine (IOM): *Committee of future health care workforce for older Americans: retooling for an aging America*, Washington, DC, 2008, National Academy Press.

Kramarow E, Lubitz J, Lentzner H: Trends in health care of older Americans 1970-2005, *Health Aff (Millwood)* 26 (5):1417-1425, 2007.

Lindau S, Schumm L, Laumann E, Levinson W, O'Muircheartaigh C, Waite L: A study of sexuality and health among older adults in the U.S. *New Engl J Med* 357(8):762-774, 2007.

Morley J: *The aging male: an issue of clinics in geriatric medicine*, Philadelphia, 2010, WB Saunders.

Masters W, Johnson V: *The pleasure bond*, New York, 1976, Bantam [classic].

Moyer VA: Screening For Prostate Cancer:US Preventive Service Task Force Recommendation Statement. *Ann Intern Med*, 2012 (epublished ahead of print) http:www.annals.org/early/2012/05/21/003-4819-157-2-2012o7170-00459.long.

National Institute of Health: *Research on aging*, 2010, from www.NIA.NIH.gov. Accessed January 2012.

Newman B, Newman P: Development through life: a psychosocial approach, ed 10, Independence KY, 2008, Wadsworth.

Paice J: Sexuality and chronic pain, *Am J Nurs* 103 (1):87, 2003.

Resnick B: Motivating older adults to engage in self-care, *Patient Care Nurse Pract* 4 (9):13-15, 2001.

Sanderson W, Scherbov S: Rethinking age and aging populations. *Population Bull* 63(4):1-6, Washington, DC, 2008, Population Reference Bureau, from www.PRB.org.

Shaie K: Willis, S: *Handbook of psychology of aging*, New York, 2008, Academic Press.

Sieck G: Physiology of aging, *J Appl Physiol* 95(4):1333-1334, 2003.

Sulmassy D, McIlvane J: Dying dissatisfied, *Arch Int Med* 162 (18):2098-2114, 2002.

Stern Y, Tang H, Albert M, Brandt J, Jacobs D, Bell K: Predicting time to nursing home admissions and death in individuals with Alzheimers disease, *JAMA* 277:806-812, 1997.

Thibodeau G, Patton K: The human body in health and disease, St Louis, 2010, Mosby/Elsevier.

Trompeter S, Bettencourt R, Barrett-Connor E: Sexual activity and satisfaction in healthy community dwelling older women, *AJM* 125 (1):37-43, 2012.

U.S. Census Bureau: *Report: "90 Plus in the United States 2006-2008*, Washington, DC, 2011, U.S. Census Bureau, from www.UScensus.gov/prod/2011/pubs/acs=17.pdf. Accessed November 2011.

Wikipedia: *Definition of older people*, 2012, from www.wikipedia.org/wiki/oldestpeople. Accessed January 2012.

Wold G: *Basic geriatric nursing*, ed 4, Philadelphia, 2008, Mosby/Elsevier.

U.S. Department of Health and Human Services (USDHHS): *Healthy people 2010*, ed 2, Washington, DC, 2000, U.S. Government Printing Office.

U.S. Preventative Services Task Force (USPSTF): *Screening for osteoporosis in postmenopausal women: guide to clinical preventative services*, ed 3, Washington, DC, 2011, Department of Health and Human Services Office of Surgeon General AHRQ Pub No 10-05145-EF-2 January 2011, 2002, Office of Disease Prevention and Health Promotion: U.S. Government Printing Office.

U.S. Census Bureau: *Profile in America: research on aging*, 2011, from www.UScensus.gov/prod/2011/pubs/acs-17.pdf. Accessed January 2012.

U.S. Census Bureau: *Report: 90 plus in America 2006-2008*, Washington, DC, 2010, U.S. Census Bureau Committee on Aging, National Institute of Aging CDC.

USDHHS: *Healthy people 2020*, Washington DC, 2011, U.S. Government Printing Office.

Waillant G: *Aging well*, New York, 2002, Little Brown.

Wikipedia: *Achievements of oldest people*, from www.wikipedia.org/wiki/oldestpeople. Accessed January 2012.

Young R: *Verified supercentenarian cases listed chronologically by death date*, from www.GRC.org. Accessed January 2012.

Online Resources

www.nimh.nih.gov/publicat/elderlydepsuicide.cfm
www.suicidology.org/older_men_and_women.htm
www.lastacts.org/files/files/misc/meansfull.pdf
www.preventiveservices.ahrq.gov

CHAPTER 15 PLANNING FOR THE END OF LIFE

American Academy of Pediatrics Committee on Bioethics and Committee on Hospital Care: Planning for the end of life palliative care for children, *Pediatrics* 106:351, 2000.

American Nurses Association (ANA): *A new code of ethics for nurses: ANA's code of ethics project task force with interpretive statements*, Washington, DC, 2001, ANA.

Archer J: The nature of grief: the evolution and psychology of reaction to loss, London, 1999, Routledge.

Associated Press: *The legality of assisted suicide around the world: patients' right society and world federation of right to die society*, published June 3, 2011, from www.Foxnews.com. Accessed January 2012.

Baldwin K, Shaul M: When your patient can no longer live independently, *Gerontol Nurs* 27 (11), 10, 2001.

Battin M, Rhodes R, Silvers A: *Physician assisted suicide: expanding the debate*, UK, 1998, Routledge.

Becvar D: *In the presence of grief: helping family members resolve death, dying and bereavement issues*, New York, 2001, Guilford Press.

Bednash G, Ferrel B: *Nursing care at the end of life*, Sacramento, 2002, California CEU course Wild Iris Medical Education inc.

Binstock R, George L: *Handbook of aging and social science*, New York, 2005, Academic Press/Elsevier.

Bluebond-Langner M: *In the shadow of illness: parents of siblings of the chronically ill child*, Princeton, NJ, 1996, Princeton University Press.

Bowden V: End of life care: a priority issue for pediatric nurses, *J Ped Nurs* 17 (6):456, 2002.

Bonanno G: Grief does not come in stages and is not the same for everyone, *Am Psychol Today* 2009, from www.psychologytoday.com. Accessed January 2012.

Catalano J: *Nursing now*, ed 4, Philadelphia, 2006, FA Davis.

Cherry B, Jacob S: *Contemporary nursing, issues, trends, management*, Philadelphia, 2011, Mosby/Elsevier.

Emanuel L: *Regulating how we die: the medical, ethical and legal issues surrounding physician assisted suicide*, Cambridge, 1998, Harvard University Press.

Enright B, Marwit S: The diagnosis of complicated grief: a closer look, *J Clin Psychol* 58 (7):747-758, 2002.

Feifel F: *The meaning of death to children: new meanings of death*, New York, 1977, McGraw-Hill [classic].

Ferrel B, Coyle N, editors: *Textbook of palliative nursing*, New York, 2001, Oxford Press.

Field M, Cassel C: *Approaching death: improving care at the end of life: report of the Institute of Medicine task force*, Washington, DC, 1997, National Academy Press.

Firestone R, Catlett J: *Beyond death anxiety: achieving life-affirming death awareness*, New York, 2009, Springer Publishers.

Forbes S: This is heaven's waiting room: end of life in one nursing home, *Gerontol Nurs* 27 (11):37, 2001.

Friedman H: *Health psychology*, ed 2, New York, 2002, Prentice Hall.

Fry V: *Part of me died too: stories of creative survival among bereaved children*, New York, 1995, Penguin Putnam.

Geiter H: The spiritual side of nursing, *RN* 65 (5):46, 2002.

Grubb L: Hearing is the last to go, *RN* 65 (1):51, 2002.

Kübler-Ross E: *On death and dying: what the dying have to teach doctors, nurses, clergy and their families*, New York, 1969, Macmillan [classic].

Lewis L, Brecker M, Reaman G, Sahler O: How you can help meet the needs of the dying child, *Contemp Pediatr* 19 (4):147-159, 2002.

Meisel A: *The right to die*, vols 1-2, New York, 2000, Aspen Law and Business.

National Hospice and Palliative Care Organization (NHPCO): *New findings address escalating end of life debate*, Alexandria, VA, 1996, NHPCO.

Nelson L: When a child dies: practical and sensitive advice for helping parents through their worst nightmare, *Am J Nurs* 95 (3):61-64, 1995.

Paice JA: Managing psychological conditions in palliative care, *Am J Nurs* 102 (11):36-43, 2002.

Periyakoil V, Hallenbeck J: Identifying and managing preparatory grief and depression at end of life, *Am Fam Physician* 65 (5):883-890, 2002.

Post S, Puchalski C, Larson D: Physicians and patient spirituality: professional boundaries, competency and ethics, *Ann Int Med* 132:578, 2000.

Potter P, Perry A: *Fundamentals of nursing*, St Louis, 2010, Elsevier Mosby.

Rivlin D: Books for children when a child's friend dies, *Contemp Pediatr* 18 (10):134, 2001.

Scanlon C: Ethical concerns in end-of-life care, *Am J Nurs* 103 (1):48-55, 2003.

Shaie K, Willis S: *Handbook of psychology of aging*, San Diego, 2003, Academic Press.

Silverman P: *Never too young to know: death in children's lives*, Oxford, UK, 2000, Oxford University Press.

Stanley K: The healing power of presence: respite from the fear of abandonment, *Oncol Nurs Forum* 29 (6):935-940, 2002.

Stephenson J: Palliative and hospital care needed for children with life threatening conditions, *JAMA* 284 (19):2437-2438, 2000.

Stroebe M, Hansson R, Stroebe W, Schut H: *Handbook of bereavement research: consequences, coping and care*, Washington, DC, 2001, American Psychologic Association.
Wold G: *Basic geriatric nursing*, ed 4, Philadelphia, 2008, Mosby/Elsevier.
World Health Organization (WHO): Cancer pain relief and palliative care: technical report series 804, Geneva, Switzerland, 1990, WHO.

Online Resources

www.lastacts.org
www.prc.coh.org
www.AmericanHospice.org
www.NPR.org/programs/death
www.soros.org/death/about_us.htm
www.aacn.nche.edu/ELNEC/index.htm

CHAPTER 16 LOSS, GRIEF, AND BEREAVEMENT

Alexander K: The one thing you can never take away: perinatal bereavement photographs, *MCN: Am J Mater Child Nurs* 26 (3):123, 2001.
American Psychiatric Association (APA): *Diagnostic and statistical manual of mental disorders*, ed 4, text rev. (DSM-IV: TR), Washington, DC, 2000, APA.
Archer J: *The nature of grief: the evaluation and psychology of reaction to loss*, London, 1999, Routledge.
Becvar D: *In the presence of grief: helping family members resolve death, dying and bereavement issues*, New York, 2001, Guilford Press.
Bonanno G: Toward an integrative perspective on bereavement, *Psychol Bull* 125:760-766, 2009.
Bowlby J: *Attachment and loss*, vol 3, New York, 1980, Basic Books [classic].
Bowlby J: Grief and mourning in infancy and childhood, *Psychoanal Study Child* 15:9-52, 1960 [classic].
Catalano J: *Nursing now*, ed 4, Philadelphia, 2006, FA Davis.
Cherry B, Jacob S: *Contemporary nursing, issues, trends and management*, ed 5, Philadelphia, 2011, Mosby/Elsevier.
Cote-Arsenault D, Bidlack D, Humm A: Women's emotions and concerns during pregnancy, following pregnancy loss, *MCN: Am J Mater Child Nurs* 26 (3):128, 2001.
Erikson E: *The life cycle completed: a review*, New York, 1994, WW Norton.
Felton B, Hall J: Overcoming adversity from illness and loss, *Gerontol Nurs* 27 (11), 46, 2001.
King A: *Suddenly alone*, Wilsonville, OR, 1994, Book Partners.
Kübler-Ross E: *On death and dying: what the dying have to teach doctors, nurses, clergy and their families*, New York, 1969, Macmillan [classic].
Leifer G: *Introduction to maternity and pediatric nursing*, ed 6, Philadelphia, 2011, WB Saunders.
Lewis L, Breckher M, Reaman G, Sahler O: How you can help meet the needs of dying children, *Contemp Pediatr* 19 (4):147, 2002.
Lindeman E: The symptomatology and management of acute grief, *Am J Psyc* 101:144, 1944 [classic].
Lipson JG, Dibble SL, Minarik PA: *Culture & nursing care: a pocket guide*, San Francisco, 1996, UCSF Nursing Press.

Ma L: Coping after loss, *Psychol Today*, from www.psychologytoday.com. Accessed January 2012.

Miller-Keane and O'Toole M: *Encyclopedia and dictionary of medicine, nursing and allied health*, ed 7, Philadelphia, 2005, WB Saunders.

Schulz R: *The psychology of death, dying and bereavement*, Boston, 1978, Addison-Wesley [classic].

Stroebe M, Hansson R, Stroebe W, Schut H: *Handbook of bereavement research: consequences, coping and care*, Washington DC, 2001, American Psychological Association.

Viorst J: *Necessary losses*, New York, 1986, Simon & Schuster [classic].

Vyieyanthi P, Hollenbeck J: Identifying and managing preparatory grief and depression at end of life, *Am Fam Physician* 65 (5):883, 2002.

Wheeler S, Austen J: Impact of early pregnancy loss on adolescents, *Am J Mater Child Nurs* 26 (3):154, 2001.

Wold G: *Basic geriatric care*, ed 4, St Louis, 2008, Mosby/Elsevier.

Wolraich M, Dworkin P, Protar D, Perrin E: *Developmental-behavioral pediatrics: evidence and practice*, St Louis, 2008, Elsevier.

Zonnebelt-Smenge S, Vries R: *The empty chair: handling grief on holidays and special occasions*, Grand Rapids, MI, 2001, Baker Books.

Zunin L, Zunin H: *The art of condolence*, New York, 1991, HarperCollins.

Online Resources

www.aarp.org/griefprograms/home.html
www.adec.org
www.aplacetoremember.com
www.compassionbooks.com
www.finalthoughts.com/rc_html
www.modimes.com
www.nmha.org/reassurance/childcoping.cfm

Index

Note: Page numbers followed by *f* indicate figures, *t* indicate tables and *b* indicate boxes.

B

D

E

F

G

I

J

K

L

M

N

O

P

Q

R

S

T